MW01093651

Diagnosis Dystonia
Navigating the Journey

A patient authored resource for
dystonia patients, loved ones, and caregivers

By Tom Seaman

www.diagnosisdystonia.com
www.tomseamancoaching.com

Shadow Panther Press

Wilmington, NC

Cover design by Yocla Designs, www.yocladesigns.com
Back cover photo by Frank Bua

ISBN: 1501004409
ISBN-13: 978-1501004407

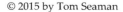

Acknowledgements

First and foremost, I want to thank my family and friends who supported me throughout the writing of this book. Without you, none of this would have been possible.

Thank you to all the people who contributed stories and testimonials. Your words will touch many lives. To everyone who encouraged me to write this book, offered insightful ideas and suggestions, and helped review my work, you are appreciated more than words can express.

Thank you to all my doctors and therapists who have worked with me over the years to help manage my symptoms and restore my life. To all the researchers, doctors, support groups, foundations, and organizations around the world who work tirelessly to increase dystonia awareness, improve treatments, and work towards a cure. Thank you also for the information you provide to help us better understand dystonia and find appropriate treatment protocols.

Thank you to my life coaching colleagues who challenge me every day to expand my knowledge and self awareness, and to my clients for sharing with me the unique dynamics of your life challenges. Your resilience and perseverance motivate me to never give up.

Thank you to all the caregivers, parents, spouses, children, siblings, and all other family members for your unwavering support under challenging circumstances. We owe you a great debt of gratitude.

Last, but certainly not least, a heartfelt tribute to all of you living with dystonia. You are a beacon of strength that helps me and so many others cope better with this life altering condition. Your determination in the face of great challenges strengthens the collective resolve of the dystonia community.

Dedication

Mom and Dad, this book is for you. You saved my life. I would not be here today if you did not step in when I developed dystonia. Without your love and support to improve my health, this book never would have been written.

Long before dystonia entered my life you were always there, sharing smiles during the fun times and tears and hugs during the difficult times. When dystonia entered my life, without hesitation you made tremendous sacrifices and did everything in your power to make my life as comfortable and tolerable as possible. You never had the retirement you planned, as the majority of your energy was put towards caring for me when I was very sick.

Your compassion and generosity are such that I could never possibly repay you for all you did and continue to do to support me. The most I can do is keep dedicating myself to being as healthy as I can be, pay forward the many gifts you have given me, and share with others the lessons you taught me.

I am so proud to be your son and hope that I make you proud to be my parents. Thank you from the bottom of my heart for your strength and all you do for me and everyone who is fortunate to be a part of your life. I am forever grateful and love you both immensely.

Table of Contents

Author's Notes

At the request of the majority of people who contributed testimonials, there are no names or other identification information. Except in cases where applicable and/or permission was granted, all personal information is kept confidential. I can disclose that the testimonials throughout the book came from both men and women all over the world from 30 to 82 years of age.

People have asked me why there is a picture of a brain on the front cover. Since dystonia affects muscles, a common mistake people make is thinking that dystonia is a muscle disorder. Dystonia is actually a neurological disorder originating in the brain which manifests in muscles. See chapter 1 for more details.

Although this book centers on dystonia, much of the information can be applied to any health condition or other life challenge. It provides useful strategies and tools for any life circumstance.

Disclaimer

The information and reference materials contained herein are intended solely for educational and entertainment purposes. The information is not intended to take the place of professional medical care; it is not to be used for diagnosing or treating dystonia, or any other health condition; it is not intended to dictate what constitutes reasonable, appropriate or best care for dystonia or any given health issue; nor is it intended to be used as a substitute for the independent judgment of a physician. If you have questions regarding a medical condition, always seek the advice of your physician or other qualified health professional.

While this book attempts to be as accurate as possible, it should not be relied upon as being comprehensive or error-free. The reader assumes all responsibility and risk for the use of the information in this book. Under no circumstances shall the author or contributors be liable for any damage resulting directly or indirectly from the information contained herein.

Reference to any products, services, internet links to third parties or other information by trade name, trademark, suppliers, or otherwise does not constitute or imply its endorsement, sponsorship, or recommendation by the author or contributors, and is not responsible for their availability, content, or accuracy.

Preface

Honesty and integrity are qualities I highly value and live life to the best of my ability with these principles intact. That being said, I need to be completely honest from the very beginning. I wrote this book for myself. At least that is how it began. It was a form of therapy.

A few months prior to putting my thoughts on paper, I noticed that my dystonia symptoms were not as well managed as they once were and in some ways I was getting worse. When I fell into holes in the past, I was always able to get out of them with different treatments, medications, and little tricks I learned over the years. This time was different. I was not able to get any lasting relief from health care professionals and my bag of tricks and tools that usually helped were not working.

Not only were my physical symptoms worse, my life in general was stagnant. It felt like time was quickly wasting away. I had recently completed my certification as a life coach, but I wasn't sure how I wanted to pursue my coaching practice. My mind was racing, I was having trouble sleeping, and I had little focus. I felt lost and was starting to wonder about the meaning and purpose of my life.

I took some personal inventory and found that I was holding onto a lot of painful things from my past that was hindering my forward progress. Some of the issues were related to the significant way dystonia impacted my life and some had nothing at all to do with dystonia. My inability to process everything was affecting my quality of life making it difficult for me to move in any direction with comfort and confidence. I was stuck and needed to de-clutter my brain. Then one day something inside me said, "Write." The voice was loud and clear. It was almost like a command.

As I began writing, I felt more liberated and clear headed. Many things changed and I found myself moving in positive directions. New doors opened that have profoundly changed my life and I began learning much more about myself and dystonia than I previously knew.

After addressing the most pressing issues, I felt compelled to keep writing and I knew exactly what it had to be about: dystonia. Not only to better understand how to live more effectively with a chronic condition, but to share with others the things I learned along the way.

Introduction

Dystonia has been the greatest challenge of my life. No past injuries, jobs, relationships, sporting events, school classes, travel mishaps, family crisis, or anything else has been as demanding and challenging on me physically and mentally as dystonia. I have endured many acute injuries throughout my life and spent almost as much time in the training room as I did on the field when playing sports, but nothing has come close to the physical and mental demands of dystonia.

The circumstances under which we all arrived at this current place in time living with dystonia are different, but we all experience many of the same things. Our personal experiences may be different in terms of how our life revolves around work, family, and friends, but most of us have had a shift in the dynamics of our lives due to dystonia to which we can all relate.

At first it may seem like we are alone in our battle, but later we learn we are not. We recognize ourselves in the stories of others and find that at the core, we are basically one in the same. We feel many of the same things. We want many of the same things. We are challenged by many of the same things. No one can share our unique experiences, but there is kinship and strength among us.

Writing a book does not mean I know more than anyone else; that I am or think I am better than anyone else; that my dystonia is better or worse than others; or I have done better or worse than others in managing my symptoms. I am no different than all of you. I am just another teammate trying to find a way to better play the game of life with dystonia. We all have a book inside of us filled with stories about our battle scars that have lessons to teach us and others. I wrote this book as a form of therapy to help heal from some wounds and I hope sharing it will help you or someone you know better deal with their life challenges.

This is not a recovery book; nor does it suggest or provide a cure. While this book does not promote or endorse a particular treatment, many treatments are discussed to show the various options available. The more substantial information provided are strategies for living with a chronic health condition. These include coping skills and mental approaches to improve your quality of life and optimize the effectiveness of your professional care and self care. Various tools and techniques for managing physical and emotional symptoms are also discussed. My goal is to provide you with as much comprehensive information as possible to make your life with dystonia easier. This book need not be read from cover to cover. It is formatted so the reader can jump to chapters and topics of relevance and interest.

There are not many books available on dystonia and most that are available were written by people who do not have dystonia. I felt there was a great need for a book from the perspective of patients, as our experiences are uniquely different than those who have never walked a day in our shoes. This book provides readers with a window into life with dystonia through the eyes of those who live with this challenging condition. I hope you find direction, inspiration, and comfort in the pages that follow.

"Great moments are born from great opportunity"

I first heard this quote watching one of my favorite movies called *Miracle* (2004). It is based on the true story of how the 1980 United States Olympic hockey team was able to defeat the Soviet Union in the semi-finals before going on to win the gold medal against Finland. Not only were the United States and the Soviet Union in the midst of a cold war and for all intents and purposes, enemies, the Soviet national team was comprised of well-seasoned players and considered the most dominant team in the world. It won four straight gold medals from 1964 to 1976; almost every world championship since 1954; nearly defeated a team of Canada's top professional players in 1972; and beat several NHL teams in exhibition games during the 1970's.

Many of the players on the 1980 Soviet team were members of the Red Army, though they had few military responsibilities. The government allowed them to devote their lives to hockey, training together year-round while retaining their amateur status. Although they were considered amateurs, the government was paying them to primarily play hockey, technically making them professional athletes. This was a loophole the Soviet government used to boost the prowess of their athletes, prior to the current rule which allows professionals to compete.

In contrast, the Americans were a collection of college students with little history of playing together. In fact, prior to becoming part of the United States hockey team, many played against each other for colleges that were bitter rivals. They now had to put their rivalries aside and become teammates.

Overcoming overwhelming odds against them to beat the Soviets was an accomplishment that no one thought was remotely possible, except the players on that team and their coach Herb Brooks. "Great moments are born from great opportunity" is supposedly what Brooks said to his team in the locker room prior to the game against the Soviets. In an unforgettable, exciting game, the United States beat the Soviet Union that evening, something the world never expected. People who never watched hockey before or had any interest in hockey were glued to their televisions watching a game that rivals most any sporting event in history. As the game clock wound down, at the final buzzer, broadcaster Al Michaels yelled, "Do you believe in miracles?!?" It is a moment that still brings me chills.

So I ask you; do you believe in miracles? Do you believe that great moments are born from great opportunity as Herb Brooks said to his team before the David and Goliath battle took place? Do you see dystonia as an opportunity or do you see it as an obstacle? If you see it as an obstacle, is it one that you can climb over or one that you allow to stand in your way and keep your life from moving forward? While you may feel that you have lost a lot because of your dystonia, what have you gained?

While I hope you are able to see dystonia as something that provides you with new opportunities, as does any event or circumstance in our lives, I also acknowledge the very dark side of this disorder. I lived it for many years. This book is an honest account of my journey which may be similar to the one you face each day. It addresses the light and dark side of this disorder in an honest manner, with the intent to acknowledge you, offer understanding, provide hope, and help you find meaning in your life living with dystonia.

Life always throws us curveballs and we have to learn to adapt to the changes. This is often when the greatest learning in our lives takes place. We can look for the opportunity or we can close our eyes and be angry, keeping us imprisoned. Dystonia has been my greatest teacher and I suspect that if you look closely, you will find it has lessons for you as well.

Whether you have lived with dystonia for years or just been diagnosed, this book is for you.

Chapter 1
What is Dystonia?

Dystonia is a neurological movement disorder characterized by uncontrollable, involuntary muscle spasms and contractions, causing repetitive movements, twitching, twisting, and/or abnormal postures. Muscle contractions can be sustained or intermittent and sometimes include a tremor. Dystonia can affect any part of the body, causing varying degrees of disability and pain from mild to severe.[1, 2] In some cases, dystonia exists without visual symptoms. Some people have muscles that involuntarily contract, but they have no change in physical appearance. Pain is almost always present regardless of physical presentation. People often describe their muscles as feeling like tightropes.

A good way of looking at dystonia is in terms of muscle pairs. During normal movement, when one muscle contracts its opposing muscle relaxes. For example, in the arm, when we contract/flex our bicep, our tricep coordinates by relaxing. When we extend our arm, our tricep contracts and our bicep relaxes. Quadriceps and hamstrings are good examples of other muscle pairs that work in the same fashion. In dystonia, opposing muscles involuntarily contract simultaneously, which is what causes awkward movements, abnormal postures, and pain. The affected muscles feel very similar to a charley horse.

Dystonia is the third most common movement disorder after Parkinson's disease and Essential Tremor. According to The Bachmann-Strauss Dystonia & Parkinson Foundation, approximately 500,000 people are estimated to have dystonia in the United States and Canada alone. This figure may be low when considering those yet to be diagnosed and those who have been misdiagnosed. There is little uniformity in how dystonia manifests, making it difficult to diagnose and treat. Many physicians are also not familiar with dystonia, as education and awareness are limited.

Dystonia does not discriminate. It affects men, women, and children of all ages and backgrounds. It does not impact cognition and intelligence, or shorten a person's life span. However, given the severity of symptoms that some people experience, quality of life can be dramatically affected. There is currently no cure available so treatments are limited to minimizing symptoms.

Characteristics of dystonia
There are multiple forms of dystonia and symptoms are highly variable (see further below for the different names and forms of dystonia). It may affect a

single area of the body or multiple muscle groups. Some people experience awkward looking fixed postures, some have sporadic and irregular movements, and some have no apparent deviation from normal. Some may feel and look symptom free at rest, but have an awkward appearance when they move or try to perform a specific task.

Early symptoms may include a cramp or a tendency for the affected part of the body to tighten and/or tilt or turn to one side, as in the neck for example. In the case of dystonia in a lower limb, a foot may curl and/or leg may drag, and coordination problems with the upper and lower torso may be evident. In the face and head, eyes may blink rapidly and uncontrollably, or close entirely. Symptoms may also include a tremor or difficulty speaking.

In some cases, dystonia is action or task specific. For example, some people may have dystonia when writing, but not when they are using the same hand to type or grip silverware when eating. Another example is a person who has neck spasms/contractions when walking or performing some other activity, but has no symptoms sitting or standing.

Dystonia tends to "disappear" when sleeping. While some have painful symptoms upon waking, for many there is a respite in symptoms. It is often referred to as the "honeymoon period" because symptoms are usually at their mildest. This period of time varies from person to person. As the day progresses, symptoms tend to increase. Symptoms may also be more noticeable after physical exertion, stress, and/or fatigue.

Although dystonia is not considered a progressive disorder, over time, early symptoms may become more severe in some people. My initial symptoms progressed over a period of six months from a minor annoyance to a severe disability characterized by forceful involuntary movements and pain unlike anything I had ever experienced. Conversely, some people have symptoms that manifest but never progress, and even improve. I attribute my steep and rapid decline to an inaccurate diagnosis and improper treatments, but I can't say for sure if my symptoms wouldn't have still progressed otherwise.

Some people have dystonia affecting one area of their body at the outset and then have other parts of their body become affected over a period of time (the time for which varies), while others have no such progression or migration. There is no conclusive evidence that symptoms plateau, where symptoms level off and remain stable, but some report such a scenario.

What causes dystonia?[1-7]

The cause of dystonia is not known in most cases, but it is thought to be due to a chemical imbalance in the brain. The origin of the chemical imbalance in most cases is unknown, but scientists believe that dystonia results from an abnormality in an area of the brain called the basal ganglia where some of the messages that initiate muscle control are processed. The cerebellum, sensori-motor cortex, and supplementary motor areas of the brain may also be involved.

In order to move muscles, messenger chemicals called neurotransmitters are released which allow nerve cells to send signals to other nerve cells. In the case of dystonia, scientists suspect a defect in the body's ability to process certain neurotransmitters that help cells in the brain communicate with each other, affecting normal muscle activity. The main neurotransmitters believed to be involved in dystonia include acetylcholine, norepinephrine, serotonin, GABA (gamma-aminobutyric acid), and dopamine.

Acetylcholine is an excitatory chemical that helps regulate dopamine in the brain. In the body, acetylcholine released at nerve endings causes muscle contractions. *Norepinephrine* and *serotonin* are inhibitory chemicals that help the brain regulate acetylcholine. *GABA* (gamma-aminobutyric acid) is an inhibitory substance that helps the brain maintain muscle control and *dopamine* is an inhibitory chemical that influences the brain's control of movement.

When these neurotransmitters are malfunctioning it can affect how the brain generates commands to move certain body parts, causing involuntary twitching, twisting, turning, spasms, contractions, curling, pulling, repetitive movements, awkward postures, pain, and tremors, the most common symptoms of dystonia. In most cases, no brain abnormalities are visible using magnetic resonance imaging (MRI) or other diagnostic imaging.

While there is currently no known cause in most cases, dystonia may be hereditary or caused by factors such as birth-related or other physical trauma, infection, exposure to toxins, reaction to recreational or pharmaceutical drugs, or a combination of things.

Dystonia classifications

Dystonia is divided into three groups: *Idiopathic*, *Genetic*, and *Acquired*. *Idiopathic dystonia* refers to dystonia that does not have a clear cause. *Genetic dystonia* refers to people who carry a defective gene from one or more parents.

However, it does not follow that if one inherits a defective gene they will develop dystonia. *Acquired dystonia* results from environmental or other damage to the central nervous system. Some causes of acquired dystonia include birth injury, such as hypoxia and neonatal brain hemorrhage, certain infections, reactions to certain recreational and prescription drugs, heavy metal or carbon monoxide poisoning, trauma, or stroke.[8, 9]

Forms of dystonia are based on the body regions affected:

- *Focal dystonia* is localized to a specific part of the body.
- *Generalized dystonia* affects more than one part of the body.
- *Multifocal dystonia* involves two or more unrelated body parts.
- *Segmental dystonia* affects two or more adjoining parts of the body such as the face and neck, neck and upper arm, and trunk and leg muscles
- *Hemidystonia* involves the arm and leg on the same side of the body.

There are several different forms of focal dystonia. Some of the more common focal dystonias are:

- *Cervical dystonia* (a.k.a. Spasmodic Torticollis) - Cervical dystonia is the most common focal dystonia. The muscles in the neck that control the position of the head are affected, causing the head to turn or pull to one side, or pull forward or backward. Some people have a combination of two or more head positions such as laterocollis and rotational collis. Movements can be intermittent or sustained (locked in position) and it is common to have one shoulder pulled up higher than the other. The images below show the four types of cervical dystonia. Not everyone has it to these extremes and some do not have any visual impairment, but still experience spasms, muscle constriction, and pain.

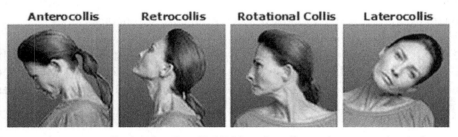

Anterocollis   Retrocollis   Rotational Collis   Laterocollis

www.dysport.com, Retrieved on June 25, 2014 from: http://www.dysport.com/cervical-dystonia-tools-and-resources

- *Blepharospasm* - Involuntary contraction of the muscles controlling eye blinks. Usually both eyes are affected. Symptoms include increased blinking and spasms may cause the eyelids to open or close completely.

- *Cranio-facial dystonia* – Forms of dystonia that affect the muscles of the head, face, and neck. *Oromandibular dystonia* affects the muscles of the jaw, lips, and tongue. This may cause difficulty opening and closing the mouth; speech and swallowing may also be affected. *Meige syndrome* is a term used to describe oromandibular dystonia accompanied by blepharospasm. *Spasmodic dysphonia*, also called laryngeal dystonia, involves the muscles that control the vocal cords, resulting in strained or breathy speech.

- *Task-specific dystonia* - Focal dystonias that occur when undertaking a particular repetitive activity. An example is writer's cramp, which affects the muscles of the hand and sometimes the forearm, and only occurs during handwriting. Similar focal dystonias include typist's cramp, pianist's cramp, and musician's cramp. Musician's dystonia is a term used for focal dystonias affecting a musician's ability to play an instrument or perform. It can involve the hand in keyboard or string players, the mouth and lips in wind players, or the voice in singers.

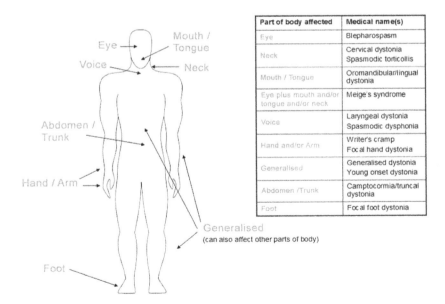

Part of body affected	Medical name(s)
Eye	Blepharospasm
Neck	Cervical dystonia Spasmodic torticollis
Mouth / Tongue	Oromandibular/lingual dystonia
Eye plus mouth and/or tongue and/or neck	Meige's syndrome
Voice	Laryngeal dystonia Spasmodic dysphonia
Hand and/or Arm	Writer's cramp Focal hand dystonia
Generalised	Generalised dystonia Young onset dystonia
Abdomen /Trunk	Camptocormia/truncal dystonia
Foot	Focal foot dystonia

Reprinted with permission from: The Dystonia Society http://www.dystonia.org.uk/, Retrieved on August 5, 2013 from: http://www.dystonia.org.uk/index.php/about-dystonia/types-of-dystonia

Dystonia and genetics

There are forms of dystonia that are known to be inherited and forms that may or may not have a genetic component. Researchers cannot confirm or rule some out at this time. Genes encode proteins, which fulfill specific functions in the body.[9] For example, *DYT1 dystonia* is a form of dominantly inherited early-onset generalized dystonia. It typically presents in childhood or adolescence and only on occasion in adulthood. The most common symptoms are contractions in the foot, leg, or arm. Dystonia is usually first apparent with specific actions (e.g. writing or walking). Over time, the contractions may become evident with less specific actions and spread to other body regions.

Dopa-responsive dystonia (DRD), also known as Segawa's disease, is another form of dystonia that can have a genetic cause. Individuals with DRD typically experience onset during childhood and have progressive difficulty walking. Some forms of DRD are due to mutations in the DYT5 gene.

While still in the preliminary stages, researchers have identified other genes that may contribute to dystonia. These include mutations in the DYT3 gene, which causes dystonia associated with parkinsonism; the DYT6 gene has several clinical presentations such as cranio-facial dystonia, cervical dystonia, or arm dystonia; DYT11 causes dystonia associated with myoclonus (brief contractions of muscles); and DYT12, which causes rapid onset dystonia associated with parkinsonism.[10]

Below is a list of DYT-designated genes associated with dystonia. This is not a comprehensive list of all genes associated with dystonia; many disorders in which dystonia is a consistent and dominant feature were described before the DYT labels came into use. [9, 11]

DYT1- Early onset generalized torsion dystonia
DYT2- Early onset segmental torsion dystonia
DYT3- X-linked dystonia parkinsonism
DYT4- Primary laryngeal and cervical dystonia
DYT5- Dopa responsive dystonia; Segawa's disease
DYT6- Adolescent-onset torsion dystonia of mixed type
DYT7- Adult onset focal cervical and laryngeal dystonia
DYT8- Paroxysmal non-kinesogenic dyskinesia
DYT9- Paroxysmal choreoathetosis with episodic ataxia and spasticity
DYT10- Paroxysmal kinesigenic choreoathetosis
DYT11- Myoclonus dystonia
DYT12- Rapid onset dystonia-parkinsonism

DYT13- Multifocal/segmental dystonia
DYT14- Dopa responsive dystonia
DYT15- Myoclonus dystonia
DYT16- Young-onset dystonia parkinsonism
DYT17- Primary focal torsion dystonia
DYT18- Paroxysmal exertion-induced dyskinesia 2
DYT19- Episodic kinesigenic dyskinesia 2
DYT20- Paroxysmal non-kinesigenic dyskinesia 2
DYT21- Late onset primary torsion dystonia
DYT23- Primary cervical dystonia
DYT24- Primary cranial and cervical dystonia
DYT25- Primary dystonia of varied anatomical symptoms and age of onset

Dystonia - disorder or disease?
There is some debate as to whether dystonia is a disorder or a disease. Some people are very passionate about using one word over the other so let's look at the both definitions.

Disorder- A disturbance in physical or mental health or functions; malady or dysfunction.[12]

Disease- A disordered or incorrectly functioning organ, part, structure, or system of the body resulting from the effect of genetic or developmental errors, infection, poisons, nutritional deficiency or imbalance, toxicity, or unfavorable environmental factors; illness; sickness; ailment.[13]

Dystonia fits under both definitions. I use both words when describing it to others, sometimes interchangeably. It is clearly a "disorder" because there is a disturbance and dysfunction in our physical health. It is also a "disease" because there is a disordered and incorrectly functioning system within the body. In addition, anytime the body is not "at ease" it is in a state of "dis-ease." Lastly, the NIH Office of Rare Disease Research lists dystonia as a disease.[14]

Unless there is a specific reason to use one word or over the other (e.g. public awareness efforts, applying for grants, speaking with doctors, social stigma) use whichever word you feel is most appropriate for the situation and audience. In most cases I call dystonia a "health condition", a "neurological condition" or simply a "condition." "Condition" is defined as, "a way of living or existing; the state of something, especially with regard to its appearance, quality, or working order; a state of health or physical fitness; an illness or

16

other medical problem; the circumstances affecting the way in which people live or work, especially with regard to their safety or well-being."[15] Clearly, a generically accurate word to describe what dystonia is and what living with dystonia is like is "condition."

Dystonic storm

It wasn't until a few years ago that I first heard the term "dystonic storm." I never understood what people were talking about because what most described is not consistent with what a dystonic storm really is. It is often used loosely and incorrectly, which could be problematic.

A true dystonic storm is a rare, life-threatening complication of severe generalized dystonia. It is characterized by relentless, sustained, severe dystonic muscle contractions that are life threatening and often require emergency medical attention. Treatment with intravenous benzodiazepines or general anesthetic agents may be required. In extreme cases, intrathecal Baclofen or even deep brain stimulation may be required.[16]

Patients with primary and secondary dystonic conditions occasionally develop severe episodes of generalized dystonia and rigidity, which may be unmanageable to standard drug therapy. This condition has been labeled as "status dystonicus" or "dystonic storm", or the patient is labeled as "desperate dystonic." The condition is quite rare.[17]

The following excerpt comes from The Dystonia Society (UK): Dystonic storms are episodes of a rare condition called status dystonicus where people develop frequent and intense episodes of severe generalized dystonia. A single episode of this severe dystonia may be referred to as a "dystonic storm" or "dystonic attack." They usually occur in individuals who already have dystonia affecting a lot of the body.

The exact origins of status dystonicus are not known. However, some cases appear to be triggered by an abrupt change in medication or by severe infections. Medications may be used to reduce or alleviate symptoms of a severe dystonic storm.

During an attack people do not lose consciousness and are aware of their surroundings, but they may not be able to communicate to others, as the muscles of the face and larynx are often involved. If breathing or swallowing is affected, emergency medical attention is required and immediate medical advice should be sought. In very rare cases, when drugs have not worked, deep brain stimulation has been successful in reversing the dystonic storms.[18]

According to the above information, dystonic storms are rare and usually associated with people who have generalized dystonia or episodes of generalized dystonia. However, many people with other forms of dystonia use this term, mainly when their symptoms become aggravated from their baseline. Most people have probably never experienced or witnessed a true dystonic storm, yet they use this term anyway. It is often used to describe a bad day or an exacerbation of symptoms that last for a few minutes to a few hours, but without need for emergency attention, as would be the case with a true dystonic storm.

People also use the term "storm" to describe an episode where they have symptoms of increased anxiety and more muscle tension than usual, often brought on in uncomfortable environments. This is not a dystonic storm. These episodes more closely resemble a panic or anxiety attack, or symptoms that get worse from stress triggers.

It is important that we use "storms" in the proper context because to doctors, a dystonic storm conveys a serious medical emergency. We don't want to overstate our symptoms and then be discounted as hypochondriacs; nor do we want to receive treatment in excess of what we actually need.

Another reason to use caution with the term "storm" is that people newly diagnosed and those still learning about dystonia may be misled about their symptoms and what they mean. Dystonia symptoms can be brutally fierce and scary, but are not life threatening, as is a storm. There is no need to lunge into fear when our symptoms act up, thinking it is something more than it really is.

Describing dystonia is difficult, let alone all of the nuances within dystonia. If we want others to listen and understand what we are experiencing, we need to use consistent terminology to describe our various symptoms and experiences. "Storm" is but one example. Work also needs to be done to clarify the meanings of other words such as "squeezing", "contracting", "pulling", "twisting", "turning", and "jerking." This is where national organizations, doctors, researchers, and patient support groups could work together to better define the terms we use and then utilize various forms of media to reach the masses. Collaboration is highly beneficial for scaling all our challenges.

18

References

1) www.wehealny.org, Mount Sinai Beth Israel, Retrieved on September 13, 2014 from: http://www.wehealny.org/services/bi_neurology/DystoniaResearch.html

2) NIH – National Institute of Neurological Disorders and Stroke, www.ninds.nih.gov, Retrieved on August 15, 2013 from: http://www.ninds.nih.gov/disorders/dystonias/detail_dystonias.htm

3) The Movement Disorder Society, www.movementdisorders.org, Retrieved on August 15, 2013 from: http://www.movementdisorders.org/disorders/dystonia.php

4) The Bachmann-Strauss Dystonia & Parkinson Foundation, Inc. Retrieved on September 11, 2013 from: http://playground.lousch.net/BS/faqs and http://www.dystonia-parkinson.org/content/how-many-people-are-affected-dystonia

5) Dystonia UK. www.dystonia.org.uk, Retrieved October 27, 2013 from: http://www.dystonia.org.uk/index.php/about-dystonia/types-of-dystonia/neck-dystonia-/the-role-of-muscles-im-neck-dystonia

6) Tyler's Hope for a dystonia cure. www.tylershope.org, Retrieved January 17, 2014 from: http://www.tylershope.org/About_Dystonia.aspx

7) www.medicinenet.com, Retrieved on August 16, 2013 from: http://www.medicinenet.com/dystonia/page2.htm

8) Dystonia Medical Research Foundation (DMRF), http://www.dystonia-foundation.org, Retrieved on April 28, 2013 from: http://www.dystonia-foundation.org/pages/genetics/87.php.

9) DMRF, Retrieved on September 13, 2014 from: https://www.dystonia-foundation.org/what-is-dystonia/genetics/gene-chart

10) NIH – National Institute of Neurological Disorders and Stroke, www.ninds.nih.gov, Retrieved on August 6, 2013 from: http://www.ninds.nih.gov/disorders/dystonias/detail_dystonias.htm

11) Canadian Movement Disorder Group, www.cmdg.org, Retrieved on September 13, 2014 from: http://www.cmdg.org/Dystonia/Dystonia_genetics/dystonia_genetics.htm

12) www.dictionary.reference.com, Retrieved on May 16, 2013 from: http://dictionary.reference.com/browse/disorder?s=t

13) www.dictionary.reference.com, Retrieved on May 16, 2013 from: http://dictionary.reference.com/browse/disease?s=t

14) NIH Office of Rare Disease Research. Retrieved December 20, 2013 from: http://rarediseases.info.nih.gov/gard/search-results

15) www.merriam-webster.com, Retrieved February 21, 2014 from: http://www.merriam-webster.com/dictionary/condition

16) Singer, H. Mink, J. Gilbert, D, Jankovic, J. (2010) Movement Disorders in Childhood, Philadelphia, PA: Elsevier, Inc.

17) Mishra, D. Singhal. S. Juneja. M. (2010) Status Dystonicus: A Rare Complication of Dystonia, *Indian Pediatrics, 15*, 883-885

18) http://www.dystonia.org.uk, Retrieved May 2, 2013 from: http://www.dystonia.org.uk/index.php/about-dystonia/symptoms/dystonic-storms

Chapter 2
My Life with Dystonia

I graduated from college with a degree in education and psychology, and went to work in a health education business. More specifically, it was a chiropractic and nutrition patient education company. Over the next five years, my partners and I developed other companies and services; a golf training and rehabilitation seminar business; a nutritional analysis service; and a fitness center. Needless to say, I was very busy. The work was fun, but I needed a change.

In August 2001 at the age of 30, I returned to school for my masters degree in counseling. The year prior to starting graduate school, I took a job as a project manager at a brand new water park and family fun center on a lake in the town where I lived. I worked very long hours at this job, but it was a relief being active and outdoors every day versus cooped up in an office or travelling the country to conferences. It was one of the most enjoyable years of my life. Little did I know it would soon be followed by some of the worst years of my life.

Shortly before I was to move into my new apartment and start school, I began to notice that my neck was a little restricted. More specifically, turning to the left was slightly difficult. I remember the first time I noticed it. I was walking past the beach on the way to lunch. When I turned to look at the beach on my left it took effort. I didn't have full range of motion and it was difficult to keep my head turned to the left. I felt it pulling back. I just assumed it was from working a lot or sleeping in a bad position, but the tightness never went away.

Within about a week, I started to feel a slight muscle pull to the right. Some days I felt fine so the pulling never lingered on my mind as being a problem. I chalked it up to the wear and tear of working long hours and several five hour car trips moving into my new university apartment. I never had much of a break between working, packing, and driving. I wasn't sleeping much either. I also had a recent fall from a bicycle and a few hard wipeouts water skiing, so there were plausible reasons for my stiff neck.

During one of those long car trips to move my belongings, it felt like my head was tilting to the right. I flipped the visor mirror down so I could take a look. My head was in fact tilting slightly to the right. Again, I chalked it up to the stress of moving and school preparations. I figured it would resolve itself.

When graduate school began in the Fall of 2001, I noticed that my neck was turning a little more, especially when I walked. It "flopped" back and forth as if my neck muscles had become weak and couldn't hold up my head. While sitting in class and at work, I often found myself cupping my chin in my hand to keep my head straight. I was not in any pain and I didn't look any different in other peoples' eyes unless I pointed it out, but to me it seemed obvious that my head was turned. I soon became self conscious in public. I began having a little anxiety which exacerbated my symptoms.

A few weeks into the semester I decided it was time to see a doctor before it got worse. Assuming it was a musculoskeletal problem, I went to a chiropractor who practiced a technique called Chiropractic BioPhysics (CBP). CBP is based on the concept that spinal curvatures that deviate from a mathematically derived "ideal" value should be corrected. Logically this seemed like the right person to see. I have also been around chiropractic most of my life and it was helpful for many other problems, so it seemed like the right doctor given my symptoms. I wholeheartedly endorse the benefits of all chiropractic techniques, but only when a patient presents with a problem that is within the scope of knowledge and practice of that particular doctor.

The initial exam consisted of x-rays and posture tests. The doctor determined that I had restricted joint movement, thoracic and cervical posture issues, and a flat curve in my neck. I was never given any diagnosis with a name; just a description of what he saw.

Treatment consisted of neck and back adjustments 3 times a week. Within about 3-4 weeks, the doctor started me on extension traction. I would sit upright in a wooden chair and lean my head back so I was looking at the ceiling. He then put a strap around my forehead with weights on the end to pull my head back even further. CBP practitioners use this in an attempt to restore the curve in people with a flat or reversed cervical curve.

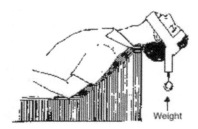

Barrett, S. A Skeptical Look at Chiropractic BioPhysics (CBP). www.Chirobase.org. Retrieved July 3, 2013 from: http://www.chirobase.org/06DD/cbp.html.

This forced hyperextension caused pain in my neck and back that did not previously exist. It was so uncomfortable that I told the doctor that I no longer wanted to do the traction and instead just stick to the adjustments. To his credit, he went against normal treatment protocol and obliged. The pain subsided.

As the first semester wore on, my symptoms ebbed and flowed. I would get a little better for brief moments and then worse again. Sometimes I thought I needed to get adjusted more and then sometimes less. I couldn't figure out what was causing the inconsistency in my symptoms. That being the case, I decided to stick to a regimen of 3 adjustments per week and just play out what I still thought was a temporary problem. I also began wearing a soft collar neck brace on occasion to reduce the uncontrollable spasms and turning/pulling. The collar helped me do some activities with more ease, but I was always worse when I took it off. My muscles felt weaker and my neck turned more. I was also starting to have pain again, and this time it didn't go away.

Nearing the end of the semester my symptoms were worse than they had ever been. I assumed it was because of the stress of final exams and all the papers and presentations I had to do. I was spending countless hours with my nose in a book or on the computer, so it seemed logical that this was why my neck was pulling to the right a bit more than usual and why I had some minor pain. It was all very tolerable; I just had a neck that turned away from center a slight amount and "flopped" a little when I walked. Granted, my symptoms had gotten worse over the past four months and my neck was starting to hurt, but I could still manage all of my activities. Looking back, I think I was in denial about how bad it had become.

After I took my last final exam, which was essay in format, my neck felt the best it had the entire semester. As silly as it sounds, I thought the way I sat while writing for three hours corrected the problem. The relief I had from being done with the semester factored in my mind as well. I was symptom free for a couple days and rejoiced by telling my family and friends that I was all better, a logical conclusion at the time since it was the longest I had gone without any symptoms.

Over the Christmas break I visited family and friends. As the days progressed my symptoms started again. I was having more pain and involuntary muscle contractions than ever before. It forced me to lie down often, but it was still pretty minor relative to how things would become.

The night I returned to school for the next semester is when things began to go downhill very quickly. I recall feeling a combination of a spasm and an itch in the middle of my back next to my right shoulder blade. I reached my arm back to scratch it and I felt an unfamiliar yank in my neck. Instantly my neck began to involuntarily pull to the right harder than it ever had before. I was terrified. Adrenaline pumped through me. I had no idea what was going on. I managed to get to sleep and the next morning I went to my chiropractor. He did his normal adjustment and there was no change. I went back almost every day the next two weeks. During those two weeks, I also saw a physical therapist and a medical doctor at the college health center. They had no idea what was wrong and pretty much dismissed me because they didn't know what to do.

Not knowing where else to turn, I continued going to the chiropractor. I kept getting worse so he referred me to another chiropractor in town who used an approach called the Pettibon System. My referring doctor felt this would be best based on my worsening symptoms. He made me feel very confident that this new doctor would fix my problem. I was in so much pain and my neck was now pulling and turning to the right, and starting to lock up. This made it very difficult to get to work and class, let alone concentrate when I was there. I could barely hold up my head without using my hand, so I was game for anything.

I saw the new chiropractor the following week. When I was in the waiting room with my neck turned and pulling towards my shoulder, a patient across from me who looked perfectly normal said, "I looked just like you two weeks ago and the doctor fixed me right up." This was the most reassuring thing I heard since my symptoms started 6 months earlier. I was so relieved and excited. I thought I finally found the doctor who was the answer to my problem. Little did I know that his treatments would be the beginning of the worst nightmare I ever experienced.

They took a series of x-rays and while I was still not given a diagnosis, the doctor determined that I would need a minimum of 6 weeks of treatments 3-4 days a week (with exercises at home as well) following the Pettibon System. Believing wholeheartedly that it would help from the glowing referral and patient testimonial, I gladly signed on to my only known option at the time.

Treatments consisted of sitting on a wobble chair, over-the-door cervical traction (Image 1), wearing a head and shoulder harness with weights in them (Image 2), and neck adjustments. I was also instructed to do over-the-door cervical traction at home and wear the weighted head harness a few times a day. The doctor gave me the most violent adjustments I ever had in my life. He literally had to put me in a headlock in order to adjust my neck. Since I saw him adjust other patients, I knew this was not his standard neck adjustment technique. He adjusted me this way because he needed extra leverage to fight the dystonic muscles that were forcefully pulling the opposite direction he wanted to move my neck.

Image 1

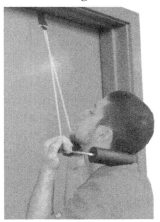

Retrieved on February 3, 2014 from: http://www.amazon.com/Repetitive-Cervical-Neck-Traction-Regular/dp/B004O83JY8

Image 2

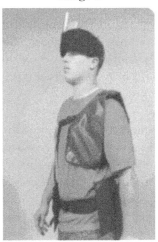

Retrieved on February 3, 2014 from:
http://backbonerestored.info/trusted%20posture%20pages/posture%204.htm

I could barely get out of bed after a few treatments. I had pain in my back, shoulders and neck unlike anything I ever experienced before. The pain to lift my head off my pillow was the worst I ever had in my life. Naively, I figured this was no different than any other kind of exercise I had done in the past where I felt pain the next day. I managed to get to the doctor that morning and he told me it was normal to feel this way. Trusting him, I continued with treatments. Each day over the next two weeks I got worse. My neck was turned and now locked to the right. I also had forceful spasms that pulled my right ear towards my now raised shoulder. I was unable to sit or stand without holding my head to relieve the pain. Again I was told it was normal and would subside.

One day my parents were visiting so they drove me to the doctor. On the way to an appointment, my head jerked and slammed into the passenger side window. I hit it so hard that it felt like I had cracked my head and/or the window. There was no damage other than a big lump on my head. My parents were taken aback at how much I had declined so quickly.

After going downhill like a runaway train, I searched the internet for answers. I was barely able to fight back tears from the pain as I sat at my computer pushing my head with one hand while typing with the other. I could only handle sitting for 10 minute intervals. During my search I came across "torticollis." Torticollis literally means "twisted neck" and is usually an acute condition that can be resolved in a short period of time. It is when a muscle, joint, or ligament in the neck is irritated. "Acute" means that the symptoms developed quickly, over a period of hours, or often overnight. This is what I think the girl in the waiting room had wrong with her and why she got better so quickly. I then came across "Spasmodic Torticollis (ST)." Spasmodic Torticollis (a.k.a. Cervical Dystonia), a problem within structures of the brain, is an entirely different beast and in most cases should not be treated the same as acute torticollis.

When I read about spasmodic torticollis/cervical dystonia, I finally knew what was wrong. The page could have literally been written by me. I told my doctor the next day what I found and he agreed that this was probably what I had. He wasn't entirely sure, but it sounded pretty close. Not knowing a lot about it, he continued with the status quo of treatments. I continued to get worse so I told him I was not coming back anymore. I wish I had done that much sooner.

I then sent out a blanket email to every doctor, nurse, and medical student at the university asking for treatment suggestions. Most who responded said I should get Botox. Others suggested physical therapy, medications, and chiropractic. I read up on Botox and was not comfortable putting a toxin in my body. I hoped to find another option. However, I did follow a suggestion to go to Duke University for a neurologist's opinion. The doctor confirmed my diagnosis as dystonia and also suggested Botox injections. I was still leery about it so I declined, but finally getting an official diagnosis was a relief.

I continued to search the internet for alternative options to Botox. I came across the ST Recovery Clinic in New Mexico. It offered a natural approach to symptom management which included things like stretching, exercise, massage, and nutrition. Everything I read and from everything the director told me over the phone made perfect sense, so I decided that this was what I wanted to do. I was able to get into the clinic a month later.

In the meantime, I spent my day on the floor rolling around in pain beyond words. I couldn't take it anymore so I went around the corner to a 24 hour medical facility for medication. I had to find some relief. I literally wanted to die. I never even liked taking over the counter medicine so this was a major thing for me to do. I begged the doctor for the strongest drugs he could legally prescribe. Whatever it was, it kicked my tail. It took away the pain and I was able to go to sleep pretty easily for the first time in months, but I woke up having hallucinations, cold sweats, and unshakable fear. Thankfully, this all dissipated in a few hours, but the pain returned. I never took those medications again. It was terrifying.

You might be thinking to yourself as you read this; why did you go to all these doctors who didn't help? Why don't you remember what medications you took? Why didn't you go back and tell the doctor what the drugs did to you? The simple answer is that the pain was such that I could not think clearly and I made poor decisions. I didn't care about anything other than how to end the pain or end my life. When someone is in this state of mind, not a whole lot of rational thought takes place. I had never experienced anything like this before. It was far worse than any broken bone or other injury I had incurred prior to this point in my life. I was in unchartered territory.

Why didn't I just try Botox you might also be wondering. Frankly, I was afraid that the side effects might be greater than the benefit. It had only been approved by the FDA just two years earlier so I didn't know much about it. At the time it sounded like a dangerous poison that I was afraid to put in my body. I had always taken a more natural approach to my health so this was a little too much out of my comfort zone.

My neck was now locked to the right and the pulling significantly worsened with any type of movement. The intense spasms felt like a freight train was pulling me over. It was a miserable existence. It felt like I was simultaneously being beaten by a baseball bat while a drill penetrated the back of my neck and skull. I began to have suicidal ideations, but loving life as I do, I couldn't and wouldn't give up. I believed there was an answer out there for me.

At times I felt like the elephant man. I was very lonely with bizarre symptoms no one really understood. For example, I showed someone close to me how my neck snapped to the right when I took my hand off my face. They said "ewww" and looked away. Still looking for compassion, I showed them again what I was living with and they said I looked gross and asked me to never show them again. They meant no harm, but hearing this felt like a kick in the gut.

During the month of February 2002 while waiting to go to the ST Clinic, I spent the day as follows: wake up, eat breakfast, lie on the floor, eat lunch, lie on the floor, eat dinner, lie on the floor, and then go to bed and try to fall asleep. In fact, I also ate lying on the floor. I would lie on my side and slide food from the plate into my mouth. I spent about 14-16 hours a day in a fetal position on my floor in tears most of the time.

I became almost totally dependent on the help of others. Everything I could do, or had to do, was with one hand because the other hand was constantly supporting my head and neck to try and alleviate some of the unbearable pain and muscle pulling. Every week, my parents drove over two hours to stay with me for a couple days to do my laundry, go food shopping, clean my apartment, and just be there with me. I was useless. I can't imagine how they felt seeing their son suffer with no idea how to help. None of us had any idea what to do.

At the end of February I made the trip to the ST Clinic in New Mexico with my father's help. To this day I am still surprised I was able to do it considering my symptoms. It was sheer will power and determination. I had to fight through the relentless pain every minute of the trip. I took any chance I could to lie down in airports, restaurants, and rental car agencies. I didn't care what people thought. I had to find a way to make it there as comfortably as possible. The hardest part was sitting upright on the plane. I can only imagine what people thought was wrong with me as they watched my neck twist and turn while I squirmed around trying to get comfortable.

When I got back from the ST Clinic (see chapter 15 to read about my experience there), I returned to the floor for most of the day. Every once in a while I would attempt a stretch or two, but that was all I could muster up the strength to do. Everything I did caused screaming pain. Anytime I would get up to eat or go to the bathroom, I would be laid out until I had to get up again to eat or go back to the bathroom.

Things like shaving and showering for me were the equivalent of working out with weights or doing high impact aerobics for an hour. Let that marinate for a moment; the strength it took to merely shave my face or shower was as physically demanding (and far more painful), than heavy exercise. This speaks volumes about how torturous dystonia can be. For those of you who experience symptoms to this degree, you know what I am talking about. You are not alone and you are not without hope.

A few more weeks passed with no relief. As much as I wanted and tried to stay on my own, I couldn't live like this anymore. I needed significant help. I gave in to pleading from friends and family to move in with my parents. I remember the day I called to tell them I accepted their offer to live with them because I couldn't carry on by myself any longer. A week later I was living in their guest bedroom. It was a very humbling experience to give up my independence.

March 9th, 2002, the day my Mom drove me to their home (a 2 1/2 hour ride), is clearly etched in my mind. Within about a mile from my apartment, I was in so much pain that I begged my Mom to take me back. The spasms, pulling, and pain were so intense that I could not keep from crying, screaming, and thrashing around trying to find some level of comfort to handle the ride. I didn't think I could make the trip. My poor Mom helplessly watched as she drove. The person next to her was being tortured by an invisible force and she couldn't do anything to stop it.

My father was in his van ahead of us with all my belongings. We thought about calling him to tell him we were turning back, but never did. Somehow I was able to grind it out, mainly with my Mom's help. She kept reassuring me that things would be okay. I still remember her repeatedly saying, "We have to keep going. The sooner we get home, the better it will all be. Hang in there. Everything will be better in a couple hours." I knew she was right, so I pleaded with her to drive as fast as she could. She never breaks the speed limit, but this day she put more pedal to the metal than I ever saw before. My pain trumped the risk of a speeding ticket.

When I got to their house I was met by several family members. Neighbors also came by throughout the day and brought food. It was really strange; as if someone just died. I don't think anyone knew what to do other than just be there for me, for which I was very grateful. Everyone thought this was going to be a temporary thing and they would be there to help me out for the next month or so while I "recovered." It was like I was recovering from surgery or an injury that required me to get a little rest and relaxation.

In the ensuing months and years when no recovery took place, it affected some of my relationships. There was an expectation from others that was not realized. The fact that I had a chronic condition that may never go away was not something some people were able to embrace. It was not something I was able to embrace, so I wouldn't expect them to either.

Some of my friends came down hard on me. The expected me to do more than I was. No matter what I told them about how I felt or how challenging it was to just get through the day doing menial tasks, it was never good enough. I felt ostracized and nothing I said or did changed their opinion.

As the weeks went by, I slowly began following parts of the program I learned at the ST Clinic in New Mexico. It was very hard because I was in so much pain, but I pushed through believing it would help. Easter arrived and I went to my aunt's house to be with the family. My Mom had to get a plate of food for me because I needed my hands to support my head. My cousin had just been in a car accident so we were joking how we were like the walking wounded. We pretty much sat there while others waited on us.

Within about an hour, my pain climbed to a level where I had to leave. When I got back to my parent's house (thankfully only a couple miles away), I laid my body down on the floor to try and reduce the pain. I was crying uncontrollably. The physical pain was brutal and the mental pain of not being able to sit and enjoy Easter with my family was gut wrenching. Not being able to handle something as simple as eating a meal at the table was very hard for me to rationalize. Less than a year ago I was able to do what I wanted, when I wanted, and how I wanted without a second thought. Now I could barely do anything without screaming pain. It was at this moment that it hit me that I had something seriously wrong with me that may never get better. Reality hit me like a ton of bricks and I was terrified.

A couple days went by and I decided I wanted to go on medication. I needed some relief. Imagine the pain I was in to come to this conclusion after the earlier episode when I took medication that I thought was going to kill me. Nevertheless, I read up on medications for dystonia. I came across Klonopin (clonazepam) which seemed like an effective and commonly used drug for dystonia. It seemed like the best option for me. Even though there is no drug specifically for dystonia, other drugs like Klonopin are used "off label", meaning that they are designed for another condition but have been found helpful for something else. I went to see a doctor that week. He was an internist who knew very little about dystonia, but he was the only doctor in town my family went to and trusted.

The doctor and I went over the literature on medications used for dystonia. I told him I wanted Klonopin. He agreed and wrote me a prescription for .5mg, 3 times a day. Within about a week or two, my pain subsided about 25%. My adrenaline that was so fired up from the pain also subsided. This minor relief made it so I could function with a little more comfort. I began to drive a little and started going to my sister's house a couple miles away to go in her family's pool. I found that submerging my body in water reduced my symptoms a little so I was there almost every day. The sunshine also helped me feel better, as I was previously holed up in the house all day long. My Mom expressed concern about me being such a hermit and suggested I sit in the sun a little each day. She was right and I made a point of reaping the healthy benefits of daily sun exposure as often as I could. However, after only an hour (often less) I would have to come home and lie in bed for several hours, if not the rest of the day on some occasions. This minimal activity wore me out.

I continued with the ST Clinic program and began to notice I was getting a little more control of my neck and I felt less twisted. Pictures proved otherwise, but I was feeling better because I had a little less pain. I began to spend a little more time outside of the house. It felt good to be out and about a little more, but the increased activity caused more pain and spasms. Finding a balance between rest and activity was tricky. To clarify, my "outside of the house" activities consisted of maybe attending a school event for one of my nieces or nephews once in a while, hanging out at the pool for an hour or two, and walking around the yard. Anything beyond that was far too painful.

A few months passed and it felt like my medication was not as effective as it once was so my doctor doubled my dose. I was now taking 1mg of Klonopin 3 times a day (at one point, for a short while, I was taking between 4-6mg a day). 3mg a day is a pretty hefty dose, but I was none the wiser about the effects of this drug and long term use. All I cared about was that it made me feel better so I could be a little more functional.

For several months I was on a good program. I did my stretching and exercising every evening, took an Epsom salt bath, and then got a back rub from my father before I went to bed. I began to notice some small positive changes. However, I was becoming very impatient. I was not getting better as quickly as I would have liked. I was tired of working so hard with such little results. I was told that I would have to be very patient and that it would take many more months to start seeing significant changes. Not being a patient person, this didn't sit well with me. I wanted faster results.

One day I was offered a beer. I was fearful about drinking alcohol while on Klonopin, unsure of how they would mix. The person who offered it to me said not to worry because if anything, it might just increase the effect of the medication. Since the medication was helping a little, I thought some added benefit would be great. As it turned out, the alcohol did enhance the benefit and I had no ill side effects. So, from time to time I had a drink or two. Little did I know that this would lead to a lot more than just one or two drinks within a couple months.

My evening regimen of stretching/exercising, Epsom salt baths, and massage began to change. I grew tired of the routine and I liked the benefit of alcohol. I started to have a glass or two of wine in the late afternoon and then do my neck stretching and exercising before dinner. I found that the alcohol loosened me up and I was able to do my stretches with greater ease. I was seeing a psychologist during this time and I told him about my routine. He didn't see any harm in me having a couple drinks if it helped me stretch. His approval was surprising to me, but I welcomed it because it gave me permission to do something I knew was probably not a good idea.

After a few weeks on this routine, I found that I needed more alcohol to assist me with my stretching. Eventually, I found much more relief just drinking alcohol than stretching. Instead of going into the garage to stretch and exercise, I went into the garage to drink.

When I emerged a couple hours later, my neck was more relaxed and I was in less pain. My improvement was apparent to my parents and anyone else in the house. They thought my neck was better from the exercises. Little did they know that I was not exercising much, if at all. It was the alcohol that was really helping my muscles relax. I pretty much replaced alcohol for exercise and deceived the people who loved me most. I felt guilty every single day, but obviously not guilty enough because all I did for my symptoms over the next 4 years was drink every day. It was the most desperate and alone I ever felt in my entire life. I used to hide cases of beer in my closet. It got to the point that I was drinking about 15 beers every night. I was literally a closet drinker. I didn't know how else to cope with the constant pain.

In January 2003, my friends and family convinced me to try Botox so I went back to Duke. I didn't have health insurance at the time so my friends graciously chipped in to pay for my treatment. Unfortunately, I didn't get any relief. More frustration led to more drinking. Occasionally I did a couple stretches, but by then, alcohol was my treatment of choice. I went back to Duke 3 months later for another round of Botox; again, no benefit. Only drinking gave me physical and mental pain relief. I don't think anyone can truly understand the mindless desire to self medicate with alcohol and drugs unless they have experienced such miserable pain. It's no excuse, but desperation can make a person do most anything. Over the next 10 years I tried Botox several more times. Unfortunately it never helped.

Pretty soon I began to put on a lot of weight from drinking. I was also eating very poorly which contributed to the weight gain. Most people thought it was just my poor diet that caused all the weight gain. My Dad tried to talk to me about my weight, but but and I didn't want to hear it. I didn't want to tell him the truth about my drinking. I was embarrassed. I also knew that if I told him he would have found a way to get me to stop, and at the time I needed my alcohol to survive. At least I thought I did. It was a terribly scary and lonely place to be. It got to the point that every day was pretty much a daze, except for the daily wake up vomit or dry heaves, accompanied with ridiculous pain during the day until I started drinking again.

Minimal activity caused horrible pain. For example, I only shaved once every week or two because it was too difficult. As for haircuts, it was too painful to sit upright to have it cut, nor could I groom it, so my Dad gave me crew cuts. I stood outside by the back porch and leaned over as he shaved my head. I begged him to go faster because my head and neck hurt so much. He did the very best he could to get it done quickly, but I know I drove him nuts rushing him. When he was done, I laid down the rest of the day. I didn't care how it looked. I just wanted it short. The less grooming the better because it hurt too much to raise my arms to my head.

I spent most of my time alone in my bedroom. I didn't like who I had become. Many of my friends didn't like me either. I was miserable and miserable to be around. I stopped calling and visiting people, and they stopped as well. Pretty soon the phone never rang. I also stopped going to my sister's pool. I never went to any family functions or holiday gatherings for several years, unless they were at my parent's house. I lived there so I couldn't avoid them. I would have left if I had somewhere else to go because I didn't want to be around anyone. I was too riddled with pain and depression, as well as embarrassment over my weight and my crooked neck. I was also experiencing significant anxiety so being around a lot of people was uncomfortable. I also had no friends because I didn't know anyone in town other than my family and I was too sick to get out and meet people. Dystonia relocated me to a town where I had no social or vocational connections, and I didn't feel well enough to get out and grow some roots. It was very lonely and I lost a lot of self confidence.

The only thing I did was go to a massage therapist a mile from the house. She worked on me 3 times a week. It was helpful, but my lifestyle was not conducive to benefitting much from the treatments. I continued to eat a horrible diet and drink myself into submission. Around this time, I began having panic attacks and was often afraid to leave the house, except when I absolutely had to. I would buy a couple cases of beer at a time so I had enough to last me a few days. Going for a massage and getting beer was pretty much the only time I left the house. It was the most pathetic time in my life.

My panic attacks were such that I would get very dizzy and weak when I was in public. My heart would beat rapidly and I would lose all sense of where I was. My mind would go blank and I couldn't think clearly. I feared passing out. I was also self conscious about how I looked. Having always been thin and athletic, it was a very different life being overweight. It felt like all eyes were on me. My twisted neck added to the embarrassment and shame.

When I hit around 240 pounds, my doctor put me on blood pressure medication. This was mind boggling to me. Never in my life did I have trouble with my blood pressure. What in the world was I doing to myself? One might think this would deter me from my unhealthy lifestyle, but the pain was still too much to handle so food and beer remained my drugs of choice, along with my prescription medications. I'm lucky to be alive considering what I was putting in my body.

Along with Klonopin and the blood pressure medication, I was now taking Baclofen (muscle relaxer) and Restoril (sleeping pill). I told people that my continued weight gain was due to side effects of my medications. I was too embarrassed to tell them the truth. When my weight reached 310 pounds, I stopped getting on the scale. I refused to look anymore. I couldn't even watch shows like *The Biggest Loser* (a weight loss show) because I felt so guilty. I tried to ignore my guilt and shame as much as I could.

I used to run from the camera. I regret it now because I don't have many pictures to compare with how I look now, but I didn't even want to look in the mirror let alone have a picture taken. On Christmas 2005, my niece and nephew stood behind me as I opened a gift from them. Before I knew what happened, my sister-in-law took a picture of the three of us. I was upset for a moment and then forgot about it.

A month went by and it was my birthday. My niece and nephew gave me a birthday card with a picture on the front of the envelope. It was a picture of them with a man I didn't recognize. I stared at the picture for a while wondering why they would give me a picture of them with someone I didn't know. Then it hit me. It was me!! I was shocked. I looked like I was blown up for a float in a parade. I then asked, "Is this me? Is this how I look? Am I really this big?" No one responded to not offend me, except my niece who said, "Don't worry about it Uncle Tom. The camera always adds 10 pounds." As sweet as this comment was, the first thought that came to mind was, "How many cameras are on me?!?"

You might think this would have turned my unhealthy lifestyle around, but it didn't. I kept drinking and eating poorly for another year. A few weeks prior to Christmas 2006, at around 330-350 pounds (I am not entirely sure because I stopped weighing myself a year earlier at 310 pounds), I came down with a stomach virus and was too sick to eat or drink anything. I spent most of the time in the bathroom with diarrhea. The rest of the time I was in bed. I didn't have any solid food for over a week and all I drank was water and ginger ale.

Of course I couldn't drink alcohol. This concerned me because I thought I would need it to curb the pain. Thankfully this was not the case. My neck felt pretty good. It was still turned and off center, but I was not in much pain. All the resting was very helpful in that regard. I also feared I had become addicted to alcohol to the point of facing difficult withdrawal. Luckily, perhaps even miraculously, I didn't have any at all and my drinking days were over. It was like turning off a light switch. I realized drinking would eventually kill me and made a conscious decision to stop. I've never looked back. I am deeply grateful that my problems with alcohol went no further.

Getting sick with the stomach virus was the best thing that could have happened to me. Those two weeks of being idle gave me time to rest my dystonic body and think about my life and what I was doing to myself. After a lot of reflection, I made the decision that I had better change my lifestyle or I might soon be dead.

I lost about 10-15 pounds while I was sick. When I was well enough to get out of bed and eat solid food again, I threw out the remaining four cases of beer I had in my closet. I put them in my car late one night when no one was around (I was still ashamed and didn't want anyone to know), drove down the road, and threw them all in a dumpster. It was such a relief to finally let go of that chapter of my life. It was an even bigger relief when I eventually told my parents about my drinking habits and why it had dominated my life. Being the saints they are, they listened and didn't judge me. They understood why I did it and felt sad that I was in bad enough shape to do that to myself. They were mostly proud of me for having the strength to overcome it.

I then began eating the way I always had previously, which was far healthier than how I was eating the past 5 years. My parents encouraged me to begin walking a little each day. I was still over 300 pounds and could only walk about 100 yards. I made it a daily practice to walk to the end of my street and back home. My parents came with me most times to make sure I didn't fall. I was dizzy, anxious, and unstable from the weight and my tight neck. I also quickly ran out of breath.

In about two weeks I was confident enough to walk by myself. It felt great. I was so excited. I remember coming in the house one day after a short walk and saying to my parents, "That felt so good! I'm going to do it again!" That day was the start of my weight loss journey. I got the fever to be healthy again and I never looked back.

Further into the book in the nutrition section you can read how I lost all the weight, but to summarize, I went from well over 300 pounds to 180 pounds in less than a year. I completely dedicated myself to changing my lifestyle to get healthy again. In the process, my dystonia also got better, which I attribute to better nutrition, stress reduction, and faithfully incorporating the ST Clinic program into my lifestyle. Unfortunately, my desire to lose all the weight pushed me past my limits. I walked too much which made my neck pull to the right again causing pain in my mid back. I backed off by walking less, but the pain was too much so I had to stop walking entirely. Thankfully, I continued to lose weight by eating properly. My neck also stopped pulling.

Each time I went to the doctor (about every 2 months) he couldn't believe how much I changed. Everyone in the office also took notice. Most people commented on the weight loss versus the change in my dystonia. That was understandable because losing 100 plus pounds was far more obvious, but dystonia symptom reduction was my main focus.

In the Fall of 2007, my doctor and I discussed reducing my medications. Considering how much my symptoms had improved, we both felt they were no longer necessary. I was already off the blood pressure medication. Now I wanted to get off Klonopin, Baclofen, and Restoril so he started to taper me down. Unfortunately, my taper plan was way too fast. Within a couple weeks I began having very bizarre symptoms. You can read more about this in the section on benzodiazepines (benzos) in chapter 15, but suffice to say, my new symptoms introduced a whole new level of horror.

In brief, I became very weak and dizzy, among many other symptoms. I was so weak and off balance that I didn't know how I was able to stand most the time. A small bottle of water felt like a 10 pound weight. I tried getting stronger using weights, but they were too much for me. I had to use soup cans and even they felt heavy. My muscles began to atrophy and I became very skinny and frail. It was very disappointing. I went from fit and athletic, to weighing well over 300 pounds, to almost sickly thin.

I became extremely sensitive to all sorts of visual and auditory stimuli, and it felt like my skin was dripping of my body. When I drove in a car it felt like I was floating on top of the seat and wasn't aware that I was even touching the steering wheel because my sense of touch was altered. In the morning and evening I also experienced full body spasticity where I could barely move.

Below are pictures of me peeling a banana, which was very difficult with the intense spasticity. To remedy this, I began taking GABA supplements (gamma-aminobutyric acid). GABA is the chief inhibitory neurotransmitter in the central nervous system and is responsible for the regulation of muscle tone. It is often called the brain's calming neurotransmitter. After about 2 weeks of taking 750mg of GABA 2x/day, the spasticity significantly dissipated, but the other symptoms continued with a vengeance.

Fall 2007

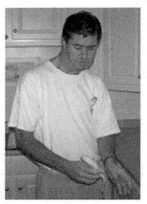 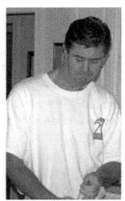

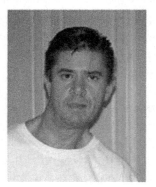

My doctor thought all my symptoms were side effects of the medications, as did other people, so he tapered me off even more! This made my symptoms worse so I started talking to other people and reading about benzodiazepines, the class of drugs home to Klonopin and Restoril. After living in confusion about my symptoms for over a year, my search was over. I discovered I was in severe benzodiazepine withdrawal.

Over time, the brain develops tolerance to certain medications. This can happen even when taking the prescribed dose, as was the case with me. When they are not increased or when they are reduced (usually abruptly), the brain can go into withdrawal, potentially causing hundreds of strange symptoms. The drugs take the place of natural neurotransmitter production so when they are removed there can be significant communication failures in the brain.

I sought out a doctor who specializes in helping people with medication addiction. Over the course of a year, he helped me reduce my withdrawal symptoms by changing my medication and taper regimen. Unfortunately, I still live with some minor protracted withdrawal symptoms, but I am so much better than I used to be. I have to be patient, as it can take time for neurotransmitters in the brain to begin working properly again.

When I was better stabilized with my medication, I had more energy which enabled me to establish an exercise routine again. After a few years of hard work I am proud to say that I am biking and swimming a little a couple times a week, I am able to lift light weights, do squats, lunges, and modified pushups. Some of these things are not dystonia friendly so I modify them to not hurt my neck and back. I am building some strength again which feels great. Past experiences have taught me to be more patient with my exercise routine.

As you can see in the photos at the end of this chapter (ranging from 2002 to 2014), I have made significant progress. My dystonia has greatly improved and my body is much more balanced and relaxed. However, I am not without challenges. While my neck and body appear straight, my cervical spine actually angles to the left and I tilt and pull to the right, particularly when I stand or walk. C1 is apparently rotated about 10 degrees from center and I also have scoliosis. I do exercises that specifically target the muscles that keep my neck and back as straight as possible. Some days these muscles have to work harder than other days to compensate for the imbalances. This can cause pain, instability, and fatigue, so I do my best to balance my daily activities to minimize these symptoms.

Some doctors suspect that I might have cervicogenic vertigo (a.k.a. cervical vertigo or cervical dizziness). This is a syndrome of disequilibrium and disorientation often associated with neck pain and/or neck trauma. It is provoked by a particular neck posture no matter what the orientation of the head is to gravity. Thus far it is only conjecture on their part based on a variety of symptoms that are difficult to understand. It is also tends to be a controversial diagnosis because there are no diagnostic tests to confirm that it is the cause of dizziness. It is very uncomfortable to put it mildly.

I also have mild anxiety doing certain things in public because I never know how my body is going to behave. I can get dizzy and have muscle contractions that come out of the blue, making me apprehensive about being in certain environments. Apprehension and fear are common for people with dystonia because we often don't know how our bodies will cooperate. Since these distressing emotional symptoms often go unnoticed, many of us are a good example of the saying, "Don't judge a book by its cover."

My visible dystonic movements are now more task-dependent, versus years ago when they were present no matter what I did. For example, my neck pulls off center when I walk, eat, shave, brush my teeth, and if I sit or stand for too long. My current symptoms are similar to when dystonia began back in 2001, but I feel different. The years of wear and tear, medications, medication withdrawal, scoliosis, compensatory muscle activity, and changes to the discs in my spine, make me less functional than I was when my symptoms first started. The difference now is that I better understand my symptoms and how to do things within my boundaries.

I follow parts of the ST Recovery Clinic program which consists of specific stretches, exercises, and lifestyle habits, all for the purpose of lengthening and strengthening muscles, and reprogramming motor areas of the brain. I do other exercising as well. I also get acupuncture treatments every two weeks and massages as often as possible. I also use various trigger point tools to relieve pain and relax tight muscles. I rest and use heat and ice as needed, and take muscle relaxants. I also pray, meditate, and do relaxation breathing exercises.

To maintain balance in my life, it is important for me to address my physical, mental, social, emotional, and spiritual needs. I exercise my body and eat healthy foods, I involve myself with positive people, I challenge my mind by learning new things, and I spend time in meditation and prayer. These all help keep dystonia from being the dominant force in my life. Dystonia may be my evil twin at times, but we have learned to work with each other and get along much better than we once did. I've had to learn to accept that life is different than it once was and most of the time I am okay with that. Adapting to change is a key component to any healthy life.

Of course I experience frustration not being able to do some of the things I love so much, but considering how sick I once was, I am doing great! I am a better person in so many ways and my life is filled with new and exciting things that were non-existent for years. Instead of living as a victim by focusing on my limitations and how life was before dystonia, I look at the many obstacles I overcame and build on those accomplishments. I am grateful for the things I could do before dystonia, but even more grateful for what I can do now.

I dedicate myself to a healthy lifestyle, body and mind. I avoid toxic food, toxic people, and unhealthy relationships. I frequently remind myself how horrible my pain and debilitation used to be and live in gratitude for everything that now occupies my life. I choose to not let dystonia get the better of me and I don't feel sorry for myself. I keep looking for solutions to challenges and new ways of doing things.

I do my best to vary my days to keep life fresh, even if I only make one tiny change. On difficult days, which I still have, I don't fight it. Fighting makes it worse. I do my best to listen to my body. When it says rest, I rest. When it tells me to be active, I'm active. I try to not beat myself up when I make mistakes or have a challenging day. I do my best to put my ego aside and take baby steps towards a better tomorrow. When I try to solve everything at once, I make life more difficult.

I don't think too much about how my life once was. I can't change the past. Now is the only moment I have. No dwelling. No regrets. I've learned and grown from it all. I value whatever is happening right now and then build on it. This is easier now because I feel much better and my mind is in a better place, but I still have to remain disciplined. I can easily get lazy and fall into negative patterns of behavior.

One of my biggest challenges was not feeling guilty for having dystonia. For years I felt like a failure not being able do more for myself and live a "normal" life. I felt guilty that people sacrificed so much to help me. I have now learned to accept help with less guilt. I let people who love me love me more. I also give myself and others more credit that we are handing things quite well despite our challenges. Everyone does what they feel they should to help me and if the roles were reversed, I would do the very same for them. We all have challenges and need help from others. Accepting help and providing help to others are important parts of the healing process.

People often ask me what prompted me to change my lifestyle to get to where I am now and how I stay motivated every day. The short answer is that I love life and want to make the biggest impact I can on others' lives for as long as I can. I want to motivate people to grow and make positive changes. I can't do that if I am sick.

In 2012, I became certified as a life coach to help others who live with similar challenges. My main focus is on health and wellness, primarily working with people who have chronic conditions, weight loss issues, and those making lifestyle changes. Living with dystonia has taught me valuable lessons that provide me with opportunities to help others in meaningful ways. What a gift!

While I don't know why I have dystonia, I refuse to go through all of this for nothing. I know great things will come of it. They already have and more great things are on the way. I believed this even on those dark days when I thought about taking my life. Maybe that is one of the reasons I never did. I knew there was meaning in all of it. Along with my love for life and the people in my life, this is what still keeps me going. I believe dystonia happened for a good reason and I'm staying around as long as possible to learn all I can from it.

2002

2007

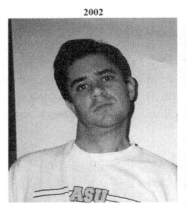
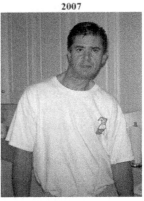

2014

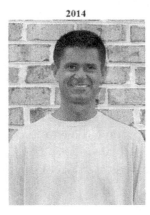

Chapter 3
The Dystonia Diagnosis

Diagnosing dystonia

Dystonia is a complex disorder that is not well known so getting an accurate diagnosis can sometimes be like finding a needle in a haystack. Except for the lucky few who stumble across someone familiar with dystonia, it can take months to years to get properly diagnosed. You may have been to numerous doctors and other health professionals, none of whom could give you answers. You may have been misdiagnosed and given harmful treatments. You may have self diagnosed, which is not uncommon for a lot of people.

Doctors, family members, and friends may have told you that your symptoms are "all in your head." This is often just another way of saying, "I have no idea what is wrong with you so you must be making it up." If the person with dystonia is unfamiliar with it or still learning about it, this might seem plausible to them as well, especially if there is no clear cause. As far from the truth this belief is, it is not uncommon to second guess ourselves and think that maybe we really are making it up or that it was our fault. This mindset is damaging. It can be a source of shame and guilt. We may internalize our guilt to such an extent that it prevents us from advocating for ourselves to pursue the care we need and deserve. Self blame can also inhibit healthy coping.

In no way are you to blame for your dystonia and anyone who puts you in a position to question yourself should be ashamed of themselves. Trust your intuition and refuse to accept subjective labeling. Your symptoms are real so don't allow the ignorance and arrogance of others prevent you from seeking a proper diagnosis and appropriate care.

A proper dystonia diagnosis is typically made by a neurologist if other doctors are unable to make an accurate diagnosis. You may hear people refer to these doctors as "movement disorder specialists" or "movement disorder neurologists." There is no single medical test to diagnose dystonia. It depends primarily on a doctor's ability to recognize the symptoms and rule out other possibilities. There is also genetic testing available for certain types of dystonia.

During your visit, a thorough medical history is taken with an emphasis on family history, head, brain or neck injury/trauma, stroke, exposure to dangerous toxins, and recreational and prescription drug use. A complete neurological exam is, or should be, given. Tests such as an MRI, CT scan and

Electromyography (EMG) may also be done. Urine and blood tests may also be done to check how well your organs are functioning and to see if you have an infection or high levels of toxins in your body. Genetic testing may also be done to see whether you have any of the genes associated with some types of dystonia. In most cases, a positive diagnosis of dystonia can be made by a visual examination of your physical symptoms by a doctor familiar with dystonia and other movement disorders.

Receiving the diagnosis

"You have dystonia" are three words that can be very confusing and frightening. Receiving the news that you have a chronic condition can bring out a lot of emotions. I felt a sense of relief. It was not because I was happy to have dystonia. I was relieved because it confirmed what I thought I had and then knowing for sure helped me pursue appropriate treatments. The diagnosis gave me direction.

People may react with fear, anxiety, anger, disbelief, a sense of loss and injustice, and depression. Some cry, scream, go numb, become very inquisitive, or feel vindicated that what they have wrong has been acknowledged. I would guess that most people experience a combination of all these things and more. I can appreciate these reactions because I experienced them all at one time or another. However, it was not when the doctor said, "You have cervical dystonia." It was in the weeks, months, and years that followed that I rode the emotional roller coaster.

If the dystonia diagnosis isn't enough, even more deflating to hear is, "there is no cure." This can cause anger, fear, and depression, to name but a few reactions. However, it is important to put this into perspective. How many diseases/disorders that people live with today, and live very well with, have a cure? I don't have the answer to this, but it is pretty low. Most diseases are managed, not cured. Just like people with diabetes, multiple sclerosis, Parkinson's disease, celiac disease, AIDS, etc., all of which have no cure, people with dystonia can live a fulfilling life with proper treatments and lifestyle changes. Please don't allow yourself to believe that you won't have a happy, functional life simply because dystonia has no cure. Many people have transformed their lives by finding successful ways to manage their symptoms.

How we respond to the diagnosis often depends on who tells us and how we find out, meaning the optimism or pessimism in the message about the prognosis. Some people are damaged by doctors who tell them that there is nothing that can be done and they will have to learn to live with it forever. This may be true for some people to an extent, but I don't believe anyone is immune to getting better. Having a genuinely positive attitude from our health care professionals about the efficacy of their treatments is paramount to our level of hope and our ability to manage our symptoms. Having a genuinely positive attitude that we will get better is just as important.

Accepting the challenge

The dystonia diagnosis is not the definition of your life. It is not the book of your life. It is just one chapter of your life among many other chapters. While it can alter the course of your life from subtle to dramatic ways, it need not be how you define yourself. It is not what happens to us in life that defines us. It is what we do with it that defines us.

Work hard every day to think about your life right now and not the life you once had. This is the way everyone should live, dystonia or not. The past is over. Also, don't predict where you might be in six months or a year. As with all of life, dystonia is unpredictable so it is best to roll with the punches versus anticipating "what might happen." Being consumed with worry can prevent you from helping yourself right now. Take each day one at a time. When I struggle in this area I say the following affirmation: "I relax into the flow of life and life flows through me with ease." I read this in a book by Louise Hay called, You Can Heal Your Life (1984), which I highly recommend.

One of my favorite quotes about dealing with obstacles is by Charles Lindbergh: "Success is not measured by what man accomplishes, but by the opposition he has encountered and the courage with which he has maintained the struggle against overwhelming odds." Dystonia is a great opposition and struggle for many people, so in order to not let it run our lives we must have the courage to keep battling. We should fully embrace even the most seemingly minor accomplishments every day and use them as stepping stones to a brighter tomorrow. Tough times don't last but tough people do.

Saying how much we hate dystonia won't make it go away. When we say we hate something we become a part of hatred. When we become a part of hatred we become the exact same thing we are trying to eliminate. Instead, find a way to cohabitate with your dystonia because no amount of anger will take it away. Fighting any adverse condition will only increase its power over us.

We have a choice to feel how we want about everything. Mindfulness tells us that there is peace in accepting things the way they are in this moment. This acceptance gives us the space to just be, and with that space, the opportunity to let go. Focus on things just as they are; not the way you think they should be. The changes that can come out of this acceptance are incredible. As Michael J. Fox says, "Acceptance doesn't mean resignation. It means understanding that something is what it is and there's got to be a way through it."

Set a course for recovery, but be prepared for life changes and different manifestations of this disorder that may come along. This is not to say they will, but the more flexible we are with the unpredictable nature of dystonia, the better we will be at managing the roller coaster ride that can accompany this condition. It is no different than how we should handle every aspect of our lives, as it is always in flux to one degree or another.

If you have a racing mind full of questions and concerns, please reach out to the many forums, support groups in your area, and dystonia organizations to talk to others who can relate. Dystonia can be distressing and exhausting. Share what you are thinking and feeling. Learn about treatment options and coping mechanisms. You need not feel any shame. You have done nothing wrong to be in this situation. Take control and do what is best for you in order to get better.

Testimonial

It's hard to look back and pinpoint a moment when dystonia began for me. I can remember having difficulty in certain situations in the early stages, but it was a gradual build up to the point where my head would involuntarily turn to my left. I hid the fact that something was wrong until it was impossible to conceal. When I couldn't talk to my own children without my head turning I knew I was in trouble. Because you don't see many examples of people with dystonia, when it develops, it's hard to know what is going on. I thought it was a psychological issue in the early stages; like I couldn't face things so I was turning away. At one stage I was told the problem was that I was depressed so I was given anti-depressants. This was the lowest point for me and gave me the spur I needed to find out what was going on.

In March 2008, my condition was such that when I walked my head would be pointing over my left shoulder and I needed to strain to look through the corner of my eye to see where I was going. When I talked to people, my head would twist away from them during a conversation. Because of all the pulling and twisting in my neck, I was getting a lot of pain. The only time I was comfortable was lying motionless on my back. Car rides were extremely painful. I had to sit with my head between my knees or lie on the back seat to get some relief from the pain. If I was walking in a crowded place I had to be led or I'd bump into people. Just walking my dog became hard because my head would twist away from people as I passed them when it was normal to utter a greeting. Work was very difficult because I'm a construction site manager for overhead lines and I have to speak to a lot of different people daily, sometimes large groups. I was embarrassed and ashamed of what was going on. Work and my social life were becoming unbearable.

At this time I decided that I needed to find out if this had ever happened to anyone else so I started searching "twisted neck" on the internet. It didn't take long before I was reading case studies that struck a chord with me and I started to see the word dystonia for the first time. Relief flowed through me as I began to realize that I had a recognized condition and I wasn't alone. There were plenty of difficult days ahead of me but at least I could put a name to what I had.

Testimonial

My emotions were up and down before I can remember getting the first visible symptoms of dystonia. To this day I don't know if that was because the condition was developing in me or if it contributed to the onset of the condition. I had higher than normal levels of stress when dystonia first kicked in, and it became worse as my condition developed.

The worst time for me was when my body started doing things I had no control over and I didn't have a clue what was going on. I kept it mostly to myself in the initial stages, blaming the symptoms on stress and hoping it would go away. As things worsened, my mood started to dip. I was on a downward spiral with my condition contributing to my mood and vice versa. I went to see the doctor for the third time to see what was happening with me. I was told I was depressed and this was the reason I had the symptoms. This was as low as I've ever been in my life; not only did I have something that was causing me pain and embarrassment, but I was causing it by being depressed. I wasn't totally convinced by the doctor though, so I decided to discard the anti-depressants I was given and tried to find out for myself what was wrong.

It only took a couple of hours in the internet before I knew what was wrong with me; that I had a recognized condition, a condition that was also affecting other people. At that moment I had turned a corner and I would never be as bad again. Relief flowed through me to know I was not alone and could maybe get some help. A few days later I was diagnosed and referred for treatment and I knew that I wasn't going crazy. I still felt embarrassed when I talked to people and my condition was evident, but I could now tell them that I had Spasmodic Torticollis.

Even though I had been diagnosed, my condition was still getting worse and I was still scared about how my life was going to pan out. I put spasmodic Torticollis into YouTube and watched other people who had it worse than me and wondered if I would get the same way. I wondered if my condition could leave me disabled and unable to provide for my family. At the same time though, I read accounts from people who had overcome their difficulties and could lead a near normal life. I decided that if others could, I could too. I sought out as much information as possible.

My condition did start to improve and I've never been as bad since that time, but dystonia is always on my mind. My social life took a nosedive, I found it very hard to sit at a table and talk to others while having a meal, even with family. I found it difficult to talk to groups of people. I disliked having the attention on me because I was embarrassed about the way I looked. As with anything else though, I gradually came to accept what I had and over time it has become a part of me, a part of me that requires constant attention.

After the diagnosis

After being diagnosed with dystonia and then learning that it is not a temporary problem, experiencing fear, anger, depression, and anxiety is normal. These feelings are also caused by loss of a valued level of functioning, such as the ability to drive, work, walk, run, and dance, to name just a few activities. It would be abnormal to deny that life has changed.

We not only experience the painful symptoms of dystonia and the loss of immediate competency, we have many questions. What does dystonia mean? How will it affect my life? Is it curable? Will it get worse? Will it get better? How is it treated? What treatments are available? What will treatments cost? Do I have to take medication or have surgery? Will the pain ever go away? Will I have it the rest of my life? Is it all in my head? How did it happen? Was it my fault? Will I still be able to work? Will I be able to take care of my family? The questions are endless and not all of them can be easily answered or answered at all. Seek answers one at a time so you are not overwhelmed trying to solve everything at once. Prioritize your concerns.

No one's future is ever guaranteed, but dystonia can deprive us of an expectable future. Most people become accustomed to looking at the odds (e.g. "If I invest my energies in a particular direction, I can be reasonably certain I'll reach a desired goal in that area"). When dystonia intervenes, all past efforts may seem irrelevant and the comfortable patterns of the past have been shattered. We have to cope with the fear of an unknown and unknowable future because it is not clear what may lie ahead.

Both mentally and physically, our energy is directed towards reducing symptoms and controlling panic about what the diagnosis means. My energy was strictly on how I could end the ridiculous pain. Literally, nothing else mattered. It was a very confusing time for me because I felt so lost and alone. What it meant for my future was very scary.

My family and friends came to my aid, but it caused an increase in their stress because they had a hard time seeing me in such bad shape. This added to my stress because it hurt me to see them worrying so much. I also felt guilty, which was silly because I did nothing wrong. We all felt helpless, but they assisted me in so many ways. They did things like cooking, cleaning, laundry, shopping, finances, driving me to doctor appointments, and most importantly, listening to me vent. I did my fair share of crying and yelling.

People around us respond the best they can. Some will abandon us while others shower us with cards, flowers, and get-well-soon wishes. Unfortunately, the idea of "get well soon" has no relevance to a person with a chronic condition. Our energy and attention are focused on responding to the onslaught of physical symptoms and the fear of the unknown. Dystonia is not like a sprained ankle or a case of the flu, both of which we heal from and return to normal. Chronic conditions are entirely different.

We are haunted by the knowledge that life may never be the same, which can cause us to become indifferent with ourselves and others. There is a belief, usually partially justified, that no one can understand the devastation of our condition. This can cause isolation which is not conducive to healthy coping.

Doctors and friends often mistake how we feel as self pity. They may say, "Just stop feeling sorry for yourself", which dismisses what we are experiencing. It is important for us to have others understand that it is difficult to have a sense of self when we lose physical competence and are afraid that we may never again be of value to ourselves and others.

In time, family and friends may give up on us because the idea of a chronic illness scares some people. After an initial burst of support, some may find it too overwhelming to continue having contact with us. Many people do not know what to do or say. This has little to do with you, unless you did something to drive them away. More than likely, they are the ones who can't handle the new dynamics. Regardless, it can be devastating to experience an apparent lack of concern shown by people close to us. I say 'apparent' because failure to be there for us often means that people care but don't know how to act. It often falls on us to keep up contact and ask for help when needed. It is important to understand that relying on other people when it is necessary does not indicate weakness or failure. Asking for help is a sign of strength.

One of the emotional barriers to asking for help is a feeling of guilt about having a health condition that puts us in a position of dependency. This can cause us to experience negative feelings about ourselves. When this happens, open communication is vital. Sharing how we feel is a way to break the guilt and isolation, or prevent them from happening in the first place. The sooner we begin talking, the better off everyone will be.

Family and friends who do well with the diagnosis and the changes in our lives understand that we are still a whole person and not a disease. They know that we are all in this together and are committed to dealing with it as well as possible. The response to my dystonia was a mixed bag. It definitely brought to surface the people in my life who truly cared. It's during the most difficult times in our lives when we usually get to see people's true colors.

Suicidal ideations
Dystonia cannot be wished away. The symptoms are there to deal with every day and the threat of an increase in symptoms may cause constant anxiety. With the feeling that the cause of dystonia cannot be solved, a lot of us experience intense fear, anger, and unhappiness. Sometimes families are unable to help because they are upset with us for being sick. Their anger is misdirected towards us and not dystonia. Even some doctors may be upset with us for having a chronic condition they are unable to cure. We may then become angry at those angry at us. We may even become angry with ourselves. It is a vicious cycle that serves no one's best interest.

Anger, which is often associated with fear, is hazardous to our emotional well being. Both are destructive emotions usually caused by a sense of loss of control over our lives, particularly in the case of dystonia where we literally lose control of body movements. Where anger and fear exist, anxiety, isolation, and depression are soon to follow. Add physical pain and a sense of helplessness and life can lose all meaning. If these feelings persist, the most perverse thought one can have is suicide.

If you have any thoughts about suicide, please speak to someone. It is not uncommon in the dystonia community to have these thoughts so please have the courage to speak about it. You will be doing yourself a big favor. You will also be doing others a big favor by opening the door for them to talk about it as well. If you are in the United States, you can also call the National Suicide Prevention Lifeline (1-800-273-8255).

I thought about suicide. I no longer do, but when my pain was severe and my neck and back muscles would not stop contracting and twisting, I considered driving into a brick wall or jumping from my balcony. I would often say that I wanted to die, but I never really talked about actual suicide with anyone. I was afraid. It seemed taboo. I wish I did talk about it because I really needed some perspective about what I was feeling. There was no shame in feeling the way I did, but in the moment I was confused and afraid. I didn't know who to talk to or what to say. Looking back, I could have talked to family members, friends, therapists, and others with dystonia. I know now that it would have helped.

The battle with suicidal thoughts was a difficult mind game for me for a long time. I thought about how good it would feel when the pain was finally gone and the depression ended. What stopped me from going through with it was the belief that I could get better (which I have done), fear of the punishment I might endure from the powers that be, and the pain it would inflict on my parents. The thought of hurting my parents by taking my life was worse than the pain I was already feeling.

Thoughts of self harm passed when I learned more about dystonia, treatment options, coping tools, and stress management techniques. It also helped when I began to focus on the things I could do versus all I had lost. It took great mental fortitude to find meaning in my life, but I did and it grew as more time passed. Talking to others with dystonia also helped and still helps to this day. It also helps to remember that suicide does not end the chances of life getting worse. Suicide eliminates the possibility of life ever getting better.

Testimonial
I used to think that suicide was the most unacceptable acts one could perform. I couldn't understand complete lack of hope given my religious background and my professional background as a mental health counselor. I had wondered as a child whether suicide might be the "unforgivable sin" that I had heard about. Then dystonia took me to the brink. I couldn't imagine living another hour or day with the pain. It felt so weird to know that I had everything to live for – children, husband, comfortable

lifestyle, extended family and friends, and talents to contribute – and yet I did not want to live due to unremitting physical pain. I have since found better ways to manage my symptoms and also come to accept my situation that I no longer contemplate suicide. To remind myself of just how close I came, on my computer I keep the searches I performed for how to access firearms.

Acknowledgement

We all have periods when we feel overmatched and not up to the struggle, but we will get through the day. If you have always been pretty resilient throughout your life, you are likely to have resilience coping with dystonia. If you did not have a resilient personality before dystonia, you will develop one.

The losses and the sadness dystonia causes may never go away entirely. There may be some anger over the things we have lost, but we should acknowledge and be proud of how we have learned to live with challenges, as well as endure treatments that can be uncomfortable, taking unwanted medications, and in some cases, surgical procedures to reduce our symptoms. However, it doesn't mean that we have to like any of it or resign ourselves to the compromises we need to make to get on with living. What is necessary for healthy living is acknowledging and accepting that changes in lifestyle must be made. It helps us learn to not waste the present because of anger about the past or fear about the future.

When family, friends, and doctors acknowledge our ability to overcome odds against us and accomplish daily tasks that are challenging, we feel more triumphant. These people (well intended) too often make the mistake of only praising us for progress without also acknowledging the difficulty of our ongoing daily battle. The latter acknowledgement is often more helpful to us.

Be realistic

When thinking about your daily activities, make your expectations realistic. For example, "Within the limits of my physical ability I will do (whatever it is) for as long as I can." Notice the use of the word "ability." It is very important that we focus on our abilities and not our 'dis'-abilities. The most important aspect of making expectations realistic is the recognition that they may be time-limited. "What can I do now based on the way I feel at this moment?" Check in with yourself to find out what you want to do and then determine if you are up to it. A chronic condition can make us feel that we must surrender all goals and all wishes, but this is not necessary at all. We can shift our plans based on what our life is like now. Not how it once was or will be, but right now.

I came from a life of hell where I could barely speak sometimes because of the breathtaking pain, to starting a few businesses, becoming a certified life coach, and writing a book. Even at my very worst, I always knew that I would write this book someday. I didn't know when, but I knew I would do it. It took 14 years after my diagnosis, but it was something I never stopped thinking about, even when I was too sick to sit at the computer to write.

Even though dystonia can rob us of many things, it does not mean that we cannot effectively manage our symptoms and live a fulfilling life. Don't ever give up on your dreams and goals, but be realistic about the time frame you set in which to do them.

Stay connected
I can't stress enough how important it is to maintain contact with the social and vocational world to the extent you are able. It will fend off depression, help improve self confidence, and create a sense of normalcy in your life. Life may not be like it once was, but our self worth is kept intact. We may still ride a roller coaster of physical and emotional symptoms, but each experience we master is a building block towards greater trust that we can safely live in this world with something "different."

Adversity and adaptation
When adversity comes our way it provides us the energy to be propelled to a higher level. This concept originally came from the Kabbalah, the ancient text of Judaism, which says, "The falls of our life provide us the energy to be propelled onto a higher path."

The more challenging and the greater the obstacles, the more potential there is for personal growth. Consider this in the context of weight training. The sole purpose is to increase strength and muscle mass. When we break down muscle and then allow adequate time for healing, we end up with increased growth, mass, and strength. It is a physiological fact that muscle must be broken down before it can be rebuilt into a stronger form than it used to be.

This is how it is with everything in our lives. There are times when we must be mentally broken down in order to rebuild to a place that is better than where we came from. As Ernest Hemingway said, "Life breaks all of us, but some of us are strong in the broken places."

None of us are immune to the challenges of life. At some time or another we all endure tough experiences. When adversity comes, how we respond to it determines what happens next. Life experiences become tragedies if we make the conscious decision to make tragedies out of them. We can either resist or we can accept challenges. If we choose to view all challenges as opportunities for personal growth, they can be a driving force for positive changes.

Instead of always fighting with what is wrong, a part of us eventually has to say, "Screw it. This is my life and I am going to live it to the best of my ability despite the challenges, and do my best to enjoy every moment. If all I do is focus on what is wrong with me, then I will live in a dark and depressing world. I accept that things are tough and it won't keep me from being happy."

It all comes down to the choice we make about how we want to live. If we want to be happy, we need to learn to be okay that things may not be the way we want them to be; that they are the way they are and we can find ways to live with it, all the while, still being committed to our search for symptom relief.

Acclimation
Being flexible and riding the fluctuating waves of symptoms will maximize the chances of acclimating to new life circumstances. This is the key to creating and sustaining a sense of inner tranquility in the face of difficult realities. To be psychologically well while physically sick involves the belief that our personal worth transcends physical limitations. This belief in our self-worth rarely emerges until what we have lost and grieved for stands second in importance to precious moments of inner peace and joy.[1,2]

Take back control in small steps. Do things that are task-oriented. For example, "Today I will walk to the end of my street, call a friend, or answer some emails." The size of the step you take doesn't matter. Each step is just as important as the others.

Don't let dystonia be stronger than you and define who you are. Flip the switch and use dystonia as a way for you to learn from it. It happened for a reason. Find the reason and your life will be transformed. If you get caught up in anger and bitterness, and let these emotions run your life, you will never see it. If you look for the lessons, your life will change. For a healthier life with dystonia, as well as anything else in life, it is better to be a student than a victim.

Success is not final, failure is not fatal: it is the courage to continue that counts.
- Winston Churchill -

Tips for dealing with your diagnosis:

- Research your area and surrounding areas for quality people who treat dystonia.
- Respect your dystonia and know your limitations. Learn to listen to your body.
- Educate yourself about dystonia as much as possible and become your own best health advocate.
- Understand that this journey requires trial and error, and patience.
- Trust that life will continue for you regardless of this challenge.
- Trust that you will get better if you are true to yourself and follow the treatment path that works best for you.
- Don't make getting better your entire life's mission to where you feel no other purpose.
- Stay connected and involved with family, friends, and community.
- Get involved with support groups. Seek help from others and learn how to help them as well. Helping others is a big part of healing.
- Stop asking "Why me?" and start asking "Why not me?" Opportunity lies in all good fortune and all misfortune.
- Spend time in prayer and meditation.
- Be kind to yourself and others.

References
1) Maistre, J. Retrieved April 28, 2013 from:
   http://www.alpineguild.com/COPING%20WITH%20CHRONIC%20ILLNESS.html
2) Maistre, J. (1995) *After the Diagnosis*. Ulysses Press.

Chapter 4
Why did I get dystonia?

"Why did I get dystonia?" is a question most of us ask ourselves. It's a natural question to ask, but one that is not easily answered. Some people can identify something specific that caused their dystonia, but many are unable to do this. If you were able to answer this question, what would or could you do differently now that would change what has already happened? The only helpful reason to ask this question is to find out if you are still doing something that exacerbates your symptoms or if your specific cause leads to a specific treatment.

I don't think knowing will change anything for me so I am not on a major quest to find out why I have dystonia. The only reason it piques my interest is to find out if I am doing something that may be causing or contributing to my current symptoms. Also, even though I can't go back and change things, the curious part of my nature wants to know why I attracted dystonia into my life.

Possible physical causes
Some of the physical things that may have contributed to my dystonia include head trauma as a child, idiopathic tonic-clonic (grand mal) seizures in college, medication for the seizures (Dilantin/phenytoin), injured joints and muscles from years of playing sports and my body compensating for the physical damage, over-taxing my body that was not prepared to handle physical activity in which I was engaged, a bike fall and bad waterskiing wipeout, both of which jarred my neck, and a major life change shortly thereafter when I left the business world to return to school for my masters degree.

Possible personality causes
I believe that people with dystonia and other disorders have personality traits that may contribute to their onset. One such trait, or rather, set of personality traits I find common among those with dystonia is HSP or "Highly Sensitive Person." An "empath" is similar to an HSP. An HSP is a person having the innate trait of high sensory processing sensitivity (or innate sensitiveness as Carl Jung originally coined it). Roughly 15 to 20 percent of the population is considered HSP.[1] In her book, The Highly Sensitive Person (1997), Dr. Elaine Aron outlines the characteristics of an HSP and how to live more easily in our often chaotic world. My use of the word chaotic is an indication that I have characteristics of an HSP. On the surface, being called "highly sensitive" could have negative connotations, but an HSP has many desirable traits.

Common traits of an HSP include great imagination, a curious mind, high intellectual abilities, creativity, conscientiousness, and compassion. They are hard workers, problem solvers, objective, and able to see the big picture. HSP's also have profound and intense sensations, and tend to process events in their lives deeper and more intensely than others. This is due to a biological difference in their nervous systems which often makes them intuitive, assertive, and strong willed. On the other hand, HSP's can take things too personally, overanalyze things, feel defensive, experience social discomfort, are easily aroused, are sensitive to subtle stimuli, shy, sensitive to the moods of other people, and hold onto intense experiences and emotions.[1-3]

Typically an HSP demonstrates greater caution and reluctance than the non-HSP population with things such as taking risks, trying new experiences, meeting new people, and venturing to unfamiliar places. Then there is the other extreme - roughly 30 percent of HSP's are thought to be extroverts and sensation seekers.[1-3]

Most people I know with dystonia have many HSP qualities. This is neither good nor bad. The important thing is being mindful of your tendencies so you can use your personality traits to your advantage to progress forward and work on those that are holding you back from where you want to be.

Whatever the cause of our dystonia, we can't undo what has happened. It helps when we accept the belief that we have health and other life challenges to teach us things about ourselves so we can grow as people. The main things I have learned and continue to learn living with dystonia include patience, persistence, perseverance, resilience, compassion, empathy, confidence, and courage.

The most difficult lesson for me has been patience. I have always been an impatient person and someone who likes things a certain way. It is challenging for me to be around people who have disorganized thoughts and don't take the bull by the horns to get things done or work to better themselves. My patience is challenged by people who waste time, leave things hanging in the air undone, and don't follow through with what they say they are going to do. Ironically, I find that there are many people in my life who are like this. To me this is no coincidence. They are part of my life to teach me patience, as well as other things where I need to improve.

Many of life's lessons are not gift wrapped in pretty packages. They often come in the form of challenging people and situations, and even a distorted body that seems to have a life of its own. We are meant to learn something from the good, the bad, and the ugly in life, and if we look at it this way, it makes whatever we are faced with easier to accept because it has a purpose.

With this in mind, how can we not look at dystonia as anything but a gift? While I have lived with great pain and discomfort like many of you, I am grateful for having been given the opportunity to learn more about myself by having to endure major struggles. Dystonia has been the greatest challenge of my life. It has also been one of my greatest teachers. If I do not choose to learn from it then I will become its victim. Although we may not write the screenplay of our lives, we direct every action and inaction which determines our mental well being.

References
1)   Aron, E. The Highly Sensitive Person. (1997) Broadway Books, New York, NY
2)   www.huffingtonpost.com, Retrieved on January 22, 2014 from:
     http://www.huffingtonpost.com/roya-r-rad-ma-psyd/highly-sensitive-people_b_1286508.html
3)   www.webmd.com, Retrieved on January 22, 2014 from:
     http://www.webmd.com/balance/features/are-you-too-sensitive

Chapter 5
Victim Mentality Reform

The term "victim mentality" refers to people who blame someone or something else for the unpleasant things in their life. Life is easier when we play the blame game. It helps us rationalize why we are not growing and moving forward. "Victim mentality" also applies to people who believe that undesirable life circumstances only yield negative outcomes.

Feeling like a victim is normal when diagnosed with a serious health condition like dystonia, but it is self destructive if we remain in this state of mind. We become isolated, depressed, bitter, angry, and resentful. Victims are only focused on themselves and upset with all the things they do not have or cannot do, whether it is because of financial constraints, health limitations, a combination of both, or something else entirely. The victim will always find something wrong and live a life of excuses. You probably know some of these people. You may be one of them.

Victims will ask "Why me?" in a sulking and moaning ("poor me") manner when something happens that they don't like. Asking "Why me?" in an inquisitive manner is more proactive and might yield more answers because it puts us in the role of an unattached observer where we can be more objective.

For the first few years with dystonia I was stuck in the "Why me, poor me" frame of mind. It got me nowhere but depressed. I had to change this question if I wanted freedom from my mental anguish. Instead of asking, "Why me", I began asking, "Why not me?", "How can I learn to live with dystonia?" and "How can dystonia help me learn and grow?" I was no better or worse than anyone else so if it happened to me, so be it. There was nothing I could do to reverse things so I needed to learn to accept it and find the good in it, even when I was in ridiculous pain and could barely function.

When we moan and groan about our problems it puts us in a hole that is difficult to get out of. We find comfort in the depressed world we mentally create and are unmotivated to find solutions. I did it and I see others doing it all the time; and it isn't just people with health issues. People complain about everything; the weather, their job, car, family, spouse, bills, yard work. What's the point? There is nothing inherently wrong with any of these things. The only thing wrong is our perception.

A big part of the victim mentality is due to being stuck in the past; how life was before dystonia. Find a way to release the past. It is not who you are. You can be whomever you want right now. You just need to make the choice, set the intention, and act it out. By no means is it as easy as I am making it sound. I completely understand that it is a process that unfolds one day at a time. We just need to allow ourselves to let it unfold so we are free to live your lives.

When I get stuck thinking about my life before dystonia it gets me down. I could be on top of the world and all of a sudden I try to do something my body won't allow me to anymore and I am reminded of how life once was. Feeling sad about it is momentary though because I don't allow myself to dwell. Instead, I think new thoughts and involve myself in other activities.

A popular quote many have heard is, "The past is history. The future is a mystery. Today is a gift. That's why it's called the present." Do your best to enjoy the gift of this moment. An affirmation I like to use to help me when I am stuck in days gone by is, "I release the past. I am free to move forward with love in my heart." I say this over and over until I feel it resonate within me.

Accepting change
My life before and after dystonia are as different as night and day. I went from a very active lifestyle to one that was extremely sedentary. For most of my life, I played organized and recreational sports all year round. My two main sports were golf and baseball. I could easily walk 18 holes several times a week and some days I played 27 holes. I played baseball from a young age all the way through college, practicing or playing games every day of the week. I loved it!

I also never passed up the opportunity to swim, bike, play tennis, racquetball, basketball, soccer, or ultimate Frisbee, to name just a few of my favorite activities. In the mid 90's, I trained to be a place kicker in the NFL. Along with working full time, I was training twice a day until a hip injury ended that dream. I then studied karate for several years and earned a brown belt. Long story short, I never sat idle for long. When dystonia prevented me from living my active life, it was a major shock to my psyche.

For the first five years I was miserable. I had a lot of negative self talk about how I could no longer do the things I loved so much. I characterized dystonia as an evil intruder that "ruined my life." I was deeply frustrated, which caused a lot of anger and bitterness. This made my dystonia worse because negative emotions cause increased muscle tension. I had to shift my thinking if I wanted to live a happier and healthier life.

It was hard work, but I eventually came to understand that change is a natural part of life over which we have little to no control. Just ask any aging person about their former abilities compared to their current abilities. Healthy aging requires accepting change just as healthy coping with dystonia requires accepting change.

I came to understand that certain things do not last a lifetime, so I thought of all the good times I had playing baseball and golf (and other sports), said thank you for all those times, and let them go. I had to say goodbye. I had to release the past so I could live in the present and focus my energy on the direction my life was heading.

Letting go of baseball was probably the most difficult. It was hard to watch a game, in person or on TV, without feeling depressed. To make matters worse, my nephew was playing Little League so I was missing out on an important part of his life. I should note that at that time my dystonia symptoms were such that it was very challenging to go to a game. I was in too much pain to sit or stand, let alone drive to get there. My inability to do something so seemingly simple added to my depression.

When my symptoms became more manageable, I watched him play his last three years of high school, never once feeling depressed while at a game. The main reason was because I stopped feeling sorry for myself. I gave into gratitude for the time I was able to play and took advantage of the opportunity to now see him play and grow as a person doing something so near and dear to my heart. I still missed an occasional game when my dystonia acted up, but I was okay with that because I learned to accept that some days are more limiting than others.

Except for a few matches, regretfully I did not see my two nieces play volleyball. It was far too uncomfortable being in the gymnasium with fluorescent lighting and loud, sharp noises. The sounds bounced off the walls and through my head as if I were inside a bass drum. It made me dizzy, caused anxiety, and exacerbated my physical pain. I wish I saw them play more and be part of that experience with them, but I had to think of my health which really took a toll in that environment. My youngest nephew is still in high school. On days I feel well enough, I look forward to watching him play soccer and tennis the next two years.

I would like to say that I freely go to sporting events and do other activities with ease, but that is not always the case. There are days when things are far too uncomfortable. Therefore, I live my life within the boundaries of my abilities and accept that I can't always do everything I want. If I don't accept this reality, I will mentally torture myself when I miss out on things. When I am able to do more, I enjoy the hell out of myself! I have finally learned to not take feeling well for granted.

It is what it is

I often think of acceptance in terms of the saying, "It is what it is." For a very long time I despised this statement. I always thought another line should be added that says, "But it doesn't have to be." Up until a few years ago, I believed that nothing had to be how it was if we didn't want it to be. When I realized that there are many things in life we can't do anything about, my egomaniacal denial disappeared.

The only thing we can change about most things is how we respond to them. When I think about life from this perspective, I really like the saying, "It is what it is." "It" truly is what it is. "It" can't be anything else. How we deal with "it" is what matters. This mindset makes it so much easier for me to accept things that come my way.

I am not resigned to think that I can't change things about myself. I have just come to better accept the challenges I live with. I have learned that each day is different and I have to roll with the punches. Every night I go to bed praying I will wake up with fewer symptoms than I had the previous day. If this does not happen, I am better at not fighting what I can't change physically about myself in the moment. I can only change how I respond to how I feel and be grateful for what I am able to do on that given day.

What helps me most are the words I use. When I say something like, "If only I didn't have dystonia I could jog again," I am punishing myself with harsh judgment. Instead I say, "I miss jogging, but I am so happy I can go for a walk today." Reframing my thoughts helps me embrace the things I am able to do with more excitement and joy.

In order to be happy, we can't dwell on what once was. All we have is the present moment so that is where our focus needs to be. When we focus on the abilities we have now, acceptance follows, giving us greater peace of mind.

Moving forward

While I am not doing things with my life I thought I would because of dystonia, I am doing other positive things with my life because of dystonia. I'm sure this is the case for many of you. I am grateful for all I have experienced because it offers me the opportunity to grow in ways I never imagined. It also gives me the opportunity to help others, either with dystonia or other life challenge. What a gift to be given a life lesson that helps others find hope and meaning in their lives. It is certainly a challenge to be in this mindset, and I am not all the time, but I know that we have to be like this if we want to find meaning in our struggle and happiness in our lives.

I once worked with a client who had mild dystonia symptoms; mild compared to many others I know, but to her it was severe. She was in her late 20's and studying to be a doctor. She complained incessantly about how her life had been ruined. She was stuck in the depressed "Why me" mode of thinking, even though she found some symptom management techniques that were significantly helpful. She just simply resented the fact that she had dystonia, regardless of how much or how little it affected her life.

I tried to impress upon her how fortunate she was to have this experience. When it came time for her to be a doctor she would be much better able to empathize with her patients thanks to having dystonia. Her patients would be so lucky to have a doctor who had the capacity to put herself in their shoes, much like the movie *The Doctor* (1991) with William Hurt. She had a choice to continue moaning about her health challenge or see the blessing in it because of the many fortunate patients with whom she would come in contact throughout her career. We lost touch, but she is a smart woman who I feel confident is now helping many people, largely in part because of dystonia.

Everything in life happens for a reason. Sometimes we can figure out the reason and other times not, but I live my life with the belief that nothing is happening TO me. Everything is happening FOR me and I am exactly where I am supposed to be at every given moment. I may not always like the circumstances, but I am here for a reason and there is something to learn. If we keep our focus on gratitude instead of bitterness and anger, life is less stressful and more fulfilling.

You may have heard the following quote: "The most beautiful stones have been tossed by the wind and washed by the waters and polished to brilliance by life's strongest storms." We will have many storms throughout our lives and they all help us grow. Instead of running from the storm, it is best to find a way to dance in the rain.

Most of us can think of a previous challenge in our lives and list things we learned from it. In most cases, we learned why we had to go through it after it happened. My suggestion is that we find the meaning as we are going through it. Instead of fighting, we should embrace the storm so we don't prolong the pain. If we can learn the lessons we are being taught, the storm will not last long. Storms in our lives help us if we let them.

Dystonia is not the most significant thing in our lives. It is how we respond to it and learn to live with it that is most significant. Remember that any setback in life is a setup for a comeback and we have the choice to become either a victim or a victor.

Heal your mind, heal your body
In chapter 3, I mentioned Louise Hay's book, You Can Heal Your Life (1984). Her belief is that we create every illness in our body. The following quote comes from one of my favorite chapters called The Body: "The body, like everything else in life, is a mirror of our inner thoughts and beliefs. The body is always talking to us, if we would only take the time to listen. Every cell within your body responds to every single thought you think and every word you speak. Continuous modes of thinking and speaking produce body behaviors and postures, and 'eases' or 'dis'-eases. The person who has a permanently scowling face did not produce that by having joyous, loving thoughts."[1]

Reading her book helped me look more closely at the mind-body connection, especially when my dystonia was severe and when I was going through some difficult challenges outside my battle with dystonia. I saw how my response to everything had a direct impact on my physical health.

I find the appendix of her book to be particularly interesting. It discusses how specific problems in certain body parts are connected to thought patterns. Take the neck for example; Louise says, "The neck and throat are fascinating because so much 'stuff' is going on there. The neck represents the ability to be flexible in our thinking, to see the other side of a question, and to see another person's viewpoint. When there are problems in the neck, it usually means we are being stubborn about our own concept of the situation."[1]

As it does me, this may describe many of you. I have always been a stubborn person. Throughout my life, whenever I felt I wasn't being heard or if I disagreed with something, I would tense up in the shoulder and neck area. I would also clench my teeth. I still do now, but to a much lesser degree thanks in part to the information in her book.

I am not claiming that dystonia is created by our behavior or thought patterns, but I am also not discounting that it does have an impact. Perhaps more than we realize. With this in mind, have you chosen to become a victim of dystonia or a curious and grateful student?

The most beautiful people we have known are those who have known defeat, known suffering, known struggle, known loss, and have found their way out of the depths. These persons have an appreciation, a sensitivity, and an understanding of life that fills them with compassion, gentleness, and a deep loving concern. Beautiful people do not just happen.
- Elisabeth Kubler-Ross -

References
1)	Hay, L. (1984) You can heal your life. Hay House Publishing. 123; 126

Chapter 6
Dystonia and Grief

Learning to live with dystonia or any chronic condition is a process. Like all processes, it has different stages with different characteristics. Each stage toward wellness usually involves loss, grief, and acknowledgment of internal pain. It may sometimes seem that you have no reason to live or that you are living only to experience pain. Even so, the reason for living and the incentive for becoming psychologically well is the potential for the future.

As with the death of a loved one, it is common for people with dystonia and other chronic conditions to go through the stages of grief. When something alters one's life to an extent that they are no longer able to do things they once could, it can cause a great sense of loss which initiates the grief cycle.

When my dystonia became severe I lost all sense of self. I didn't know where I fit into the world anymore. I was no longer a student, an employee, a businessman, an athlete, a traveler, a friend, a brother, an uncle, a son, or an active member of society. I was a guy who lived on the floor in writhing pain who basically did nothing but eat and sleep. I was like a child going through the egocentric stage of development. This may sound melodramatic, but that truly was my existence. I was grief stricken. I had an identity crisis and felt a deep sense of personal loss.

It was important for me to understand grief so I was better able to process the significant changes to my life and accept new challenges that dystonia added. Grief is an important process that many of us need to go through in order to be mentally healthy.

Stages of grief
The information below is a compilation of the work done by Elisabeth Kubler-Ross, M.D. The late Kubler-Ross was a Swiss-born psychiatrist, a pioneer in near death studies, and the author of the book, On Death and Dying (1969), where she first discussed what is now known as the Kubler-Ross Model. In this work, she proposed the five stages of grief as a pattern of adjustment. People experience most of these stages, though in no defined sequence.[1]

Kubler-Ross did not intend this to be a rigid series of sequential or uniformly timed steps because people do not always experience all of the grief cycle stages. Some stages might be revisited and some stages might not be experienced at all. Rather than a steady progression, people tend to ebb and flow between stages. The five stages are also not linear or equal in their experience. Grief and other reactions to emotional trauma are as individual as a fingerprint.

The grief model is perhaps a way of explaining how and why 'time heals', or how 'life goes on.' If you don't go through some or any of the stages it does not mean that you are going through grief "incorrectly." We all experience loss in different ways.

While Kubler-Ross' focus was on death and bereavement, her grief cycle model is a useful perspective for understanding emotional reaction to personal trauma and change, irrespective of cause.

1. *Denial* - Denial is a conscious or unconscious refusal to accept facts, information, and reality relating to the situation concerned. It is a defense mechanism and perfectly natural. Some people can become locked in this stage when dealing with a traumatic change that can't be ignored. A chronic condition, especially when pain is involved, is certainly not something that can easily be avoided or ignored, so denial in the literal sense is probably not very common. Rather, we know something is wrong, but we may ignore the extent to which it affects us, wishing it would go away. Some days you may be tempted to pretend you never received your diagnosis. However, facing your diagnosis head on is the best way to cope.

2. *Anger* - People dealing with emotional upset can be angry with themselves or with others, especially those close to them. Knowing this helps us keep detached and non-judgmental when experiencing the anger of someone who is very upset. I have experienced anger plenty of times, all to varying degrees. It may spark from my symptoms, my frustration with doctors and ineffective treatments, indifference or lack of acknowledgement from others about my situation, or the frustration of not being able to do some things I enjoy. Sometimes anger feels like the only appropriate outlet. I am far less prone to anger now than I once was, but the challenges of living with dystonia engulf me from time to time.

3. *Bargaining* - The bargaining stage is characterized by attempting to negotiate with a higher power or someone or something you feel has some control over the situation. You might make promises in return for the painful situation not to occur or for things to go back to how they were before the loss or change.

You may find yourself intensely focused on what you or others could have done differently in order to prevent the loss or change. You may also think about how life could have been if not for this unpleasant situation. While these thoughts may help you begin to accept the loss or change, bargaining rarely provides a sustainable solution.

4. *Depression* - Although this stage means different things depending on who it involves, it is sort of an acceptance with emotional attachment. It's natural to feel sadness, regret, fear, and uncertainty. It shows that the person has begun to accept reality. Although, this reality can often keep people stuck, especially those with chronic health issues. When we are constantly reminded of our pain and how life once was, it is challenging to break away from depression. If you live with depression, it would be wise to seek out a trusted friend or therapist. Please also see the section on depression in chapter 7.

5. *Acceptance* - Acceptance is one of the greatest challenges for individuals and also one of the most important to achieve for progress to be made towards living a fulfilling life. This stage varies according to the person's situation, although broadly it is an indication that there is some emotional detachment and objectivity. People dying can enter this stage long before the people they leave behind, who must also pass through their own individual stages of grief.

When it comes to chronic illness, this is usually the stage we reach and retreat from more often than the others. When we are having a good day acceptance is easier, but on tough days, it can be a roller coaster ride where we may fluctuate through all the stages. What we resist persists so accepting our current situation is essential for forward progress. Without acceptance, the fight with pain can end up in a battle with ourselves that we will continue to lose. Everything we fight weakens us and everything we embrace strengthens us.

It was very hard for me, but I had to learn to accept that there were things I was no longer going to do; some by choice because of how they make me feel and some because my body does not allow me to do them. Several formerly important parts of my life were gone. I couldn't bring them back so there was no point fighting any of it. Perhaps as I continue to get better I will be able to do some or all of those things again, but for now I have to accept that they are not part of my life. It has taken me years to get to this point and I still need to work hard to detach myself from what life once was so I can embrace what life is now.

As Rosalind Joffe (www.cicoach.com) points out, chronically difficult health issues often leave us making choices based on events we have no control over, and the choices we have are limited. This can be profoundly disappointing and sad. But consider this: when we accept that we are doing the best we can, isn't that the best choice we've got?

One of the keys to acceptance is learning how to accommodate our dystonia. Too often we fight against it rather than embracing it as a part of our lives. Not unlike having to walk on crutches when we sprain an ankle, when our body has limitations from dystonia we need to learn to accommodate it as best we can. We have to find a way to make dystonia our friend. Yes, you read correctly. Learn to treat it as your friend so the inner battle and turmoil you are experiencing will end. This may sound like a crazy concept to some of you, but it truly is the secret to living a meaningful life with a chronic condition. If I heard this at a different time on my dystonia journey I would have shot the messenger. Now I better understand this concept and it has served me well. Work on accepting dystonia as part of your life so you can move on, similar to the way practicing forgiveness sets us free from past events.

It took me years, but I now choose to accept dystonia and embrace the things I have and can still do with passion and excitement. I don't have time or interest in being depressed about all the things I have lost and find challenging. Neither do you. Life moves by too quickly to wallow for too long. If you are able to get up after getting kicked in the gut, regardless of how many times, you have more than a fighting chance at a quality life. Let the process of grief play itself out and do your best to roll with the stages. Your internal strength and perseverance increase every time you rise from falling.

If you want to make peace with your enemy, you have to work with your enemy. Then he becomes your partner.
- Nelson Mandela -

References
1) Based on the Grief Cycle model first published in *On Death & Dying*, Elisabeth Kubler-Ross, 1969. Interpretation by Alan Chapman 2006-2009. Retrieved on April 21, 2013 from: http://www.ekrfoundation.org/five-stages-of-grief/

Chapter 7
Depression and Anxiety

Dystonia and depression

Sudden and unexpected changes to our health can alter our lives in many ways. Feelings of shock, anger, grief, loss, and sadness are common. These feelings usually pass with time. However, if they cause ongoing stress, we are at risk of developing depression and anxiety, two of the most common complications of a chronic health condition like dystonia.

Living with dystonia requires us to adjust to the demands of the symptoms, as well as to treatments, medications, lifestyle changes, and in some cases an uncertain future. It may affect our independence and change the way we live, how we see ourselves and how others see us, and how we relate to others and how others relate to us. Dystonia can also create a social stigma where we may be embarrassed by our appearance and/or inability to control body movements. This can cause seclusion and disinterest in activities that previously brought us joy or entertainment. The inability to perform work or tasks as we once did may cause feelings of worthlessness or helplessness. This is a heavy burden so it is not uncommon to experience a roller coaster ride of emotions which can be exhausting and very distressing.

This stress can cause despair or sadness which is normal. However, if it persists, it can turn to depression. The challenge for you and your doctor is to decide whether symptoms of depression are just a normal reaction to the stress of having dystonia or so intense and disabling that you require specific treatments for the depression itself.

Not everyone with dystonia will experience depression, but it is common so it is important to recognize and understand the symptoms. Be open and honest about your feelings and share them with your family and health care team. Depression is not a weakness. It is just an obstacle to overcome.

Common symptoms of depression:
- Irritability and restlessness
- Apathy
- Feelings of guilt, worthlessness, and/or helplessness
- Feelings of hopelessness and/or pessimism
- Overeating or appetite loss; significant weight changes
- Insomnia, early-morning wakefulness, or excessive sleeping

- Difficulty concentrating, remembering details, and making decisions
- Fatigue and decreased energy
- Thoughts of suicide; suicide attempts
- Loss of interest in activities or hobbies once pleasurable, including sex
- Cramps or digestive problems that do not ease, even with treatment
- Persistent sad, anxious, or empty feelings

We and our family members often overlook the symptoms of serious depression, assuming that feeling depressed is normal for someone struggling with a chronic condition. Symptoms of depression such as fatigue, pain, anxiety, and insomnia are also common features of dystonia, adding to the difficulty of deciding whether they are due to depression or from the challenges of living with dystonia.

Situational depression

Always be on your toes mentally because sometimes when things begin to look brighter, we are tempted to relax and might be caught off guard when a bout of depression recurs. Dystonia can be unpredictable, so be prepared that one day of feeling well may not transfer over to the next day. Also, the excitement associated with mastering new living skills can give way to new feelings of despair when we begin to recall how much simpler it once was to do routine things. Nostalgia may bring on sadness and discouragement. If something reminds us of what life was like before dystonia or what life would be like if we never got dystonia, depression is likely. This is the main ongoing mental battle that a lot of us with dystonia live with.

While I am now in a better place mentally and physically, and proud of the things I am able to do again because of all my hard work learning to manage my symptoms, I am often reminded of things I used to do and how easy they were compared to now. This can be frustrating, but I have to remind myself that I am doing the best I can. This is all I can ask of myself. If I don't reframe my accomplishments based on my abilities then I am not living in reality. The more I focus on the life I have created for myself now versus the one I used to have, the more upbeat I am. The more I involve myself in new ventures and new ways of living, fun events take the place of unhappy memories. Everyone, dystonia or not, has to do this. Changing and adapting is universal to life.

Thinking our way into depression

Having gone through long and short bouts of depression after developing dystonia, I fully acknowledge its presence and the reasons for its occurrence.

The way we process life conditions affect us emotionally. Our emotions then affect our thoughts which play a significant role in our state of mind. When my symptoms were more severe I dove deep into the pits of despair, largely in part because I didn't have the tools I do now.

This may offend some people, but in most cases I believe depression is a choice; not always a conscious choice, but a choice nonetheless. Like me, it may be from a lack of strategies for dealing with challenges, but it can also be from low levels of perseverance in the face of a challenging situation. For some, it is a way to garner attention. It is also a way to validate physical symptoms and illustrate to others in a dramatic way how much dystonia really affects us. In the name of depression, we also sometimes excuse ourselves of responsibility in certain areas of our lives.

While I acknowledge the seriousness of depression, there are times when we falsely classify what we are feeling as depression, when in fact we are simply experiencing the challenges that are part of the process of living. This can lead to a self fulfilling prophecy so be careful how much power you give to depressing thoughts.

While it is normal to go through bouts of depression at times, we have the ability to ward off chronic depression; we even have the ability to avoid bouts of depression. If we can recognize the signs, we can to shift our thinking to change our mood. That is basically what depression is; a temporary mood that engulfs us because of thoughts we are generating.

It is important to understand that dystonia does not cause depression. No health condition causes depression. We have been conditioned to think that poor health causes depression, but this is not true. What causes depression is how we respond to our dystonia. It is no different than any other life experience. We can let life events bring us down or we can choose to rise above them and continue to find joy and meaning in our lives.

If it is true that in most cases we choose to be depressed, at least to some degree, it must follow that we can also choose to be happy. We all have visceral (gut) reactions to things that include fear, worry, anger, and sadness, but it does not mean that we have to live with chronic fear, worry, anger, or sadness. We are in charge of our emotions. We choose every feeling in all circumstances in our lives. No person or any life condition can make us feel a certain way unless we allow it.

I understand and appreciate that depression is painful and real. It is a biochemically-based physiological reality that exists in the body and what needs to be understood is that there are toxic chemical consequences of thinking any stressful thought that exacerbates depression. When we think positively, the pituitary gland disperses endorphins which are effective in releasing energy that eases healing and relieves pain. However, when we have negative thoughts, noradrenaline (a stress hormone sometimes referred to as norepinephrine) is dispersed.

Thoughts like "I am depressed", "I am fat", "I am in pain", "I can't get out of bed", "Life is terrible", "I hate dystonia", power up the chemical factory in the brain causing it to turn out buckets of stress chemicals. This causes the brain to become more chemically imbalanced, plunging us deeper into depression. These thoughts may be true, but we are better off not replaying them over and over in our head.

Depression is really a complicated mind trick. Since the mind can only think one thought at a time, we have only one attention. Since the pain of depression is so persistent, we give it our one attention. Since our feelings are located in a separate part of the brain from our cognitive area, we are temporarily disconnected from the totality of our experience. We feel lost, helpless and powerless, but in reality, we are not helpless and powerless at all.

Since we can only think one thought at a time we can think any thought we want. This principle is based on neuroscience and is also the basis for transcendental meditation and hypnosis. If this principle was not true there could be no such thing as medical hypnosis for brain surgery or how we form a new habit. We are not forced to feel painful feelings like depression. It is caused by a chemical imbalance in the brain that we have the ability to change by changing our thoughts.

We don't have to give a thought attention merely because it pops into our brain. Nothing is actually forcing us to think them. We can force ourselves to think neutral thoughts long enough for the chemical brain factory to power down and balance out. Depression is not really a terrible illness. Depression is really a terrible mindset. It is dependent upon our rapt attention to it. When we focus our attention on something other than our depression, it recedes or disappears.

We are free to direct our thoughts the same way we direct the cursor on our computer to tell it what to do. When most of us think of tasting a lemon we salivate. Salivation is a biochemically-based physiological reality that exists in the body just as depression is a biochemically-based physiological reality. We don't have to cut out our tongue to stop salivating. We just have to stop thinking about lemons. Thoughts cause salivation and thoughts can un-cause salivation. Likewise, thoughts can cause depression and thoughts can un-cause depression.

We don't have to ignore our feelings, but we don't have to needlessly suffer from them either. When we switch from our thoughts of depression to new thoughts and new behaviors, it creates new feelings; less stressful feelings. When our stressful thoughts stop, our brain is no longer in a state of alarm and good feelings can once again return.[1, 2]

I invite you to look at the work done by Dr. A.B. Curtiss who helps people with depression using a technique called "Directed Thinking" which is designed to change neural programming in the brain by changing harmful thought patterns.[3]

Managing depression
The stigma that depression carries drives many people to hide it, try to tough it out, or self-medicate with alcohol and drugs. To effectively treat/manage depression, it is important to seek care from a licensed mental health professional and get a correct diagnosis and treatment plan. Many treatments for depression are available and typically include a combination of therapy and medication. However, it should be noted that anti-depressant medications may contribute to the onset of dystonia and/or exacerbate existing symptoms, so please exercise caution. See chapter 15 for a complete list of medications that medical experts believe may contribute to dystonia.

Along with counseling/therapy and medications, other ways to reduce depression include getting adequate sleep, eating a healthy diet consisting of an abundance of fruits, vegetables, proteins, and omega 3 fats, social support, stress reduction, massage, acupuncture, yoga, and tai chi. Other lifestyle changes that may help include getting into a regular routine, setting goals, taking on responsibilities, challenging negative thoughts, doing new things, and being socially active. It is not necessary to implement all of these things at once. Find one or a few things that work and then implement others as needed when you are ready.[4-10]

Regular exercise has also been shown to increase the effectiveness of multiple organs that are critical for mood regulation. Exercise has also been shown to have an anti-inflammatory effect. This is important because inflammation can often accompany depression. Combining music with exercise is also effective for battling depression. According to a Cleveland Clinic research study, listening to upbeat music can ease symptoms of depression up to 25%. Music can also make people feel more in control of their pain and less disabled by their condition.[11]

Tips for coping with depression:
- Get help as soon as symptoms of depression appear.
- Learn about your condition so that you can better manage it. Don't be afraid to ask for help. If you believe your medication is causing your depression, speak with your doctor about alternative treatments.
- If possible, stay involved in activities you enjoy and learn new skills.
- Maintain a daily routine as best you can.
- Keep your support network active. Whether it is friends, family, church, golf or another activity, connections to others are very helpful to fight depression and isolation.
- Take proper care of yourself. Eating well, exercising, and quitting smoking and drinking can reduce the risk of depression and reduce negative effects of chronic illness.
- Become more involved with your health care team in your treatment decisions.
- Maintain emotional balance to cope with negative feelings.
- Maintain confidence and a positive self-image, understanding that you are no less of a person because of your dystonia.
- Get involved with support groups.
- Do for others, especially when you are feeling down.

Dystonia and anxiety
Like depression, anxiety also affects many people with dystonia. Anxiety is the apprehension, uncertainty, and fear one feels when he or she is anticipating a threatening event or situation, whether the threat is real or imagined. Anxiety is not the same as fear. There are subtle differences. Fear is an emotional response to a known or definite threat; something realistically intimidating or dangerous. It is an appropriate response to a perceived threat. Anxiety can occur when there is no present threat. It is an over-reaction to a situation that is subjectively seen as dangerous. It is often accompanied by restlessness, fatigue, problems concentrating, and muscle tension. Put simply, it is an unpleasant

state of inner turmoil often accompanied by nervous behavior. However, the two are related as fear can cause anxiety and anxiety can cause fear.

Anxiety is actually a normal human emotion that everyone experiences at times. Many people feel temporarily anxious or nervous when faced with a problem at home or work, before taking a test, making an important decision, etc. For people with anxiety disorders, worry and fear are constant and overwhelming, which can be crippling. They can cause so much distress that it interferes with a person's ability to lead a normal life.

While the person living with it may realize their anxiety is too much, they may have difficulty controlling it which can negatively affect their day-to-day living. There are many types of anxiety disorders that include panic disorder, obsessive compulsive disorder, post-traumatic stress disorder, social anxiety disorder, specific phobias, and generalized anxiety disorder.

Anxiety can reduce or eliminate self confidence, especially if you also have to deal with disability, job loss, marital problems, and chronic pain, things that are not uncommon when you have dystonia. Anxiety can cause us to excessively worry, sometimes to the point of paranoia.

An elephant can be tethered by a thread if he believes he is captive.
If we believe we are chained by habit or anxiety, we are in bondage.
- John H. Crowe -

Panic attacks
I often hear people with dystonia talk about having panic attacks. I used to be one of them. Panic attacks are the sudden onset of intense anxiety. They are characterized by feelings of great fear and apprehension, and are often accompanied by heart palpitations, shortness of breath, sweating, and trembling. Panic attacks are usually accompanied by avoidance, anticipatory anxiety, and worrying about the consequences of a panic attack.

Heightened apprehension to the point of panic or terror and fear striking when no threat is present is an inappropriate response to the environment. If your attempts to avoid fear begin to dominate your life, seek professional help. Treatments include medication, stress reduction techniques (breathing re-training, exercise, guided meditation, deep muscle relaxation), and cognitive behavioral therapy (and other forms of therapy that your doctor deems appropriate).

I know all too well what panic attacks are like. One of my former triggers for a panic attack was driving, even around my own town, let alone long distances. I used to panic at a red light if I was not the first car at the light and didn't have a way to turn off the road. I felt like I was going to have a heart attack or pass out. My heart wound pound and my hands would sweat. I was claustrophobic. I would also feel very weak and my legs would tremble. My breathing also became shallow.

After a few years, I had to do something about it. I knew I couldn't live like that anymore. I had to force myself to deal with the anxiety if I wanted to live a fuller life outside of my home. I knew I had to face my fears head on.

For the next couple of weeks, I put myself in situations that created anxiety and panic. I purposely drove in congested areas of town during afternoon rush hour where I was certain to get caught at red lights and slow moving traffic. Previously, if I saw that I was not going to catch a green light at an intersection, I would turn off the road, make a u-turn and then catch the green light from another direction. As long as I kept the car moving I could avoid a panic attack. Within two weeks of exposing myself to heavy traffic and red lights, my panic attacks ended. It was a process, but I managed to overcome them in a shorter period of time than I expected. I overcame something in two weeks that I lived with for over 2 years.

I then approached my next driving fear which was going over bridges. Anytime my field of vision expanded to wide open spaces, which is typically what happens on bridges, along with being high up, panic would set in. Just as I did with heavy traffic and red lights, I chose to face this anxiety head on by driving over a bridge we have in town that takes you over a river. I avoided it for years, even as a passenger. The first few times I drove over the bridge by myself I was dizzy, my hands were sopping wet, and my body was trembling. I also felt like I was floating on top of my seat as if I was not part of the car. I had white knuckles from gripping the steering wheel so hard.

I did my best to focus on the music I had playing in the car. I specifically chose it to distract me. It took about a minute to get over the bridge, but it seemed like 20 minutes. I had such a feeling of relief to be safely on the other side, but then I had to return! Worrying about the return trip, I missed my turn around exit. I found myself on a highway travelling at speeds I hadn't driven in 10 years. My anxiety skyrocketed trying to keep up with other cars. I finally came to the next exit and had to park for a little while to calm down before I got back on the road to head back.

Anxiety crept back in when I got back on the highway and onto the bridge again. When I got across safely I wanted to get home immediately. Instead, I stopped myself, did some slow, rhythmic breathing, turned around, and drove back over the bridge again. Even though I just did it, I was not satisfied with how I felt. I was concerned that the high anxiety I experienced would prevent me from coming back so I had to do it again. The second time was a little better so I went home after I was done, proud of my accomplishment. I then did the same thing every day for the next week.

Each time I was on the bridge and the highway I had anxiety, but it was less and less every day. My confidence grew which gradually reduced my anxiety. After about a dozen times over a period of a week, I no longer had anxiety driving on this bridge or any other bridge. Nor did I have anxiety being on the highway. Another plus is that my dystonia symptoms did not get worse, which was a big concern of mine. In fact, my neck was looser than it usually was. All that tension I was holding onto released.

Shortly after I conquered my fear of heavy traffic, red lights, and bridges (March 2013), I was invited to visit a friend who was on vacation about an hour and a half from where I lived. It was also in another state. I hadn't driven that far on my own or been out of my state since March 2002! I was invited to go to this vacation destination by different people several times in the past and always said "no." It was my immediate response without any thought whatsoever. It was automatic because I "knew" I couldn't do it without experiencing the physical consequences and terrible anxiety.

This time something was different. While I had some trepidation about the trip (a road trip I had done many times before dystonia and before my anxiety disorder), I said "yes." I had to. I knew this invitation was a test. It was the next step towards expanding my boundaries. Even though I conquered going over that bridge and driving on a highway, I was still only 20 minutes from home. If I was to progress further out of my comfort zone and reduce my anxiety, I had to drive further beyond my boundaries.

Long story short, not only was the trip free of any anxiety or problems with my dystonia, I actually felt better and my confidence soared. I drove on highways by myself that I hadn't in over a decade. I went over bridges, adapted to wide open spaces that normally caused me to get dizzy and anxious, and dealt with traffic in unfamiliar places. I found myself not thinking at all about my dystonia. I was enjoying the ride and all the fresh sights. I was in the moment not thinking about anything other than the pleasure of being on the open road on my own. When I crossed the state border I cheered in celebration. It was a huge accomplishment.

I didn't have a GPS and my map was outdated. Part of this was by design. I purposely made it a little more difficult to find my destination than I had to so I could really test my anxiety to strengthen my resolve. It worked and I did great. I also had a great time. I did have to spend a few days recovering from all the activity when I got home, but it was not as bad as I thought it would be.

I now had much more confidence to do things I previously feared, as well as try new things. This boost in confidence was the most significant part of the experience. I began doing other things I was avoiding which opened my world and made life interesting and exciting again. Instead of worrying about all the bad things that might happen before I did an activity, I started to look forward to them. A huge burden was lifted and I was living again.

It is so important to test our boundaries and re-evaluate our limitations (or limiting beliefs) to avoid over-protecting ourselves and missing out on the richness of life. Asserting control over our lives by putting anxiety into perspective can give us a tremendous sense of accomplishment and confidence, two things that are missing when we have a life filled with worry.

The key to switching out of an anxiety state is to fully experience and accept all of the uncomfortable feelings, and allow time for them to pass. Let it come. Let yourself feel all of it. Then breathe and let your rational mind enter. Speak to your anxious thoughts with that rational mind, understanding that these are just harmless thoughts. Don't judge them as good or bad. Just let them come and let them go. Accepting anxiety helps it disappear. Fighting it will make it worse. The acronym, AWARE, from the book Anxiety Disorders and Phobias: A Cognitive Perspective (2005), by Aaron Beck and Gary Emery, is a helpful reminder for how to cope with anxiety.

A: Accept the anxiety. Welcome it. Don't fight it. Replace your rejection, anger, and hatred of it with acceptance. By resisting, you are prolonging the unpleasantness of it. Instead, flow with it. Don't make it responsible for how you think, feel, and act.

W: Watch and Wait. Look at your anxiety without judgment. It's neither good nor bad. Become detached from it. Remind yourself that you are not your anxiety. The more you can separate yourself from the experience, the more you can view it as a third party observer.

Even though there is a powerful urge to run away to try and escape anxious situations, postpone that decision for a little bit. Stay in the situation. Don't tell yourself you can't leave. Keep that option open so you don't feel trapped, but remember that you don't need to run away to get relief. Let relief come to you.

A: Act with the anxiety. Act as if you aren't anxious. Function with it. Slow down if you have to, but keep going. Breathe normally. If you run from the situation your anxiety will go down, but your fear will go up. If you stay, both your anxiety and your fear will eventually go down.

R: Repeat the steps. Continue to accept your anxiety, watch it, and act with it until it goes down to a comfortable level.

E: Expect the best. What we fear rarely happens. Recognize that a certain amount of anxiety is a normal part of life. Understanding this puts you in a good position to accept it if it comes again. You are familiar with it and know what to do with it.

Our minds are amazing. We can use them to our advantage or to our detriment. Along with using the AWARE strategy above, when I feel nervous or am losing confidence I recite the following:

Until one is committed there is hesitancy,
The chance to draw back; always ineffectiveness.
Concerning all acts of initiative (and Creation) there is one elementary truth,
The ignorance of which kills countless ideas and splendid plans:
That the moment one definitely commits oneself, then Providence moves too.
All sorts of things occur to help one that would never otherwise have occurred.
A whole stream of events issues from the decision,
Raising in one's favor all manner of unforeseen incidents
and meetings and material assistance, which no man
could have dreamt would have come his way.
Whatever you can do or dream you can, begin it.
Boldness has genius, power and magic in it.

- Johann Wolfgang von Goethe -

Here are some questions to ask yourself about your fear and anxiety:

- What fears do you have that prevent you from taking part in different activities?
- What beliefs do you hold onto that create self fulfilling prophecies?
- To what extent have you challenged your boundaries?
- How willing are you to take a step, however big or small, towards overcoming a fear?

Defeat isolation

Anxiety can often lead to isolation. Dealing with others can be challenging because there is a belief that no one can understand our devastation. People who had previously been very independent might even be more prone to isolation, as they might see themselves as significantly more inadequate or irrelevant to the world. We also don't like to attract attention to something we view as negative or different, or maybe what we think makes us less of a person, especially when our symptoms are noticeable.

However, even if they are not noticeable to others, we may feel different to such an extent that we think others can see what we feel. This is distressing and can make us very self conscious, which erodes self confidence. However, I think our efforts make us stronger in many ways. The awareness that we are living quite well despite great challenges can be a catalyst for boosting self confidence, if thought of this way.

I cannot stress enough the importance of learning to become comfortable where you are uncomfortable. We have to dig deep to avoid isolation that is associated with depression. Human interaction is very important to our well being. If only once or twice a week you meet with friends or volunteer in your community, for example, it can do wonders for your mental stability.

Worrying

Do you worry a lot? Do you ever find yourself worrying about worrying? How many of the things that you worry about actually come true? More than likely, most things you worry about never happen and it ends up being time wasted. There is a misconception that worrying protects us, but no matter how much we worry, we cannot change the outcome of most things. Worry is like a rocking-chair; it keeps us busy and gets us nowhere.

I am a worrier; much less of one now after doing lots of work to get over my anxiety that caused me to worry, but I still fall into the trap from time to time. I also feel a need to be in control, which got much worse after developing dystonia. When my body began doing things out of my control, it increased my need to find some way to control my surroundings in the hopes it would reduce my symptoms. This led to obsessive compulsive disorder (OCD), which impacted my life to such an extent that I had to seek therapy. Thankfully, with a lot of hard work I have learned to manage it.

There was/is also the worry that I will get worse, to which I am sure many of you can relate. This is reasonable to think about from time to time so we can remain diligent in our symptom management efforts, but to constantly do health checks and worry about the unknown is damaging. It can exacerbate physical symptoms and exhaust our minds, making us worry more. Worrying prevents us from living and enjoying the moments. Worrying about something that might happen may also become a self fulfilling prophecy.

When I let go and just live my life, my symptoms calm down. Doing things I enjoy and engaging in life versus worrying about how I feel always decreases my anxiety. It often comes down to a conscious decision to either worry and live in fear or take a leap of faith and live life to the fullest in the moment, rolling with the punches. Once we realize that worrying is the problem, not the solution, we can regain control of our anxious mind.

Remember that in life we are only guaranteed moments; this very moment. Once this moment is over, we are only guaranteed the next moment until all our moments are used up and life is over as we know it. I suggest we enjoy our time here as much as we can. Worrying is wasteful and leads to unhappiness.

As Ferris Bueller said in the movie, *Ferris Buellers Day Off* (1986), "Life moves pretty fast. If you don't stop and look around once in a while, you could miss it." It might do us well to get out of our own way and enjoy the life we have, no matter what might be "right" or "wrong" with us. "Right" and "wrong" are just words. How we perceive them is what matters most. Many of us need to stop worrying, wondering, and doubting, and have faith that things will work out. Maybe not how we planned, but just how it is meant to be.

Tips for coping with anxiety:
- Recognize false alarms. A rapid heartbeat does not mean you are having a heart attack. It's your body's natural response to arousal. Many thoughts and sensations that we interpret as cues for concern or panic are just background noise. Notice them and let them pass.

- Repeat your worry until you are bored. Face your fear head on and repeat it over and over until it no longer bothers you, similar to how I approached my fear of driving.
- Allow time to pass. When we worry, everything can feel like an emergency. This is all about anxious arousal, which is temporary. Every feeling of panic comes to an end; every concern wears itself out; and every so-called emergency evaporates.
- Make your anxiety worse. When you try too hard to control your anxiety, you only heighten it. Instead, exaggerate it and see what happens. This is similar to getting over my fear of red lights and heavy traffic. I purposely put myself in the worst traffic possible. When I was able to deal with the worst, I could drive anywhere with ease.
- Eat a balanced diet of healthy carbohydrates, proteins, and fats. Avoid caffeine, sugar, and white flour products.
- Distract yourself with work and fun activities.
- Deep breathing and progressive muscle relaxation.
- Prayer, meditation, counseling, life coaching.
- Exercise regularly.

References
1) www.healthcentral.com, Retrieved January 14, 2014 from: http://www.healthcentral.com/depression/c/84292/112118/depression/
2) www.depressionisachoice.com, Retrieved January 14, 2014 from: http://www.depressionisachoice.com/depressionisachoice/interview.html
3) Curtiss, A.B. Depression Is a Choice: Winning the Battle Without Drugs, 2001, Hyperion; New York, NY.
4) www.cdc.gov, Retrieved October 29, 2013 from: http://www.cdc.gov/pcd/issues/2005/jan/04_0066.htm
5) www.clevelandclinic.org, Retrieved October 29, 2013 from: http://www.clevelandclinic.org/health/health-info/docs/2200/2282.asp
6) www.beyondblue.org.au, Retrieved October 29, 2013 from: http://www.beyondblue.org.au/resources/for-me/men/what-causes-anxiety-and-depression-in-men/serious-health-events-and-chronic-illness
7) www.webmd.com, Retrieved October 29, 2013 from: http://www.webmd.com/depression/guide/detecting-depression
8) www.spasmodictorticollis.org, Retrieved October 29, 2013 from: http://www.spasmodictorticollis.org/index.cfm?pid=298
9) www.infodystonia.com, Retrieved October 29, 2013 from: http://www.infodystonia.com/post/32254759204/living-with-dystonia-disability-distress-and-despair
10) www.helpguide.org, Retrieved January 26, 2014 from: http://www.helpguide.org/mental/generalized_anxiety_disorder.htm
11) Good, M., Siedlecki, S. (June 2006). Listening to music can reduce chronic pain by up to 21 per cent and depression by up to 25 percent. Journal of Advanced Nursing. Vol 54. Issue 5. 553-562. Retrieved October 29, 2013 from: http://www.jbmusictherapy.com/wp-content/uploads/2010/11/Seniors.pdf

Chapter 8
Stress and Stress Management

As we all know, stress and dystonia do not mix. It can have a negative impact on our symptoms, such as increased spasms, twisting, pulling, pain, anxiety, headaches, physical weakness, increased tension, sleep interference, and many other problems. A dystonic body is under significant stress during normal circumstances, making our response to additional stress potentially catastrophic. Stress can affect us to such an extent that our nervous system is always aroused, keeping us trapped in chronic fight or flight mode because our body is conditioned, particularly if we are in pain, to always be on guard.

What is stress?
Stress is our body's reaction to an internal or external stimulus that disturbs its physical or mental equilibrium. When we are stressed, our body responds as though we are in danger. Our sympathetic nervous system is activated which increases hormones such as adrenaline and cortisol that surge through our body, initiating the fight or flight stress response. The fight or flight response becomes activated when we believe there is a chance we can outfight or outrun a perceived threat or stressful situation.[1]

Stress experts around the world are now adding the word "freeze" to the fight or flight response with respect to the fact that instead of fighting or fleeing, we might sometimes freeze (like a deer in headlights) in painful or traumatic situations. This is very intriguing as it relates to dystonia, as well as other chronic conditions, which is discussed in more detail below.

A little stress, known as acute stress, can be of great benefit to us. It keeps us active and alert, raising levels of performance during critical events, such as a sports activity, an important meeting, or in a dangerous situation or crisis. However, long term, or chronic stress, can have detrimental effects on our health and can diminish our quality of life. It can play a part in problems such as headaches, high blood pressure, heart problems, asthma, arthritis, depression, anxiety, pain, and muscle tension. Emotions such as anger, frustration, bitterness, and fear can exacerbate muscle tension. We also increase tension by closely monitoring our symptoms and having an over awareness of just how tight or sore we are.[2]

If stress is prolonged, adrenaline and cortisol maintain tension in the body. Over time, muscle tension can become habitual which pulls the body further away from relaxation. You may reach a point where you are no longer aware how constricted your muscles have become, and relaxing them can be very difficult. In fact, if you try to relax, your muscles may tighten even more because they have forgotten what letting go and relaxing feels like.

Keeping muscles tense drains much more energy than keeping muscles relaxed, which is one reason so many of us with dystonia experience pain and fatigue. Hence the importance of practicing relaxation techniques because it is only when the body finds relaxation can it reverse the damaging effects of stress.[3]

Since muscle tension and pain is a common feature of dystonia, many of us are living in stressed out bodies with heightened nervous systems, even at rest. It then takes only minimal stimuli for our system to become overloaded, causing an increase in symptoms. We are like a full glass of water where it takes only a few drops before it spills over.

My nervous system is highly sensitive, as I am sure is the case with many of you. It takes very little to overload my system, even in some of the calmest environments; environments where I never had any problems prior to developing dystonia.

Examples of things that threaten my nervous system include certain colors, lights, sounds, groups of people where it is noisy and there is activity, listening to the TV and someone talking at the same time, talking on the phone for too long, some HD televisions, movie theatre screens, and loud music. They cause anxiety, a racing mind, dizziness, headaches, muscle tension, and physical weakness. My brain tries so hard to keep up that I am sometimes unable to think clearly. I want to run away because I feel like I am in danger.

This all may sound extreme, especially to someone who does not have dystonia, but this is how it is for many of us which illustrates how fragile a dystonia body and mind can be. Oddly, there are times when none of these things bother me and I can even handle more than this, such as being in a busy restaurant, concert, or crowded party. The nature of dystonia is such that we do not often know where or when something will trigger stress and an increase in symptoms.

Before dystonia my stress shield was strong like a layer of metal through which little could penetrate. Since having dystonia and from taking medications, my stress shield has weakened to the strength of saran wrap. Knowing this, I do my best to avoid things that cause me stress. When I am unable to avoid them, I do my best to process it in a way that doesn't activate the fight or flight response. It is imperative for me to practice things such as mindfulness meditation and other mind calming activities. The more I practice and learn to accept the things that cause me trouble, the easier it is to deal with them.

Since stress and pain deplete our energy which reduces our ability to cope, identify your stress triggers and do your best to limit them or find new ways to respond to the trigger. Avoiding stress entirely is very difficult so the best thing we can do is learn how to better deal with it. We may not be able to eliminate the stressors in our world, but we can change our reaction to them so we are not so dramatically affected.

Fight, flight, and freeze response
As mentioned earlier, the fight or flight stress response becomes activated when we believe there is a chance we can outfight or outrun our attackers (or any perceived danger and stressful situation). The freeze response differs in that it gets activated due to a perceived or real inability to take action. In essence, one feels helpless to fight or flee the threatening, painful, or stressful experience. Doesn't this helpless feeling sound similar to living with dystonia? As you continue reading, consider the connection between dystonia and the fight, flight, and freeze response; in particular, the freeze response.

The sympathetic branch of the nervous system activates the fight or flight response. It tells the heart to beat faster, the muscles to tense, the eyes to dilate and the mucous membranes to dry up; all so we can fight harder, run faster, see better and breathe easier than we would without this response. This response kicks in for real and imagined threats in as little as 1/20th of a second. The parasympathetic branch calms us down to rest, telling the body that the danger has passed and it can relax. The parasympathetic branch also coordinates the freeze response.

During the freeze response, the body becomes both tense and paralyzed at the same time. The thoughts, sensations, and emotions of the stressful experience become suppressed or internalized, not only in the mind but in the tissues of the body. This is called somatic memory (body memory) and can have damaging effects if the event or trauma experienced is not processed in a healthy way. Somatic memory is used by trauma therapists to describe symptoms that don't seem to have a physical cause, but can be related to trauma, perhaps in childhood for example, and then forgotten by the mind but not by the body.

Trauma may begin as acute stress from a perceived life-threat or as the end product of cumulative stress. Both types of stress can seriously impair a person's ability to function with resilience and ease. Trauma may result from a wide variety of stressors such as a health condition, accidents, invasive medical procedures, sexual or physical assault, emotional abuse, neglect, war, natural disasters, loss, birth trauma, or the corrosive stressors of ongoing fear and conflict. Experts believe that trauma is not caused by the event itself, but rather develops through the failure of the body, psyche, and nervous system to process adverse events.[4]

As described by Jonathan Tripodi, author of <u>Freedom from Body Memory</u> (2012) & Founder of the Body Memory Recall (BMR) Approach, consider the interplay of a cat and mouse. When a mouse is approached by a cat it will run away. If cornered, the mouse might try to fight back. Once the mouse realizes that it can't win by attack and can't run away, it becomes paralyzed with fear (freeze response). The cat might swat at it with its paws and may even bite it, but the mouse remains frozen with tension. The cat will eventually interpret the mouse's frozen state as a sign that it is dead and will leave it in search of more stimulating prey.

Once the threat is over and if the mouse lives, it will come out of the freeze response by spontaneously discharging excess energy through involuntary movements including shaking, trembling, and deep spontaneous breaths. This discharge process resets the autonomic nervous system, restoring equilibrium. Body memory (or somatic memory) from the attack is released and the mouse walks away as if nothing ever happened. The mouse has effectively survived and released the traumatic experience. It does not carry any tension from the attack and its body is again at ease. This is similar to a deer that freezes at the sight of headlights. When the threat has passed, it trembles violently which "shakes off" the freeze response and then goes about its business without lasting impairment. This shaking is called neurogenic tremor.[5]

Neurogenic tremor is the natural response of a shocked or disrupted nervous system attempting to restore the neuro-physiologic homeostasis of the body. The tremor (vibrations) restores a relaxed muscle state in order to prevent the development of joint pain and physical constraints. The tremors/vibrations signal the brain to release tension to return to a resting state. This helps us better adapt to our environment and this process of adaptation makes us stronger and more prepared to deal with difficult future experiences.[5-7]

The primary difference between animals and humans is that humans do not tend to go through the instinctual discharge of the freeze response, leaving us vulnerable to constriction and pain. Through rationalizations, judgments, shame, and fear of our bodily sensations, we may disrupt our innate capacity to self-regulate, functionally "recycling" disabling terror and helplessness.

Think of this in terms of the rhythm of breathing. We breathe in and we breathe out. Imagine what it would be like to inhale and then hold it. To a certain extent, this is what is happening while in the freeze response. Experiences go in but they don't come out.

When the nervous system does not reset after an overwhelming experience, sleep, cardiac, digestion, respiration, and immune system function can be seriously disturbed. Unresolved physiological distress can also lead to an array of other physical, cognitive, emotional, and behavioral symptoms. Trauma experts believe that the interruption of the freeze response (which animals rarely experience) contributes to what is called "kindling" in humans.[5]

Kindling is a process of over-firing chemicals in the nervous system that triggers symptoms of post traumatic stress disorder, chronic pain, and other health problems. Kindling has been compared to spontaneous combustion, a chemical reaction that occurs when objects reach a certain temperature. In neurology, kindling is a term used to explain how over-firing or neural excitability in the nervous system becomes self perpetuating without additional external triggering. Doesn't this sound familiar to life with dystonia?

Ideally, humans should respond to trauma the same as the mouse and deer. However, the release of the freeze response and the associated tensions and fear from the overwhelming event may instead occur gradually over time or not at all. With repeated unresolved trauma, syndromes can develop or existing syndromes can persist. Perhaps kindling is why some of us developed dystonia and/or why symptoms persist. Perhaps kindling is also why people with dystonia are so dramatically affected by seemingly innocuous stimuli.

Think about the common symptoms of dystonia which include contractions, stiffness, and rigidity. Don't these symptoms sound similar to an organism stuck in the freeze response? Out of fear, many of us also live in protection mode where we consciously restrict our movements (to the best of our ability) to try and decrease pain and/or involuntary movements. Purposely restricting our movements, avoiding activities that *may* increase our symptoms, and holding ourselves in postures to prevent further pain and involuntary movements is similar to the freeze response. This adds more stress than already exists. We rarely to never let our bodies "be" in pain or move as it wishes, so we keep ourselves stuck in crisis.

What would happen if we just allowed our symptoms to be what they were without mentally or physically trying to fight them? Easier said than done of course, but think about the possibility of just letting go and embracing the pain and involuntary movements. Perhaps some of the tension in our body is from our intellectual brains keeping the symptoms of dystonia stored in memory. Since relaxation and self-healing are prevented when the freeze response remains active, if we get our mind out of the way, we might be able to reduce our symptoms. It certainly merits consideration because the body is better able to remain balanced, vital, and adaptable to new experiences when we don't fight what is "wrong" with us so much.

I remember the day my Mom received a call from her doctor telling her she had breast cancer. She got the call while we were driving home from one of my doctor appointments. When she got the news I was amazed at how calm she was. It was probably because we were still in the car and she had to focus on driving, the news didn't hit her yet, or she went into the freeze response to some extent. When we got home, which was only about five minutes from the time she received the news, she stood in the kitchen completely numb with tears in her eyes and unable to speak. She then began to shake uncontrollably for a couple minutes. When the shaking stopped, she was able to clearly articulate the diagnosis, treatment, and prognosis. If I understand the freeze response correctly, this is what she went into and came out of.

That was over five years ago and I am happy to report that she is cancer free. I often wonder if she would have gone through surgery and radiation treatment as well as she did had she not experienced neurogenic tremors and instead, held onto the shocking news that caused her such fear. Perhaps if she held onto the news instead of "shaking it off", her recovery would not have gone so smoothly. When I speak with her about it now, she views her cancer as something she had, was treated for, and it is over. She doesn't hold onto any of it. It was taken care of and she has moved on with her life. She has no attachment to it, similar to the frightened mouse that "shook off" the attack from the cat.

Her attitude was and is amazing, which contributed greatly to her successful recovery. The more I think about how she handled the entire experience and how she views it to this day as a temporary thing, unlike others who are "married" to their past or present health condition (like many of us with dystonia where it becomes part of our identity), the more I am convinced that the way we process bad news, a challenging circumstance, an acute or chronic health condition, or a frightening situation, affects how our illness manifests and either progresses or improves.

Unlocking the freeze response

A method used to unlock the freezing and hypersensitive responses of the nervous system is called pendulation. Pendulation is the movement between dysregulation (trauma) and regulation (healing) within the body. It is the natural rhythm of movement between constriction and release inherent to all physical systems. It helps activate basic regulatory rhythms and stops nervous system rigidity and random responses, interrupting all kinds of traumatizing pain, including nerve pain.

Pendulation is an aspect of a therapy called Somatic Experiencing which was introduced by Dr. Peter Levine in 1997. Somatic Experiencing is a form of therapy aimed at relieving and resolving the symptoms of post-traumatic stress disorder (PTSD), rape, auto accidents, post surgical trauma, chronic health conditions, etc., by focusing on the client's perceived body sensations (or somatic experiences). It is a body-awareness approach that restores self-regulation and returns a sense of aliveness, relaxation, and wholeness to traumatized individuals. It is based upon the realization that human beings have an innate ability to overcome the effects of trauma.

Pendulations are done with the help of a Somatic Experiencing Practitioner. They help clients move to a state where he or she is believed to be somewhat dysregulated (aroused or frozen from past trauma) and then helped to return to a state of regulation (loosely defined as not aroused or un-frozen). This process is done in small doses called titrations, with progressively more levels of dysregulation as the client successfully progresses through pendulations.[5, 8]

Stress management

When Dr. Peter Levine, author of the 1997 book, <u>Waking the Tiger</u>, gives lectures on surviving trauma, he shows a video of a lion chasing a baby gazelle to demonstrate how the freeze response works. He explains that the video is short because the average time for a lion attack from start to finish is about 45 seconds. He makes the additional point that this is how long the victim's stress response (and our stress response) was designed to be activated; not hours, days, weeks, or years.

Unfortunately, those with chronic stress, pain, or illness live in a body with a heightened nervous system that does not know how to turn off the stress response, even under normal conditions. This can have harmful effects and keep us in our chronic unwell state. There is good news however; we can learn stress reduction techniques and make lifestyle changes to better cope with stress and recover from the fight, flight, and freeze response. This is very important for us, as the constant release of stress hormones can slow down or prevent relief and recovery from the symptoms associated with chronic health conditions.[9]

General health and stress maintenance can be enhanced by regular exercise, an anti-inflammatory diet (see www.deflame.com), and by avoiding excessive alcohol, caffeine, and tobacco. Instead of relieving stress and returning the body to a relaxed state, these substances tend to keep the body aroused. People also resort to abnormal eating patterns and passive activities, such as watching television.

Physical activity, such as aerobics, walking, swimming, biking, yoga, Pilates, tai chi, stretching, and weight/resistance training, are all helpful for reducing stress. These activities also serve as effective distractions from stressful events. Physical activity may also blunt the harmful effects of stress on blood pressure and the heart. Just be sure that all your physical activities are dystonia friendly. Symmetrical activities (cycling, rowing, walking, swimming) are usually safer than one sided activities (golf, tennis, bowling). Be careful about the intensity of your exercises. Some people with dystonia find the increase in adrenaline from aerobic activity to be problematic, so exercise within comfortable boundaries.

Working with a counselor who uses cognitive behavioral therapy (CBT) can also be an effective way to reduce stress. A typical CBT approach includes identifying sources of stress, restructuring priorities, changing one's response to stress, and finding methods for managing and reducing stress.

The benefits of talking to a therapist, CBT or otherwise, is that the act of verbalizing our feelings helps us release tension, sort through problems, and gain new perspective. Feelings such as anger and frustration that are not expressed in an acceptable way may lead to hostility, a sense of helplessness, and depression. Expressing feelings does not mean venting frustration on others, boring friends with emotional baggage, or wallowing in self pity. The primary goal is to explain and assert your needs to a trusted individual in a positive way.

Stress can also be managed by writing in a journal, writing a poem, or composing a letter that is never even mailed. Along with expressing our feelings, learning to listen, empathize, and respond to others with understanding is just as important for maintaining strong relationships necessary for emotional fulfillment and reduced stress. Music is also an effective stress reducer. It can reduce heart rate, blood pressure, and feelings of anxiety.

Removing ourselves from a stressful environment and listening to guided relaxation/meditation programs can also be helpful. Spend time focusing on your breathing and visualizing peaceful settings, such as floating on a raft on a lake in the mountains or lying on a private, white, sandy beach. If you are able, take a slow walk and pay attention to the sounds of nature around you. Try to zone everything out except for the sights and sounds.

Limit the amount of time you spend on the phone, computer, and other forms of technology when possible. People may not be aware how significantly stressful they can be. If you are not sure how much technology is affecting you, turn everything off for a few hours and/or just leave your phone at home for the day. I bet just the thought of doing this causes discomfort for many of you. If it does, you are probably overusing your gadgets. Allow your mind time to rest. The instant message world we live in promotes anxiety so it is important to balance our usage.

By following the above ideas, over the years I have learned to better deal with stress and anxiety. One of my biggest keys to managing stress is allowing myself to acclimate to an environment or situation that is uncomfortable. Rather than finding a way to escape, I let time pass which lets my body and mind adjust and relax. I allow all the uncomfortable feelings come over my body with as little judgment as possible. The longer I allow myself to acclimate to the environment or situation, reminding myself that I am safe, the more my stress and anxiety dissipate which prevents my symptoms from getting worse.

Dr. Claire Weekes, author of Hope and Help for Your Nerves (1990), talks about this in the context of first fear and second fear. Some people who experience a flash of fear and anxiety from stress often fear that initial feeling which adds a second fear; in other words, fear on top of fear. This is what causes us to panic and keep us in fight or flight mode. If we instead practice complete acceptance and allow the first fear to happen without adding second fear to it, it is significantly much easier to handle uncomfortable situations. It takes practice, but the more we do it, the easier it becomes.

Stress reduction techniques:[4]
- Slow and deep breathing. Stop what you are doing. Breathe gently but deeply from your abdomen. On the out breath say to yourself, "Be calm. Be peaceful."
- When you are rushed, say, "There is plenty of time. Stay calm."
- When things don't go your way, say, "Everything is happening perfectly. It will all work out for the best."
- If you're feeling angry, anxious, or depressed, it is best to acknowledge the feelings and say, "Okay, I recognize this. I feel bad at the moment, but it will pass just as it has before."
- Instead of focusing on all that you are not and cannot do, try focusing on all that you are and can do.
- Talk to your family, friends, therapist, or support group about the situations you find stressful.
- Replace negative thoughts with positive thoughts.
- Write down your feelings.
- Utilize visualization techniques.
- Spend time in prayer and meditation.
- Get outside and be among nature. It can be very grounding.

Using various relaxation techniques and changing our mindset about our life situation can reduce added tension that is created beyond what is part and parcel of dystonia. With enough work, we can even reduce the involuntary tension of dystonia itself. Relaxation does not come naturally to a lot of people. Learning (or re-learning) how to release tension and relax is a practice. When you become skilled at body/mind relaxation, you will better recognize when tension is building up and be able to shut it down. It is crucial that we learn to release tension because it is only when our body finds relaxation that we reverse the damage of stress, which can then reduce pain. Find what works best for you and put it to practice.

Tension and Trauma Releasing Exercises (TRE)
A technique called Tension and Trauma Releasing Exercises (TRE) is being used by thousands of people around the world as a tool for releasing chronic stress, physical tension, and emotional trauma. It is also a popular way to release the everyday stress from the daily pressures of life. TRE uses specific exercises to release stress tension from the body and may be helpful to certain people with dystonia and other conditions where their nervous system is compromised.

The exercises used in TRE help release deep tension from the body by evoking neurogenic muscle tremors (self-controlled muscular shaking process in the body). These gentle tremors reverberate outwards along the spine releasing tension from the sacrum to the cranium. The exercises are a simple form of stretching and are used to gently trigger these voluntary muscle tremors.

Once the technique is learned and mastered after several sessions, the warm-up exercises can be accelerated or replaced with your normal exercise activity like walking or yoga, and the technique then becomes a quick and effective method for consistent relaxation. Eventually, these tremors will evoke themselves naturally in a rest position to reduce any stress or tension that was accumulated over the course of the day.

Since this shaking mechanism in the muscles is part of our natural behavior as humans that we can cultivate more effectively with practice, you might benefit from TRE. This shaking of the muscles (neurogenic tremors) increases the resiliency of the body because it causes deep relaxation that naturally reduces stress levels. It can release emotions ranging from mild upset to severe anxiety whether it is caused by work stress, excessive worry, conflict in relationships, and physical stress or trauma from accidents. Additionally, TRE has been reported to reduce pain, increase mobility, and aid in healing past injuries.[10]

While I enjoy doing TRE, my concern for some is that it is designed to induce neurogenic tremors which may or may not be good for people with dystonia. I have not had any setbacks from the times I have used TRE, but some may. I think the exercises and the reasoning behind them makes great sense, but I am still at a crossroads about inducing tremors to a neurological system that already experiences tremors and spasms. Then again, if the goal is to release tension in the body by systematically and voluntarily introducing tremors, it may have health benefits for some with dystonia. If you are interested in learning more about TRE, please do some investigation before hand to see if it is something you feel is right for you.

Emotional Freedom Technique (EFT) is another tool you might find helpful for managing stress. EFT is discussed in chapter 15.

Put the glass down
A clinician walked around a room while teaching stress management. As she raised a glass of water, everyone expected they'd be asked the "half empty or half full" question. Instead, with a smile on her face, she inquired, "How heavy is this glass of water?" Answers ranged from 8 oz. to 20 oz.

She replied, "The absolute weight doesn't matter. It depends on how long I hold it. If I hold it for a minute, it's not a problem. If I hold it for an hour, I'll have an ache in my arm. If I hold it for a day, my arm will feel numb and paralyzed. In each case, the weight of the glass doesn't change, but the longer I hold it the heavier it becomes."

She continued, "The stresses and worries in life are like the glass of water. Think about them for a while and nothing happens. Think about them a bit longer and they begin to hurt. If you think about them all day, you will feel paralyzed, incapable of doing anything. Remember to put the glass down."[11]

Testimonial
My cervical dystonia (CD) started right after a very stressful situation in my family...the death of my mother and sister within three months of each other and a year of round the clock care for both of them prior to that. It is my belief that stress brought on CD for me and others I know with this condition. I would therefore suggest that as much stress as possible be eliminated in one's life.

I have learned to say "no" on many occasions. I was lucky that I sold my business while my loved ones were sick. After their passing I retired. It was early, but I knew that my personality would force me to jump into work again too deeply if I tried another business. My husband insisted that I just take it easy and manage the household. I was fortunate with the timing because even volunteer work had become stressful. I stopped going to some meetings because they were too much for me. Not everyone in the group understands, but I really can't care. I am doing only what my mind, body, and heart allows. I recently took up Nordic Pole walking and I am enjoying it so much. I feel very

94

normal when I walk. It keeps me straight. I am actually practicing to do the Camino walk in Spain next year!

There are times in life when things happen that we can't control. But there are other times when we can excuse ourselves from stressful situations to look after our health. Some people might not understand or like our decisions, even family members, but we need to be okay with that. We all know what pushes our stress buttons so we can't allow ourselves to go there. Be kind to yourself, body and mind.

References
1) Psychology Today, Retrieved April 29, 2013 from: http://www.psychologytoday.com/basics/stress
2) WebMD, Retrieved April 29, 2013 from: http://www.webmd.com/mental-health/effects-of-stress-on-your-body
3) Phillips, M. (2007) *Reversing Chronic Pain*. North Atlantic Books: Berkeley, CA
4) www.painsupport.co.uk. Retrieved on August 19, 2013 from: http://www.painsupport.co.uk/pages/stress.asp
5) www.traumahealing.com, Retrieved March 29, 2014 from: http://www.traumahealing.com/somatic-experiencing/
6) http://www.bodymemory.com, Retrieved August 30, 2013 from: http://www.bodymemory.com/article_habit_to_freeze.html
7) Feldman, S., (2004). Biomechanical Stimulation Web by Spencer Feldman. Retrieved August 30, 2013 from: http://www.vibraboard.com/research_study and http://traumaprevention.com/2009/06/27/neurogenic-tremors-the-bodys-natural-response/
8) Phillips, M. (2007) *Reversing Chronic Pain*. Berkeley, CA: North Atlantic Books: 59-60
9) http://www.stressstop.com, Retrieved August 27, 2013 from: http://www.stressstop.com/stress-tips/articles/fight-flight-or-freeze-response-to-stress.php
10) http://traumaprevention.com/, Retrieved August 27, 2013 from: http://traumaprevention.com/2009/12/31/what-is-tre/
11) Lindsey Biel, OTR- Retrieved August 13, 2013 from: http://sensorysmarts.com/

Chapter 9
Pain and Dystonia

As most of us are well aware, pain is a significant part of living with dystonia. Most people can relate to acute pain or some form of temporary limitation when they are sick, but life offers a whole new set of challenges when the condition is chronic, particularly for those who were once in good health. As Bonnie Prudden said, "Pain, not death, is the enemy of mankind."

Acute pain
Acute pain is of sudden onset and usually results from something specific such as an injury, surgery, or infection. It is immediate and usually of short duration. Acute pain is a normal response to injury and may be accompanied by temporary anxiety or emotional distress. The cause of acute pain can usually be diagnosed and treated.[1, 2]

Chronic pain
Chronic pain, ranging from mild to severe, is continuous pain that can persist for weeks, months, years or even a lifetime; in other words, beyond the time of normal healing. The cause of chronic pain is not always evident, although it can be due to many conditions such as arthritis, fibromyalgia, peripheral neuropathy, low back pain, and of course dystonia.[1, 2]

Chronic pain can often interfere with quality of life, as it tends to permeate every aspect of our lives. Losing one's identity, abilities, and choices that many often take for granted is the reality of chronic pain. It can be a life altering experience. While life is ever evolving for each and every one of us, adapting to a life filled with pain and debilitation (mental and/or physical) is a situation that offers many challenges. You are almost always being tested to the limits.

When my symptoms first began up to a few months before being diagnosed, I had little to no pain in my neck or back. Over a period of about 8 months my pain increased exponentially to the point that I could barely function (you can read more about this in chapter 2). It felt like there was a power drill continuously going into the base of my skull which radiated down my neck into my shoulders. It was a miserable existence. I didn't know pain like that was possible. It reminded me of how it felt at the exact moment when I sprained my ankle, stubbed my toe, or jammed a finger, for example. Unlike those instances where the pain subsided in a short period of time, the pain from dystonia never left. It was like I was experiencing an injury over and over.

I used to listen to people complain about an ache or pain and say to myself in anger and frustration, "If they only knew what real pain was like." I understood what pain was like from many sports injuries and other aches and pains throughout my life, but pain from dystonia was a different beast altogether. It took me a while to appreciate that pain is relative to everyone's own experiences (we only know what we know) and pain of any kind can have an affect on quality of life. I no longer compare my pain with someone else's pain. I no longer scoff at other's pain just because I might perceive that my pain is more severe and they have no right to complain until it gets as bad as mine. That is and was very thoughtless of me. Pain is the great equalizer when it affects your quality of life.

As Maggie Phillips writes in her book, <u>Reversing Chronic Pain</u> (2007), the common denominator for people in pain is the longing for relief and a permanent end to pain. We hold out hope for a magic bullet, which is essentially an all or nothing approach. When those hopes go unmet, we are often plunged into the depths of despair, making it difficult to remain optimistic.[3]

As humans, we don't just have physical pain; we agonize over painful memories, uncomfortable emotions, and difficult self-evaluations. We worry about them and engage in all kinds of activities to avoid them. We do not merely value feeling better. We value a productive life much more than simply a lack of suffering. We want to feel well and make the best of our time.[3]

A comment about the word "suffering"; you might notice that I do not use the word suffering or dystonia sufferers very often. Instead, I use the term "living with" or "experiencing" when I refer to different symptoms and circumstances. Suffering is a negative perspective and mindset. It is a perspective which feeds the victim mentality that we need to get away from so we can better learn to live life to the best of our ability given our circumstances.

I experienced a lot of horrible symptoms as many of you do. At my worst and even my best, I fell into the trap of using the word suffering too much which was counterproductive to a healthy mental state. I became a victim, and a bitter one at that. Calling myself a sufferer caused me to become a suffering person, even when I got my symptoms under much better control. Calling myself a sufferer made me more attached to my dystonia as well as to my "suffering." It negatively impacted every aspect of my life. It validated my existence which made me feel better about my "suffering", but it didn't make me feel better about my life. It made me feel worse. It validated my miserable existence and confirmed that dystonia defined who I was.

Changing the words to "living with" or "experiencing" helped me get out of the dark hole I was in. I now describe myself as a healthy, functional, compassionate, hard working person who lives with a condition called dystonia. It is not my life. It is a part of my life. I know how horrible the mental and physical pain is, and it can often seem like dystonia is your life, but if we change our words and reframe our perspective, it lessens the grip it has on us.

Effects of chronic pain

People with chronic pain not only live with unrelenting sensation of pain, but they may also have trouble sleeping, become depressed, experience anxiety, and have difficulty making decisions. Not only does chronic pain interfere with day to day activities, research has shown that chronic pain may actually damage the brain and destroy brain cells. Chronic pain has also been linked to high blood pressure.[4]

Researchers have reported that brain activity in patients with chronic pain is different from those who do not have chronic pain. In a 2008 study at Northwestern University, Feinberg School of Medicine, investigators identified a clue that may explain how long-term, chronic pain could trigger other pain-related symptoms. The study was supported by the National Institute of Neurological Disorders and Stroke (NINDS).[5]

In a healthy brain, all regions are in a state of equilibrium. When one region is active, the others quiet down. In people with chronic pain, the prefrontal cortex, the location for cognitive, emotional, and behavioral functioning, is always active. When this region is stuck in full throttle, neurons can change their connections with other neurons or die prematurely. It was hypothesized that these changes make it more difficult for people to concentrate, solve problems, make decisions, or be in a good mood. A person in chronic pain is impaired in a similar manner to those who are multi-tasking without ever getting a break.[5, 6]

Another common problem for people with chronic pain is an inability to sleep. Areas of the brain responsible for sensory stimulation are also responsible for controlling our sleep and wake cycle. When there is overstimulation, it makes it difficult for the brain to rest.

Another symptom frequently experienced by those in chronic pain is anxiety. Researchers observed that patients in chronic pain have reduced brain activity in the areas of the brain that control the human response to pain. They believe that reduced control over pain signals causes the brain to become extremely vigilant in anticipating future pain. This helps explain the heightened levels of anxiety frequently experienced by those living with chronic pain.[7]

Researchers also believe that reduced control over pain signals contributes to depression. It causes increased emotional reaction to future experiences of pain which contributes to a sense of hopelessness in being able to overcome pain. This research is consistent with other research that has found that people who are depressed have reduced ability to control their emotional state. It also supports studies indicating that 30 to 60 percent of patients with chronic pain also develop depression.[7]

Describing your pain
There is no medical test that can measure or convey the level of pain one is feeling. We can only describe our pain. In order to provide an accurate description of your pain, it may be helpful to share answers to the following questions with your doctor:

- Where is the pain located?
- How long have you had pain?
- Does the pain come and go or is it continuous?
- What makes the pain better or worse?
- What medications or treatments have you tried for the pain?

A convenient way to organize questions and answers about pain is to think of the letters of the alphabet from **P** through **T**.[8]

P: What **P**rovokes my pain? What **P**alliates or relieves my pain?
Q: What **Q**ualities does my pain have? For example, is it burning, aching, electric shock-like, sharp or dull?
R: What **R**egion of my body is involved with pain?
S: What is the **S**everity of my pain? Mild, moderate or severe?
T: What **T**ime of day is my pain worse or is it independent of time and more activity related?

Pain scale
When we visit the doctor, we are usually asked to rate our pain level on a scale of 1-10 (1 being no pain and 10 being the worst pain possible). I think this scale

is too subjective. Pain is relative to the individual so using a generic scale can be misleading. Furthermore, I can't recall a doctor or nurse ever asking what those numbers mean to me, so how can they tell what my pain level really is? The numbers mean something different to everyone. For example, what I consider to be a 4 or 5 someone else might consider an 8 or 9. I have become more tolerable to pain so I might assign lower numbers than someone with the same kind of pain who is less tolerable. Much of my pain is also activity/task dependent so my pain level on the 1-10 scale doesn't accurately depict what I experience because it fluctuates. It may be more or less when I am at the doctor which doesn't address my overall pain condition.

My treatment or treatment plan has never changed no matter what number I write down. It makes me wonder why the current pain scales are used, particularly for chronic pain patients who have pain that is so variable. If we are being treated for an acute injury or other ailment for which there is an expected recovery, I can see the benefit of this pain scale because it is actually measuring progress towards a desired goal of recovery or cure. In dystonia and other chronic pain conditions, the rules for "recovery" are different because there is rarely a clear or quantifiable end goal in sight.

Taking all of this into consideration, it would probably be wise to create your own personal pain scale to better communicate with doctors about how you feel. The number 1, or "no pain at all", is the only number that is quantifiable. At the other extreme, 10, or "pain as bad as it can be" is relative to what a person perceives as the worst pain possible for them. Before dystonia, my worst pain possible paled in comparison to the pain that came with dystonia. In other words, my pain scale, or perception of pain, has changed over the years.

I prefer to assign a descriptive word, phrase, or picture to each number to describe my pain. I also like to assign activities to the different numbers. For example, a 2-3 might mean that I am having a great day and am able to do x, y, z activities with more comfort than on a day I rate a 5-6. A 7-8 means I am in shutdown mode and have to lie down most of the day and a 9-10 means that I am about to hit speed dial for Dr. Kevorkian. Some days can be so random that I fluctuate between a 1 and a 10.

A word of caution regarding that last description about Kevorkian; as true as it may be to want to die because of the pain we are in at the moment, we have to be very careful what words we use. If we say we are in so much pain that we want to die, it might be misconstrued as a psychiatric condition, a cry for help, or a perceived suicide threat. It puts doctors in a position where they have to alert the appropriate authorities. Unless you really mean it, explain that your pain is such that it is near impossible to function at the moment and that the pain is currently intolerable; not that you actually want to kill yourself.

Instead of a standard 1-10 pain scale, create a personal scale that accurately paints the picture of your pain. You are different than every patient who walks into a doctor's office so be creative when communicating with your doctor.

Chronic pain management
There are many ways to treat/manage chronic pain including, but not limited to, surgery, medications, nutrition, acupuncture, chiropractic, massage therapy, cranial sacral therapy, physical therapy, behavior modification, biofeedback, prayer, meditation, and rest/relaxation therapies. Another important component to pain management involves regulating your daily schedule so that you have the right balance of activity, rest, social interaction, quiet time, and energy-giving activities.

When choosing your method of pain relief, an interesting fact to keep in mind is that neutral or positive sensory messages travel through the nervous system faster than painful messages. For example, soothing sensations travel up to seven times faster than sharp or burning pain. This means that if soothing sensations and painful sensations reach the "pain gate" at the same time, the pleasant sensations will prevail, blocking the slower, painful ones. Thus, one of the main ways of reversing the course of pain is to find what creates consistently reliable pleasant body experiences that compete successfully with pain. This might include massage, acupuncture, a good movie, quality time with family and friends, sex, a good book, meditation, prayer, exercise, and music; whatever you find to be a pleasant experience.[3]

Testimonial
There was a time when my symptoms were such that I wanted to end my life. The big difference between then and now is that I learned not to fight so much. I was fighting dystonia with my mind and my body. I fought dystonia mentally with constant anxious thoughts. What is this? Will this ruin my family? Is my life over? How much worse will this get? Why me? Where can I find a doctor to help? The constant mental anxiety tensed my body. Slowly I learned that tension makes my dystonia worse. I learned to redirect my mind away from my body. I now pour myself into a new professional focus that keeps my mind off my pain. Dystonia didn't disappear but it is much more manageable from a pain standpoint with acceptance and preoccupation elsewhere.

Secondly, I stopped trying to force dystonia out of my body with exercise. I learned about an exercise program to help dystonia, but I followed it anxiously with tension and gripping. That didn't work because, again, tension makes my neck muscles worse. I now try to avoid driving too much, which creates neck tension. I even have to watch how I do yoga because a boot camp approach makes things worse. In general, I let gravity due the work with gentle, passive stretching.

Third, I got off the merry-go-round of drugs. I was on such an anxious quest to find the right pharmaceutical cure. Thankfully, through outreach via the Internet, I got tipped off to the dangers of benzodiazepines. I now see that my constant seeking for drug relief was heading down a terrible path of addiction and anxious preoccupation.

Fourth, philosophically, I answered the question of "Why me?" with "Why not me?" Everyone has something. This is one of mine. I can see how having it has aided my development as a compassionate being. I have a special strength to help others with chronic illness due to my own walk with it. I can be sensitive to the emotional toll that difficult to diagnose diseases have on individuals and families. Don't get me wrong, I wouldn't choose this path. Nevertheless, it is also true that meaningful, deep and highly valued connections often seem to come from sharing compassion and support with others about this and other physical difficulties.

References
1) www.medscape.com, Retrieved August 19, 2013 from: http://www.medscape.com/viewarticle/465355_2
2) http://www.medicinenet.com, Retrieved on August 29, 2013 from: http://www.medicinenet.com/script/main/art.asp?articlekey=40842
3) Phillips, M. (2007) *Reversing Chronic Pain.* North Atlantic Books: Berkeley, CA
4) www.conquerchiari.org. Retrieved August 19, 2013 from: http://www.conquerchiari.org/subs%20only/Volume%203/Issue%203(3)/Chronic%20Pain%20Hypertension%203(3).html
5) Paul, M. (2008) Chronic Pain Harms the Brain. Retrieved September 2, 2013 from http://www.northwestern.edu/newscenter/stories/2008/02/chronicpain.html
6) www.wellescent.com, Retrieved September 2, 2013 from: http://wellescent.com/health_blog/the-damaging-effects-of-chronic-pain-on-the-brain
7) www.wellescent.com, Retrieved September 2, 2013 from: http://wellescent.com/health_blog/the-damaging-effects-of-chronic-pain-on-the-brain/2\
8) Serdans, B. www.care4dystonia.org. Retrieved on August 19, 2013 from: http://www.care4dystonia.org/treats/painmgmt.pdf

Chapter 10
Coping with a Chronic Condition

Living with dystonia can be an overwhelming task. It is often accompanied by exhaustion, frustration, depression, and despair. Some days you may wonder if it is possible or even worth getting out of bed. Other times you may wake up with minimal symptoms and energy and excitement to take on the day. Since each day is so different, it's important to make thoughtful choices about your daily activities so you can do all you can and want to within the scope of your abilities.

Daily coping

The key to coping successfully with any chronic condition is to acquire the right mixture of practical skills and mental attitudes. By combining these, you can promote a positive, realistic approach to your condition. Maintaining a positive attitude may seem inappropriate or even infuriating when you are in pain or exhausted. However, there are certain attitudes and beliefs associated with people who cope well with chronic conditions.

- Live for today; one day at a time; not in the past or the future.
- Treat problems as challenges to overcome.
- Take pride in your achievements in overcoming challenges.
- Accept the illness and reject "why me?" questioning.
- Learn about your condition and take responsibility for it.
- Be willing to use all available resources for help.

Being organized, setting realistic goals, and prioritizing activities will go a long way to helping you cope well on a day-to-day basis. Decide what is really important and what can slide. Then live your life as fully as you can. Don't try to do too much and don't feel guilty for tasks not completed.

- Seek help as soon as you feel unable to cope.
- Allow flexibility and extra time in your plans.
- Find things you enjoy and find the time to enjoy them.
- Get your medicines and routines organized and written down.
- Do your most difficult tasks at the time of day you feel best.
- Recognize that your capacities may vary. What is possible one day may not be another.

To stay as healthy as your dystonia allows, watch for warning signs. Stop and rest as soon as you begin to feel tired or more pain coming on. Learn to read your body and its messages. Keeping a journal of physical symptoms, emotions/feelings, and activities will help you better understand your body and its patterns. A symptom journal will also help you better explain your condition to your doctor so he or she can most appropriately treat you. We go through so much that it is often difficult to remember things unless we write them down.

Emotional health

Dystonia can damage self-image, leading to stress, anxiety, withdrawal from society, isolation, and depression. You may become anxious and uncertain about the future, worrying about physical or financial difficulties down the road; or it may stop you from doing what you once found important or enjoyable, causing grief for the changes in your life. For some, emotional issues can be just as significant as physical symptoms, if not more.

It is not uncommon to experience feelings of denial, anger, worthlessness, resentment, and loss of control as you come to terms with your dystonia. The first step in avoiding or reversing emotional health problems is to accept these feelings as part of the process and reject any negative thoughts that you may be having about them. You are entitled to feel all of it.

A careful examination of your condition will show that you are still a valued person with lots to offer, despite dystonia. Positive, reasoned self-talk can help you overcome negative thinking.

- Don't blame anyone for your dystonia.
- Define success as taking good care of yourself.
- Enjoy small pleasures when you recognize them.
- Know that you are not defined by what you can or cannot do.
- Know that your value and worth have not decreased due to dystonia.

Self empowerment

Remember that you are the only one with unique self-knowledge about your condition and how it affects your life. You are the one who can and should make the major decisions about your life. Only you know how you feel at any given time, what you are capable of, and what your limitations are. Don't allow feelings of guilt push you into doing something you know your body will pay for, either during or afterwards. Be careful about being a people pleaser. It often means jeopardizing your health for the sake of others, an attribute that may have and may continue to contribute to your dystonia. Do what you can and know your limitations. Others can adapt to you.

Be sure to find doctors you trust. This is often a difficult task. Dystonia is such a misunderstood condition that finding the right doctor who understands your specific needs might take some shopping around. To assist in this process, educate yourself as much as possible about your condition so you are able to better screen your health care team. I wasn't educated nearly enough in the beginning and I paid the price because some of the doctors I saw made me worse. Don't forget that your doctor works for you. Don't let their busy schedule force you out of the office before you feel he or she has met all your needs. Your doctor is there to serve you; not the other way around. Together, you and your doctor can map out the best plan for your care.

Make wise decisions about your priorities. On your best days you may find you can do more things with relative ease. Other days, a single task might wipe you out for the rest of the day or even several days thereafter. Plan ahead so you can prepare yourself prior to an activity and rest time afterwards if necessary.

Take personal time for yourself, whether to relax or have fun. Don't forget how important it is to let go and enjoy life. It is far healthier to focus on all you can do versus all the things you can't do or choose not to do. Dwelling on problems can make you forget how to have fun. There is joy all around you and there are ways to let go of fear and anxiety, and other problems associated with any chronic condition. Take a walk in the park. Go to a movie, concert, play, or sporting event. Treat yourself to a massage or other way of pampering yourself. Remove toxic people from your life. Do whatever you can to create peace in your life. You deserve it!

Learn how to ask for help without guilt. We all need help. Let someone else take care of cleaning the house or shopping. Let friends or family members take care of your kids every now and then so you can get some rest. When you feel well enough, pay the favor forward.

Dystonia is survivable. You can still have a high quality life regardless of your symptoms. Do whatever it takes to make it work. You can get through the hard times and come out on top. Just keep in mind what's really important in your life and then go for the fullest life possible. It's yours to live, one day at a time.[1]

Relationships
For relationships to be successful and satisfying, you must be prepared to give others what they need and be willing to ask others for what you need. You may dislike feeling like a burden, but let willing friends and family take the strain

and give you a break, especially when it comes to family responsibilities. Also be sure to ask them what their boundaries and limits are so they do not become overwhelmed. According to Dr. Micah Sadigh, having good relationships with people who don't judge or criticize us is a great buffer against stress.

- Get help from as many resources as you can.
- Educate your friends and family about dystonia and related conditions.
- Seek out and enjoy the company of others.
- Make your expectations realistic. "Within the limits of my physical ability I will do whatever it is I want to do for as long as I can."

Smiling and laughter

Please remember Rule #6. If you have ever read the book, The Art of Possibility (2002), by Rosamund Stone Zander and Benjamin Zander, you know what this means. You may have also seen this in other places. For those unfamiliar with Rule #6, here is an excerpt from the book:[2]

Two prime ministers are sitting in a room discussing affairs of state. Suddenly a man bursts in, apoplectic with fury, shouting and stamping and banging his fist on the desk. The resident prime minister admonishes him: "Peter," he says, "kindly remember Rule Number 6," whereupon Peter is instantly restored to complete calm, apologizes, and withdraws.

The politicians return to their conversation, only to be interrupted yet again twenty minutes later by a hysterical woman gesticulating wildly, her hair flying. Again the intruder is greeted with the words: "Marie, please remember Rule Number 6." Complete calm descends once more, and she too withdraws with a bow and an apology.

When the scene is repeated for a third time, the visiting prime minister addresses his colleague: "My dear friend, I've seen many things in my life, but never anything as remarkable as this. Would you be willing to share with me the secret of Rule Number 6?" "Very simple," replies the resident prime minister. "Rule Number 6 is 'Don't take yourself so damn seriously'." "Ah," says his visitor, "that is a fine rule." After a moment of pondering, he inquires, "And what, may I ask, are the other rules?" The prime minister responds, "There aren't any."

When I first heard this story I realized how seriously I took so many things and made a point of remembering Rule #6 as much as possible in all my personal and interpersonal interactions. I began to laugh and smile more which made a huge difference in my level of happiness. We tend to be our worst enemy by taking ourselves and things in general too seriously. Dystonia is a serious condition that needs our attention, but there is no reason why we can't approach it with a little less angst. Angst is only going to make our symptoms worse. We all know this. We just don't practice it enough.

When is the last time you laughed and could not stop; one of those belly laughs that kept you laughing on and off all day long? You probably felt pretty good that day. Within humor is great peace.

Benefits of laughter
- Decreased muscle tension. Laughter exercises the diaphragm, contracts the abdominals and also works out the shoulders, leaving the muscles more relaxed.
- Improved sleep.
- Increases endorphins.
- Distraction. Laughter takes the focus away from pain, anger, guilt, stress and negative emotions.
- Change in perspective. Our response to stressful events can be altered by our reaction to them. Humor can give us a more lighthearted perspective, making stressful events less threatening.
- Socially beneficial. Laughter connects us with others and is often contagious.

Laughter is also thought to have an affect on physiological functions such as lower blood sugar levels, healthier arteries, reduced stress hormones, and a stronger immune system.

Where to find laughter
- Rent a movie or go to a movie or comedy club.
- Tell jokes. If you don't know any, learn some.
- Go to a party or have friends over for a party or game night.
- Spend time around babies and animals.
- Watch something funny on television or the computer. There is no shortage of opportunities to laugh all over the place, whether in person or in front of a screen. A stroll through YouTube videos can keep you laughing for hours.

Benefits of smiling
- Improves immune function. When we smile we are more relaxed.
- Helps us stay positive.
- Lowers blood pressure.

- Relieves stress.
- Lifts the face and makes us look (and feel) younger.
- Makes us feel and appear more confident.
- Smiling makes us attractive and more appealing to others. People are drawn to us when we smile, just as we are drawn to them. Frowns, scowls and grimaces all push people away, but a smile draws them in.
- Smiling improves our mood. Smile the next time you feel down. There's a good chance your mood will change for the better. Smiling can trick the body into helping you change your mood.
- Smiling is contagious. When someone is smiling they lighten up the room and change the moods of others.
- Smiling puts others at ease and makes them more comfortable. Take flying for example. When there is heavy turbulence, a smile from another passenger or a flight attendant always puts me at ease.

I know how difficult it can be to laugh and smile when dealing with dystonia, particularly when it is accompanied by pain and self conscious thoughts about how you look. However, even just the act of forcing a laugh or smile has benefit. Some studies have shown that we can gain the positive effects of forced laughing and smiling just as much as the real thing. The body does not know how to distinguish between real and fake laughs and smiles.

With this in mind, force a smile and a laugh more often. It certainly can't hurt. You might even find that fake expressions of joy lead to real smiles and laughs. Plus, if you bring more laughter into your life, you will most likely help others around you laugh more. By elevating the mood of those around you, you can reduce their stress levels, and perhaps improve the quality of social interaction you experience with them, reducing your stress even more.

If something is frustrating or upsetting, realize that you can look back on it and laugh. Think of how it will sound when you tell others down the road, and then see if you can laugh about it now. You may find yourself being more lighthearted and silly, giving yourself and those around you more to laugh about. Despite the pain, approach life in a more joyful way. You will find that you are less stressed about negative events.

Since we don't have a choice what our muscles are going to do often times, I think it is very helpful to joke about it. There is no point in making matters worse by torturing ourselves trying to hide what is there. Laugh, joke, and talk about it. Get rid of the stigma about being "different." Everyone is different and the more we can embrace our uniqueness, no matter what it is, the more at ease we are and the more at ease others become. Have you ever made fun of yourself before anyone else had the chance? More than likely you all had a good laugh and whatever tension that existed was diffused. Instead of being the recipient of someone else's ribbing, beat them to the punch. This always lightens an uncomfortable situation.

If you have heard of or seen the stand-up comedian Josh Blue you know what I am talking about. Josh has cerebral palsy and much of his comedy routines are about his condition. He makes fun of himself and talks about what is probably on everyone's mind, but they are afraid to say. He allows himself to laugh about how he looks and moves, and welcomes others to do so as well. He has embraced his condition and is better for it. The same applies to all of us.

Happiness isn't a state, it's a skill. It's the skill of knowing how to take what life throws your way and make the most of it.
- Gary Null -

Additional coping tools:[3]
- Seek out the best medical care you can to fit your specific needs. Don't give up until you find the right health care team that fits you best.
- Keep a folder of all your medical treatments.
- Keep a journal of how you feel, noting any changes in symptoms and mood.
- Have a list of friends and family you can call for support when needed, as well as emergency numbers for your doctors and other medical personnel.
- Avoid isolation. When we lose connection with others it can intensify depression, helplessness, loneliness, fear, anger, and bitterness.
- Connect with a dystonia support group in your area or online.
- Accept help when it is offered and ask for help when you need it.
- Look into assistance programs for which you may qualify including government programs, relief programs by local community organizations, and medication discounts.
- Incorporate stress reduction activities into your daily routine.
- Get outdoors and spend time surrounded by nature.
- Exercise if you can. Modify activities to accommodate your symptoms.
- Get involved with groups that give you a sense of belonging and engage in activities that give you a feeling of accomplishment. Create new ways of doing things you enjoy that have become difficult.

- Get involved with the dystonia community. Share your experience with others and learn from them. Everyone has something to offer. Become an advocate for dystonia in whatever way you feel you can best contribute.
- Do not argue about things that are not productive.
- Avoid people who cause you stress.
- Find rewarding things you can do to increase your self image/esteem.
- Don't waste time worrying about what could have been. The past is over. Focus on the present moment.
- Simplify your goals.
- Pamper yourself.
- Eat well.
- Pace yourself.
- Engage in fun, pleasurable activities as much as possible.
- Keep busy learning new things.
- Take charge of your health care. Make informed decisions about your body. Be smart, if not smarter than your doctor.
- Find comfort in your discomfort. A happy life is not contingent on our health status.
- Stop feeling guilty for what you can't do and praise yourself for what you do get done.
- Learn how to say "No" without guilt.
- Don't compare yourself to other people.
- Don't give up your aspirations and goals. Make them realistic.
- Accept, trust, and love yourself no matter what is "wrong."

Testimonial

About 3 weeks before I get my Botox injections the pain is severe. That's when I get the feeling of falling into the black hole of, "Can I cope with the pain anymore?" Then the injection takes 3 weeks to kick in. So, if I'm lucky I have 6-7 weeks where I feel a little better. I have the strength to hang on, but I'm not sure how sometimes. The pain I live with never lets up and limits what I can do. But I must say I give it my all! I do quite a bit for someone with dystonia, like go to gym daily (even though I may have to hold my head while on the treadmill), hula dancing, belly dancing, and on and on. I'll be damned if I allow dystonia to get a hold of me. Life must go on.

Testimonial

Living with dystonia has been very challenging. One of the things that made the most impact on how I choose to think about living with this condition was meeting Nick Vujicic. Nick was born with tetra-amelia syndrome, a rare disorder characterized by the

110

absence of both arms and both legs. Nick has overcome so much and now travels the world as a motivational speaker. He is also the author of several books. I met him when he came to Indonesia to promote his book, "Give me a Hug." His main lesson for me was when he said, "I am grateful for what I have instead of being angry for what I don't have." I took these words to heart because the more grateful we are, the happier we become.

The way Nick lives his life is amazing. If someone like Nick has such a beautiful spirit and can be so optimistic about his life, there is no reason for any of us to not have hope or be pessimistic about our life. No matter our situation in life, we all have to be thankful for what we can do versus being angry over what we can't do or what has become difficult. We should exercise as best we can, eat properly, love and care for one another, and make peace with our condition to be happy. We will all face difficulties in life, but if we don't give up, if we try to do things in a new way, if we take a different view of things, everything is possible.

References
1)   Adapted from "Coping with Illness", www.care4dystonia.org, Retrieved August 21, 2013 from: http://www.docstoc.com/docs/158457339/Coping-with-illnessdoc---Care4Dystonia
2)   Zander, R., Zander, B. (2000) The Art of Possibility. New York, NY, Penguin Putnam
3)   Modified from: DMRF, Dystonia Dialogue, September 2013, p. 22 and Dystonia International Support Group on Yahoo

Chapter 11
Healthy Living and Self Care

Living well with dystonia requires that we be disciplined in taking good care of ourselves. Some people rely solely on their doctors for their health care. Unfortunately, except for suggestions, doctors can't do much for us beyond providing treatments. We have to do more for ourselves. We are ultimately responsible for our well being which is done by practicing "self care."

Self care involves many things, but generally speaking, it is the ability to deal with all that a dystonia entails, including symptoms, treatments, and lifestyle changes. With effective self care we can monitor our condition and make whatever physical, behavioral, and emotional changes necessary to maintain a high quality of life.

An important component of self care is being educated. In fact, self-efficacy, the belief in our ability to accomplish a specific behavior or achieve a reduction in symptoms, is an underlying theory of patient education. Studies show that when we increase our knowledge about our health and the care we receive, it improves clinical outcomes. Increased self care and self management also reduces hospitalizations, emergency department use, and overall managed care costs. Studies also show that educated patients are more compliant and satisfied with treatments across a broad range of conditions and disease severities, resulting in a significant improvement in health behaviors and health status. Being well educated also improves coping skills because our involvement gives us greater control over the decisions made about our health.[1-4]

Self care for me includes eating well, exercise, quality sleep, stress management (see chapter 8), massage, acupuncture, listening to music, resting by the pool or at the beach, meditation, prayer, avoiding toxic people, refraining from activities and events that overtax my body, shutting off my computer and phone, walking in the park, reading inspirational books, watching my favorite movies and TV shows, and spending time with people who lift me up. There should be no guilt or shame for anyone to do what they need to take care of themselves. We are no good to ourselves or anyone else when we do not practice mind and body self care on a regular basis.

I like to be active, but I also like and need to rest. For years I felt guilty resting during the day because I felt like I was wasting time. I was not comfortable doing what I perceived as "nothing." I felt like I was being lazy. It was not until I changed how I looked at it and realized that doing "nothing", like lying by the pool for an hour or so, is a form of self treatment and care that is vital to my health. I also realized that it is far from nothing or being lazy. It is something rather significant. My dystonic body requires that I rest so I can have more functional hours during the day. Thus, I give it what it needs by resting in a peaceful setting to relax my body and mind. This might be at the pool, beach, my yard, a park, or somewhere in my home. I schedule it into my day and call it "purposeful resting" because it serves an important need.

When I realized the benefit of my self care activities and by renaming them to things such as "purposeful resting" and "self treatment", the guilt went away. I am now more comfortable doing these things because I value how much they improve my life. With the guilt gone, my self treatments are more effective in helping me manage my symptoms and interestingly, they make the treatments I receive from my health care team more effective. It just required me to shift my thinking so I was able to accept that doing "nothing" from time to time was actually a form of loving, personal care that enhanced my overall well being.

If you are struggling with taking time to care for yourself, whatever that means to you (taking a nap, getting a massage, going to the gym, reading a book, meditating), change how you look at it and/or what you call it.

When you're good to yourself, you're being good to everyone around
you because when you feel good, you'll only react well to other people.
At the same time, it's very easy for you to do things for other people
when you know that other people are just an extension of yourself.
- Anita Moorjani -

Listen to your body
Our body is always talking to us. Pay attention. Listen to what it is telling you. With practice, you will begin to notice subtle signs that things are improving, getting worse, or something might just be more on or off than usual a particular day. Use these cues to restructure your activities.

When you notice something starting to feel worse than usual or something different than you are used to, take a moment and assess the situation. Ask yourself what you need right now to prevent things from getting worse. Do you need to lie down, put ice or heat on the affected area, exercise, meditate, pray, or talk to someone? If you need to go somewhere, can you get a ride from someone? Over time you will begin to know what you need to better manage your symptoms and keep them from getting out of control.

If you notice a pattern of feeling better for a period of time during the day or perhaps several days on end, take note of it by writing it down. Figure out what you did or did not do that helped you feel better. When you journal, it is important to include positive things as well as things that are bothering you. With a chronic condition like dystonia, it is easy to focus on all the things wrong with us which can make journaling counterproductive. Acknowledge the good things. They are very important to our mental health.

Our bodies have voices. They are often drowned out by the constant babble of the world we create for ourselves, but they are there waiting and willing to tell us what they need. Most often subtle and quiet, the voices get louder as we refuse to listen.
- Dr. Judith Petry -

Exercise
Exercise or "movement" is an essential part of healthy living. It improves circulation, reduces blood pressure, promotes weight loss, improves sleeping patterns, reduces stress, relieves symptoms of depression and anxiety, increases muscle strength, improves joint structure and joint function, and helps manage pain, among other things.

There are so many forms of exercise that it is not possible to say what would be right for you. Your symptoms may be such that you can comfortably do things such as yoga, walking, running, tennis, biking, golf, swimming, weight training, etc. For those who are unable to exercise on their feet, there are exercises designed for sitting in a chair and even lying down. The key thing to remember is that some form of movement, whether sitting, standing, or lying down, is the most important thing. There are days when dystonia gets the better of me and I need to rest and move very little, but I usually feel my best when I incorporate some form of exercise into my day.

Through trial and error (I prefer saying "trial and success"), I find stretching and light weight work to be most beneficial in helping to control my symptoms. Strong muscles support and nourish bones and joints, and hold them in good alignment. Weak muscles are more prone to injury. I also enjoy biking around my neighborhood and swimming in a pool on occasion. I modify my posture when I ride and swim so I don't aggravate my back and neck. Most of the stretching and exercising I do is from the ST Recovery Clinic program, but I have added additional things over the years.

Finding what best suits you is the key. Tailor it to your needs. There is no cookie cutter approach to exercise. Do whatever you enjoy if it does not make your symptoms worse. Even if it does make your symptoms worse, do it anyway if you find it pleasurable.

Sleep

A very important part of self care is adequate sleep. Rest and sleep help relax muscles and reduce pain, among other things, so it is especially crucial for us. Unfortunately, many people with dystonia have difficulty sleeping. This comes as no surprise considering how challenging it is to relax when your body is moving uncontrollably, is in pain, or both. Many have to use over the counter or prescription sleep aids. I used to take Nyquil to help me sleep until my doctor prescribed Restoril (temazepam). I was prescribed a whopping dose of 60mg. Over several years, I was able to slowly reduce it in small increments and am happy to report that I no longer take it.

Even with medication I had a terrible time sleeping for several years. I experimented with different pillows, mattresses, sleeping positions, etc. I didn't even sleep in a bed for a couple years. I slept on a mat on the floor. I would have preferred sleeping in bed because the mat was in the way during the day and it hurt my neck to roll it up and put away each morning, but I couldn't get comfortable in bed. I was so distressed that some nights I would go back and forth from the mat to the bed. This would often go on for hours and I always ended up on the mat. Although I slept better on the mat, it caused me more pain and stiffness during the day so I forced myself to only sleep in my bed. I put the mat in storage so it wasn't even an option. It took about 4 months before I began to feel somewhat comfortable in bed. Within about 8 months my body fully adapted.

According to medical experts, dystonia "disappears" when we are sleeping. Apparently our symptoms go dormant for that period of time. This is a huge plus for us because our bodies need that break for healing and rejuvenation. Sleep requirements vary; 6-8 hours is sufficient for me and I also take rest breaks throughout the day if I am able. If I can take a quick nap as well, it helps keep my mind and muscles calmer, and gives me more energy.

There are many other benefits to sleep. When we are sleeping, our body releases hormones that help repair cells and control the body's use of energy. During sleep, the body is also doing most of its detoxification. Researchers have also discovered that sleep plays a critical role in immune function, metabolism, memory, and learning. Chronic lack of sleep is linked to colds and flu, hypertension, diabetes, heart disease, mental health, and even obesity.[5]

Sleep is also necessary for our nervous system to work properly. Too little sleep effects concentration, memory, and physical performance. If sleep deprivation persists, mood swings may develop. Sleep gives neurons used while we are awake a chance to shut down and repair themselves. Without sleep, neurons may become so depleted in energy that they begin to malfunction. This is vital for those of us with dystonia. Our neurons are already malfunctioning, so the more restorative sleep the better.[5]

Tips for better sleep[6-9]

Boost melatonin production

Melatonin is a hormone in the brain that helps regulate other hormones and maintains the body's circadian rhythm. When it is dark, our body produces more melatonin. When it is light, the production of melatonin drops. When it is time to go to bed, turn off your computer and television. Light suppresses melatonin production and television can stimulate the mind rather than relax it. Don't read from a backlit device at night (such as an iPad). Read from something that requires a light source such as a bedside lamp. Use a low-wattage bulb so you can avoid bright lights. Make sure the room is dark. Cover electrical displays, use curtains or shades to block light from windows, and wear a sleep mask to cover your eyes.

Increase light exposure during the day

Remove your sunglasses in the morning and let sunlight hit your face. Try to take work breaks outside, exercise outside, and walk during the day instead of at night. Also let as much light into your home/workspace as possible.

Sunshine affects the brain via the interaction of the chemicals melatonin and serotonin, as well as vitamin D. When sunlight hits your eyes, your optic nerve sends a message to the pineal gland in the brain that tells it to decrease its secretions of melatonin until the sun goes down again.

The opposite happens with serotonin, a hormone connected with feelings of happiness and wakefulness. When we are exposed to sun, our brain increases serotonin production. When sunshine touches our skin, the body produces vitamin D, which helps us maintain serotonin levels. When melatonin and serotonin production are properly balanced, we feel energized during the day and a slowing down during the dark hours. Some find vitamin D supplements helpful for maintaining this hormonal balance, especially during the colder months when we spend more time indoors.

Stick to a sleep schedule
Maintain a regular bedtime and wake time schedule. A regular wake time in the morning strengthens the circadian function and can help with sleep onset at night.

Pay attention to what you eat and drink
Don't go to bed hungry or full. Also limit how much you drink before bed to prevent trips to the bathroom. Avoid nicotine, caffeine and alcohol. The stimulating effects of nicotine and caffeine can wreak havoc on quality sleep, and even though alcohol might make you feel tired, it can disrupt sleep.

Create a bedtime ritual
Establish a regular, relaxing bedtime routine each night to tell your body it is time to wind down. This might include taking a warm bath or shower, reading a book, or listening to soothing music. Relaxing activities ease the transition from wakefulness to drowsiness.

Make your bedroom more sleep friendly
Make your bedroom reflective of the value you place on sleep. Check your room for noise, light, temperature, or other distractions, including a partner's sleep disruptions such as snoring. Keep your room temperature less than 70 degrees Fahrenheit. Consider using shades that darken the room, a sleep mask to cover your eyes, earplugs, recordings of soothing sounds, and a fan or other device that creates white noise.

Make sure your bed allows enough room to stretch and turn comfortably. Experiment with different levels of mattress firmness, foam or egg crate toppers, and pillows that provide appropriate support. If you share your bed, make sure there is enough room for two. If you have children or pets, set boundaries for how often they can sleep with you or have them sleep in their own space.

Include physical activity in your daily routine
Regular physical activity can help you fall asleep faster and enjoy deeper sleep. Find a time to exercise that works best for you. Shortly before bed is usually not the best time of day as it can cause you to be too energized to fall asleep.

Napping
Take a nap if you didn't sleep well during the night or if your dystonia is such that you are having a day where more rest and sleep is required. If you need to make up for a few lost hours, opt for a daytime nap rather than sleeping late. This helps make up for lost hours without disturbing your sleep-wake cycle. I find that a good power nap during the day revitalizes me.

Reserve your bed for sleeping and sex
Use your bedroom only for sleep and sex to strengthen the association between bed and sleep. Take work materials, computers and televisions out of the bedroom. If you only use your bed for sleep and sex, when you go to bed, your body gets a powerful cue: it's time to either nod off or be romantic.

I hope this information leads you to better sleep. Many of these suggestions have significantly improved my quality of sleep. If you still have trouble falling asleep, maintaining sleep, awaken earlier than you wish, don't feel refreshed after sleep, or suffer from excessive sleepiness during the day, please consult your doctor.

Nutrition and dystonia
Nutrition is probably one of the most controversial, confusing, and emotional topics next to politics. We are bombarded with so much information that it can be difficult to really know what is best to eat.

One way of eating isn't the only way, especially when it comes to the strange symptoms of dystonia and how each of us responds so differently to things. However, there are some basic eating guidelines for a healthy life in general, and one that may also help with dystonia symptoms. There are so many ideas and opinions about diet that it is hard to know where to begin, so the best thing I can do is tell you what has worked for me and what the consensus is about nutrition and dystonia.

I am a caveman. No, I don't carry around a club to fight off bears or whack women over the head and drag them back to a cave. I don't have a scraggly beard and long hair. Although, at one point in time when my dystonia was severe, I looked a little like a caveman. I rarely shaved or got a haircut because it was too painful. When I did, that was about all I could handle the entire day because grooming was incredibly difficult.

I eat a caveman diet, more commonly known as the hunter-gatherer diet or Paleo diet. Our genetic profile was emerging and being formed during Paleolithic times, hence the name Paleo, so our bodies are designed to thrive on the food that was available at that time. In other words, our bodies are not genetically adapted to eat much of the foods we consume today. The Paleo diet consists primarily of lean meats, fish, grass-fed pasture raised animals (free range), eggs, vegetables, fruit, and nuts. It excludes grains, legumes, dairy products, potatoes, refined salt, refined sugar, and processed oils.

With all the research available to us on nutrition and disease, it is hard to argue that this is not a wise way to eat. Of course there are exceptions, especially for people with a particular health condition where they can't tolerate certain foods, but our focus is on dystonia and general health maintenance.

It is widely accepted that refined sugars, sugar substitutes, white flour and white flour products, refined omega-6 oils, too much alcohol, caffeine, preservatives, and foods with a high glycemic index should be avoided in general (glycemic index is discussed below), but especially if you have dystonia. Most of these foods are inflammatory and may trigger dystonic activity in our muscles. They also promote other health problems.

Sugar
Sugar and sugar substitutes should be avoided. They are poison to our body. Sugar consumption has been linked to numerous physical diseases, as well as mental illnesses such as depression, depersonalization, anxiety, ADHD, etc., which some who have dystonia already suffer. With this in mind, it makes little sense to consume sugar which may worsen these conditions.

To examine the hold sugar can have on us, substance-abuse researchers have performed brain scans on subjects eating something sweet. What they have seen resembles the mind of a drug addict. When tasting sugar, the brain lights up in the same regions as it would in an alcoholic with a bottle of whiskey. Dopamine, the reward chemical, spikes and reinforces the desire to have more.

When the pancreas senses sugar, the body releases insulin. This causes cells in the liver, muscle, and fat tissue to take up glucose from the blood, storing it as glycogen for energy. If you eat too much at once, insulin levels spike and then drop. The aftermath is you feel tired and then crave more sugar to perk up and the cycle of addiction continues.

Artificial sugars don't help. They travel to the part of the brain associated with desire, but not to the part responsible for reward. Nor do they trigger the release of the satiety hormones that real sugar does, so you're more likely to consume more calories.

Sugar also forms free radicals in the brain's membrane and compromises nerve cells' ability to communicate. This could have repercussions in how well we remember instructions, process ideas, and handle our moods. Sugar also causes premature aging. When sugar travels into the skin, its components cause nearby amino acids to form cross-links. These cross-links jam the repair mechanism and, over time, leave you with premature wrinkles.[10]

If you think about it, it makes sense that our bodies do not handle refined sugar very well. For the majority of human existence, there was no such sugar. We were endowed with a sweet tooth so that we would crave fruits. With the advent of processed sugar cane, our adaptive sweet tooth turned into somewhat of a curse, causing us to crave foods that our bodies are not designed to process. In other words, our bodies are not designed to process refined sugar.

Grains
Grains include rice, amaranth, barley, rye, millet, bread, pastries, pasta, cereal, crackers, chips, pizza, and pretzels to name a few. There is a popular misconception that grains should be a regular part of our diet. This is not necessary, as grains are not as healthy as often promoted. Most are high in carbohydrates, they contain ingredients that strip us of important nutrients, they are difficult to digest, and they are not as nutrient dense as other options. Just because some people seem to have no immediate negative physical effects from grains, it does not mean our bodies can function optimally while consuming them.

Grains, including whole grains, contain gluten (discussed in more detail below), lectins (cause intestinal damage such as leaky gut), and phytates (mineral blocker that prevents the absorption of calcium, magnesium, copper, iron, and zinc), all of which are pro-inflammatory. They also have a high ratio of omega-6 to omega-3 fatty acids and promote an acidic pH. Most grains and foods made from grains also contain a high glycemic index. Glycemic index measures how fast and how much a food raises blood glucose levels. Foods with higher glycemic index values raise blood sugar more rapidly than foods with lower glycemic index values, which promote inflammation. This is

120

important because a dystonic body is already inflamed from the wear and tear on our muscles and joints. There is no need to eat foods that increase inflammation.

People might read that grains should be avoided and then wonder where they will get their fiber. The answer is simple; fruits, vegetables, and nuts. Green vegetables, for example, contain substantially more fiber than whole grains on a calorie by-calorie-basis.[11]

Gluten
Gluten is a protein composite found in foods processed from wheat and related grain species, including barley, rye, spelt, kamut, and oats. It is in pizza, pasta, bread, wraps, rolls, and most processed foods. It gives elasticity to dough, helping it rise and keep its shape, and give foods a chewy texture. Gluten is also found in condiments, salad dressings, soups, processed meats (cold cuts, hot dogs, sausages, etc.), ice cream, reduced fat products, gravy and cream sauces thickened with flour, soy sauce, hydrolyzed vegetable protein, yeast extract, malted drinks, beer, ale, gin, and whiskey.

The body is not designed to digest gluten. It is a foreign protein to human physiology, as it has not been part of our diet for most of our existence. There are some people who have celiac disease, a condition that results in damage to the lining of the small intestine when foods with gluten are eaten; and there are those (I believe most) who have gluten sensitivity to varying degrees (non-celiac gluten sensitivity). This is important to appreciate because gluten sensitivity creates inflammation throughout the body, including our brain, heart, joints, and digestive tract.

Since gluten may promote a host of unwanted health conditions, ranging from mental health issues to headaches to neurological disorders, all of which can exist without digestive problems, it is in our best interest to avoid foods containing this substance. Anything that has the potential to affect brain function in negative ways should be avoided, especially by those of us with a condition like dystonia that originates in the brain. It just makes good sense.

Blood sugar
It is important that every snack and meal contain protein so our blood sugar can remain as stable as possible. When we eat something high in carbohydrates, the effect on our blood sugar level is immediate. This is because carbohydrates are quickly converted into glucose which enters our bloodstream

quickly and gives a quick burst of energy. Soon afterwards, our pancreas releases a spurt of insulin to rush in and clear out the glucose and regulate blood sugar. This is how it should work, but if we mainly eat carbohydrates, we overproduce insulin, blood sugar falls, energy level plummets, the more carbohydrates we crave, and the cycle starts all over again.

Any extra glucose that is not used up gets stored as fat for future use. If it is not used up and we continue to consume high amounts of carbohydrates, fat accumulates. If carbohydrate consumption remains excessive, the body increases cortisol and adrenaline production to handle the extra load. This does a number on the endocrine and immune systems, creating excessive inflammation in the body. Eating a diet high in carbohydrates also causes our energy levels to rise and fall.[12]

Protein converts to glucose more slowly than carbohydrates. It also helps slow the absorption of carbohydrates, keeping blood sugar under control. Protein is also important because the amino acids they contain are the building blocks of our brain's network. Most neurotransmitters are made from these amino acids and proper neurotransmitter function is crucial for people with dystonia. The body also uses protein to build and repair tissues, which is also very important for those of us with dystonia because our muscles are so overburdened.

People who do not eat enough good sources of protein (and healthy fats) are essentially starving their brain and body. With this in mind, be sure to eat protein throughout the day. Breakfast is especially important, preferably one that consists of a combination of carbohydrates (preferably plant based), protein, and healthy omega 3 fats. It is called "breakfast" for a reason. It 'breaks' our 'fast' that takes place between the last time we ate before going to bed and when we wake up. Our brain and body need to be properly re-fueled, not unlike a car needs gas and oil in order to run properly.

Water consumption
Drinking plenty of water to keep the body hydrated is also critical. Water plays an important role in digestion, blood circulation for carrying nutrients and oxygen to cells and removing toxins, regulating body temperature, protecting the movement of joints, and helping metabolize fat. A widely accepted standard for daily water consumption is to divide your weight in half and drink that may ounces of water. For example, at around 180 pounds, I consume at least 90 ounces of water day which is around 11 cups.

Changing how we eat

A good way to go about changing what we eat is to slowly replace bad foods with good foods. It may take time to adjust, so allow yourself the time you need. Also change the way you shop. It is best to shop the perimeter of the grocery store because this is where all of the healthy, fresh foods are located. Aside from a few things, the aisles are where they stock most of the foods we want to avoid. Shop "around" the store to find the best foods. This will also condition you to think more about healthier foods to help you to make better choices.

For many, eating is an emotional activity, as it is often a coping mechanism or an escape in search for comfort, which is all too common when living with a chronic health condition or any other significant life challenge. Food does more than fill our stomachs; it also satisfies feelings. When we quench those feelings with comfort food, it can be a very satisfying companion. However, most comfort foods are unhealthy which will cause overeating because they increase cravings for sugar, salt, and fat laden foods.

If you are an emotional eater, you may find yourself using food as a reward when you are happy and craving sweets or unhealthy snacks when stressed. By eating healthier, we can reduce cravings for these foods and then begin to seek or crave healthy foods, such as fruits and vegetables versus chips and ice cream, for example. This is a liberating experience. Exercise is also very helpful for reducing cravings.

Eating well can give us more energy, reduce our risk for diseases, reduce inflammation and pain, and help us lose weight and/or maintain a healthy weight. It may also help reduce dystonia symptoms, and a way to do this is to eliminate sugar, sugar substitutes, fried and processed foods, caffeine, soda, and alcohol from our diets. If you are unsure if what you are eating is causing problems with your dystonia or overall health, eliminate something from your diet for a couple weeks and see if you notice a difference. Try this with a variety of foods and food groups.

Changing the way we eat requires us to change the way we think about eating so we need to ask ourselves some important questions. Are we eating to satisfy cravings or to satisfy hunger? Are we eating foods that make us feel good emotionally or physically? Are the foods we eat causing unwanted dystonia symptoms or other health problems? Is what we eat going to be healthy in the long term or disease promoting? Your answers to these questions will determine what kinds of food fill your plate.

How I lost 150 pounds

Prior to the onset of dystonia, I lived an active, healthy life involved in many sports and activities. When dystonia hit, chronic pain caused me to be very sedentary and I no longer took proper care of my body like I used to. I began eating fatty foods and drank beer to numb the pain. While I did not eat dessert type foods, I consumed lots of fatty meats, cheeses, pasta, fried and processed foods, bread, sandwiches, crackers, chips, dips, etc. I went from an athletic 190 pounds in 2001 to around 330 pounds in 2006. I actually may have weighed more than 330 pounds. I don't really know my top weight because I stopped looking at the scale after I hit 310, and I was still rapidly climbing. At around 240 pounds, I was put on blood pressure medication for hypertension.

Ironically, prior to developing dystonia and gaining weight, I was a partner in a nutrition education company! What was I thinking you might ask; simple, I wasn't thinking because I was in too much physical and mental pain to care what I was doing to myself.

I was never overweight my entire life, let alone obese, so it was a brand new experience for me. I was very self conscious. It felt like every set of eyes was on me. I think people looked at me more because of my weight than they did my dystonia, even though dystonia caused me to have distorted body postures that attracted attention. Whatever the case, it was not an appealing combination. I felt and looked awful, but in all honesty, I really didn't know how I looked because I rarely looked in the mirror and avoided having pictures taken. I regret that now, but I didn't want to see my exterior because it was a reflection of how unhappy I felt on the inside. It was also a reminder of the pain I was in that was the main contributor to gaining all the weight. I retreated from the world as much as I could.

As mentioned in chapter 2, in December 2006, 5 1/2 years after my dystonia began, I caught a stomach virus. During those two weeks I spent all day in bed and the bathroom. It was one of the greatest blessings because I was too sick to engage in self destructive activities. Not being able to eat any solid food or drink alcohol turned my life around. Being so idle also gave me time to think about what I was doing to myself and what I could do to change.

While I was sick, I lost a little weight and my dystonia slightly improved, allowing me to be a bit more active when I got better. I knew that this was my opportunity to make lifestyle changes. If I did not take advantage of this opportunity I was potentially facing life threatening health problems. I began walking a little each day and returned to a healthy way of eating by following practices I ignored for over 5 years. I started by walking about 100 yards to the end of my street and back. Every week or so I would go a bit further. I eventually got the strength to walk 2-3 miles twice a day and lost most of my excess weight in 10 months. It was an incredible feeling!

Unfortunately, I pushed the envelope and walked too much, aggravating my dystonia to the point of injuring my back. I had to stop walking completely. The pain on my entire right side at that point was such that I was unable to even hold a pen in my hand to write. When I stopped walking, my weight was 210 pounds, but by eating well I continued to lose weight. At 6' 2", I am back to a healthy 185 pounds. My driver's license pictures from 2006 and 2012 speak volumes. I wasn't ready for the 2012 picture…hence no smile. Believe it or not, I was trying to smile in the 2006 picture. This was the best I could do.

Driver's License 2006   **Driver's License 2012**

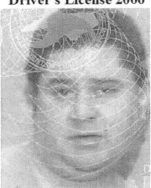 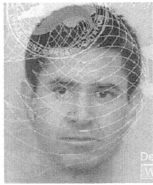

It has been over 7 years since I stopped "exercise" walking and I have not gained any weight. I find it both interesting and important to note (particularly because many with dystonia are not able to be as active as they once were) that I continued to lose weight months after I stopped walking, which I attribute to eating well.

I still don't do much aerobic exercise and am able to maintain my weight. I might bike or swim a little on occasion and do light weight bearing exercises a couple times a week, but I mainly do stretches that target my dystonia.

Flexibility combined with strength is very helpful for me, but I have to be careful with what I do and how much I do so I don't aggravate my dystonia. Too much activity can be detrimental so it is a delicate balance.

While it is possible to lose weight and maintain a healthy weight by eating properly and being moderately active, we should try and do some form of aerobic exercise if it does not make our symptoms worse. Listen closely to your body and do what is best for you and your specific situation. Exercise has many health benefits. Just make sure it is dystonia friendly. I pushed the envelope too far and paid the price. Now I know my limits and exercise within those limits. Please do the same so you don't aggravate your condition.

I primarily eat fresh fruits and vegetables, lean meats, fish, eggs, and raw nuts (Paleo diet). I do not eat dairy, grains, pasta, bread, cereal, crackers, chips, desserts, fried or processed foods, sugar or sugar substitutes, and all I drink is water. This way of eating may sound extreme, but it only sounds extreme because we have become so accustomed to eating poorly.

I don't like to call what I eat a "diet" because it is more of a lifestyle. The distinction between diet (temporary) vs. lifestyle (long term) are very important. Calling what we eat a "diet" often creates expectations and pressure, which can be self defeating and result in failure.

We need to use terminology that triggers the right attitude towards food because if we change how we look at eating, we can change what we eat. When we change what we eat, we can change how we feel. When we change how we feel, we make more thoughtful choices about what we put in our bodies, resulting in better weight management and overall health promotion.

While the years of being overweight were very painful, I am grateful I went through the experience. I now have a much better appreciation for how food and drink can become our best friends. I better understand the feelings that cause people to eat poorly and become overweight and obese, and how it feels to have a negative self body image and be uncomfortable around others. I also understand how people can escape this self-imprisonment and live a healthier, happier, higher quality life.

Take baby steps by making small changes at a time. Then build on each step to a healthier you. We all travel this road differently, so find what works best for you and put it to practice.

126

2003   **2005**   **2014**

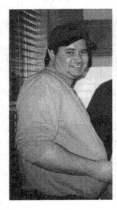 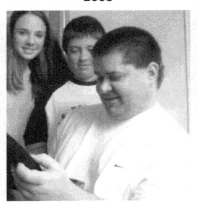 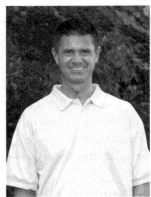

References
1) Gold DT, McClung B. Approaches to patient education: emphasizing the long-term value of compliance and persistence. Am J Med. 2006 Apr;119(4 Suppl 1):S32-7. Retrieved on November 15, 2013 from: http://www.ncbi.nlm.nih.gov/pubmed/16563940
2) American Family Physician, Retrieved October 18, 2013 from: http://www.aafp.org/afp/2005/1015/p1503.html
3) Bodenheimer T, Wagner EH, Grumbach K. Improving primary care for patients with chronic illness. JAMA. 2002;288:1775–9
4) Whitlock WL, Brown A, Moore K, Pavliscsak H, Dingbaum A, Lacefield D, et al. Telemedicine improved diabetic management. Mil Med. 2000;165:579–84
5) www.clevelandclinic.org, Retrieved September 3, 2013 from: http://www.clevelandclinic.org/health/health-info/docs/1000/1064.asp
6) www.helpguide.org, Retrieved September 3, 2013 from: http://www.helpguide.org/life/sleep_tips.htm
7) www.curiosity.discovery.com, Retrieved September 4, 2013 from: http://curiosity.discovery.com/question/affects-of-lack-of-sun
8) www.sleepfoundation.org, Retrieved September 3, 2013 from: http://www.sleepfoundation.org/article/sleep-topics/healthy-sleep-tips
9) University of Maryland Medical Center, www.umm.edu, Retrieved September 4, 2013 from: http://umm.edu/health/medical/altmed/supplement/melatonin
10) Chen, J. (2012) Effects of Sugar Consumption - How to Eat Sugar Healthily, Retrieved October 23, 2013 from: http://www.marieclaire.com/health-fitness/sugar-effects
11) Seaman, D. Nutritional Wellness, www.nutritionalwellness.com, Retrieved September 14, 2013 from: http://www.nutritionalwellness.com/columnists/seaman/
12) www.wellnessmama.com, Retrieved on July 11, 2014 from: http://wellnessmama.com/575/how-grains-are-killing-you-slowly/

Chapter 12
Mental Well Being

Dystonia not only affects our body, it also affects our state of mind which can alter how we deal with and in the world. Sometimes the emotional and psychological impact can be just as bad, if not worse, than the physical symptoms and can affect every aspect of our lives. Everyone handles the emotional and psychological side of dystonia differently, but we are all affected to some degree with many of the same concerns, fears, and worries.

Mind-Body connection
Every feeling we have affects some part of our body. Even if we are doing everything "right" (exercising, eating well, managing stress, etc.) our emotions can affect how we feel physically. To achieve emotional balance it is necessary to uncover and express emotions such as anger, resentments, frustrations, and fear, and replace them with forgiveness, love, joy, and hope. Negative emotions will negatively affect our health.[1, 2]

Some scientists are reluctant to embrace this mind-body paradigm. One of the factors is that you cannot see or measure emotions inside the body. However, just because we do not have the technology to see the mind-body connection does not mean it is not real. Those of us with dystonia know first hand that there is a connection.[1, 2]

While the mechanics of mind-body links are still being unraveled, it is known is that our thoughts and emotions do play a role in our experience of physical pain (see chapter 9 for more on pain) and may play a role in the development of chronic disease. In a study published in the Proceedings of the National Academy of the Sciences, researchers in Finland showed that emotions tend to be felt in the body in ways that are generally consistent from one person to the next, irrespective of age, sex, or nationality. For example, those suffering from depression will often experience chest pains even when there is nothing physically wrong with their heart.[3]

"Our data show bodily sensations associated with different emotions are so specific that, in fact, they could at least in theory contribute significantly to the conscious feeling of the corresponding emotion," says Dr. Lauri Nummenmaa, assistant professor in Cognitive Neuroscience at the Aalto University School of Science in Finland. From an evolutionary perspective, "Emotions developed as a way to draw organisms either away from trouble or towards positive, pleasurable events."[3]

Consider the words and descriptions we use to describe how we feel. Is your "head spinning" with everything you have to do and you find yourself with dizzy spells from time to time? Is discomfort in your stomach trying to give you wisdom about something your intuition knows on a "gut level?" Maybe work isn't going well and there are things you "don't want to hear." Could there be a connection between that and the tinnitus (ringing in the ears) that you've been experiencing lately?

These subtle language clues may offer insight and help you view your health in a new and unique way, and you may feel your body moving forward or "stepping out" into new levels of wellness and vitality.[4] For more on the mind-body connection, see You Can Heal Your Life (1984) by Louise Hay.

Forgiveness
After mentioning Louise Hay, it is appropriate to follow up with a section on forgiveness since this is a cornerstone of her book, as well as an important part of healthy living. Forgiveness is the intentional and voluntary process by which people undergo a change in feelings and attitudes regarding an offense and let go of negative emotions such as resentment and revenge.

Nearly everyone has been hurt by the actions or words of another. Some of you may have been hurt by someone because of your dystonia. You may also be hurt by what dystonia has done to your life. These wounds can leave us with feelings of anger, bitterness or even vengeance if we don't practice forgiveness.

Whoever or whatever hurt or offended us might always remain a part of our lives, but forgiveness can lessen its grip on us and help us focus on positive parts of our lives. Forgiveness helps us move away from the role of a victim by releasing the control and power the offending person or situation has on us. As we let go of grudges, we no longer define our life by how we've been hurt. Forgiveness can even lead to feelings of understanding, empathy, and compassion for whom or what hurt us.

Forgiveness does not mean that we condone, excuse, or forget what happened, or deny the responsibility of whom or what hurt us, and it does not minimize or justify it. We can forgive without excusing the act or the situation. We forgive so we can detach ourselves, bringing a sense of peace that helps us get on with life and live in the present. In many instances, we come to realize that the situation(s) we felt hurt us the most actually made us a better and stronger person. In its finality, we can learn to appreciate the "harm" that was done without spite or negativity.

When we look at the word forgiveness it is comprised of the words "for" and "give." It is an act of grace. It is more than just a positive attitude. It helps us see everything in a different way without our ego interfering. As Mark Twain said, "Forgiveness is the fragrance that the violet sheds on the heel that crushed it." It is better to look at "wrongs" that are perpetrated as lessons for us to learn from to help us in the future.

Forgiveness can set us free from emotional baggage. The less baggage we store in our mind and body the better. Living with dystonia is tension filled as it is. There is no need to add more. Dystonia may in fact be something that we need to forgive for intruding in our life. By forgiving dystonia, perhaps we can better learn to cohabitate with it and find the meaning and purpose for its presence.

If we are unforgiving, we might bring anger and bitterness into new relationships and experiences. Our life might become so wrapped up in the wrong that we can't enjoy anything else. We might become depressed or anxious. We might feel that life lacks meaning or purpose and lose valuable and enriching connections with others. Work on forgiving those who may have wronged you. Forgive dystonia as well. If you allow it to have a firm hold on your life, the only person it hurts is you.

Affirmations
Most people have probably heard the saying, "Change your thoughts, change your life." There is great truth to this. There are chemicals produced in the body when we have different thoughts and emotions. When we are happy, chemicals are produced that are beneficial to the body. When we are angry or sad, chemicals are produced that are harmful to the body. Consider the power of a placebo. It is not the placebo that heals a person but the person's belief that does the healing. When the mind thinks healthy thoughts, the body finds it easier to be healthy.

Affirmations are positive, specific statements that can condition the subconscious mind to develop a more positive perception of ourselves. Affirmations can help us change harmful thoughts and behaviors, and accomplish goals. They can also help undo damage caused by negative things we repeatedly tell ourselves (or what others repeatedly tell us) that contribute to a negative self-perception.

If you believe the phrase "you are what you think", then life circumstances truly stem from thoughts. However, we cannot rely purely on thoughts. We have to translate thoughts into words and eventually into actions in order to manifest our intentions. This means we have to be very careful with our words, choosing to speak only those which work to our benefit and cultivate our highest good.

Affirmations are like exercises for our mind that can rewire our brain. Look at them the same way as repetitive exercises that improve your body's physical health. Positive mental repetitions can reprogram our thinking patterns so that we begin to think and act in a new way. They play an integral role by breaking patterns of negative thoughts, negative speech, and negative actions. The spoken word is very powerful. When we say "I can't", the energy of those words will repel against us. If we say "I can", we will be better able to manifest all that we desire.

Write down the areas in your life or behaviors you want to work on. For each, come up with a positive, present-tense statement you can repeat to yourself several times a day. It is important that your affirmations are credible, believable, and realistic. Below are some health related affirmations. Even if some of them are not true at the moment, but how you want things to be, say them anyway. We can manifest anything with the right mindset.

- My ability to conquer dystonia and other challenges is limitless.
- I am free of dystonia, free of pain, and free of fear.
- It doesn't matter how dystonia started because it is reversing its course right now. I gently release dystonia.
- My only work is to relax and breathe.
- Everything that is happening now is for my ultimate good.
- Though these times are difficult, they are only a phase of life.
- I am at peace with what has happened, is happening, and will happen.
- I sleep in peace and wake in joy.
- Every day in every way I am getting healthier and feeling better.
- I love and care for my body and it cares for me.
- My body is a safe and pleasurable place for me to be.
- I am in control of my life and health.
- I choose to be beautiful, joyous, healthy, and prosperous.

- I value my time and energy.
- My mind is calm and peaceful.
- I allow myself to play and enjoy life.
- My body is strong and healthy.
- My body is flexible.
- Every cell in my body is alive with health and energy.
- My body has a remarkable capacity for healing.
- I am full of energy and vitality.
- Every day is a new day full of hope, happiness, and health.
- I am perfectly healthy in body, mind and spirit.

Affirmations should use positive language and clearly express what you desire. It is important to use affirmations with "I", "I am", and "I will" statements, affirming that you will use your abilities to achieve your goal. Close your eyes, shut out the rest of the world, and repeat the words, thinking what they mean to you. Feel the emotions that the affirmations evoke.[5-9]

Life can be distracting so it is easy to forget our affirmations or forget saying them. Leave reminder cards in various places. Use index cards or post-it notes to write your affirmations and put them where you will see them, such as the kitchen table, refrigerator, bathroom mirror, car dashboard, desk drawer, computer monitor, purse or wallet.

An affirmation I like to say is, "My mind is clear and calm. My body is balanced and strong. My heart is loving and pure." These are all areas where I feel the need to focus my attention to achieve balance in my life. The more I repeat this, the more it becomes part of my everyday life, positively impacting everything I do.

Developing a positive mindset is one of the most powerful life strategies at our disposal. With positive affirmations and visualization, it is possible to transform our life and our health, and renew joy and passion.

Mindfulness
The words "mindfulness" and "mindfulness meditation" are talked about a lot these days. It is becoming a common practice for many as a means to find peace of mind. A simple definition of mindfulness is, "a practiced skill of non-judgmental awareness and acceptance of our present-moment experience, including all of our unwanted thoughts, feelings, sensations, and urges."[10] Mindfulness teaches us to accept all of our unwanted internal experiences as a

part of life, regardless of whether they are "good" or "bad." As meditation teacher James Baraz says, "Mindfulness is simply being aware of what is happening right now without wishing it were different; enjoying the pleasant without holding on when it changes (which it will); or being with the unpleasant without fearing it will always be this way (which it won't)."

The first time I heard about mindfulness was when I was going through horrible benzodiazepine withdrawal several years ago (read more about this in chapter 15). Someone suggested I look into the work done by Jon Kabat-Zinn to help me get through that experience.

Jon is Professor of Medicine Emeritus and founding director of the Stress Reduction Clinic and the Center for Mindfulness in Medicine, Health Care, and Society at the University of Massachusetts Medical School. The program he developed with his colleagues is called Mindfulness Based Stress Reduction (MBSR). His practice of yoga and studies with Buddhist teachers led him to integrate their teachings with those of Western science. He teaches mindfulness meditation as a technique to help people cope with stress, anxiety, pain, and illness.

Jon has written several books and created audio programs that provide great information for integrating mindfulness into your life. The program I suggest, especially for those new to this concept, is Mindfulness for Beginners (2006). In this two CD program, Jon gives a great overview of what mindfulness is all about and also provides a few mindfulness meditation exercises that you can begin practicing right away. Among the great books he has written, I highly recommend Full Catastrophe Living (1990), which applies to many of the things we face with dystonia.

Jon felt that the phrase "full catastrophe" captured something positive about the human spirit's ability to come to grips with what is most difficult in life and to find within even the most difficult trials room to grow in strength and wisdom. Thus, practicing mindfulness helps us more effectively and joyfully live in the moment no matter what is "right" or "wrong" with us.[11]

Jon defines mindfulness as, "Paying attention, on purpose, in the present moment, as if your life depended on it, non-judgmentally." This is one of my favorite descriptions of mindfulness. It is easy to understand, making it easier to put into practice. Jon continues, "Mindfulness is basically just a particular way of paying attention. It is a way of looking deeply into oneself in the spirit of self-inquiry and self-understanding."[11]

Mindfulness is not something one masters overnight. It is a journey that requires effort, commitment, and dedication. While mindfulness may provide relatively rapid relief to one's distress in certain situations, it is perhaps better conceptualized as a long-term shift in perspective that allows us to better manage the complexity of human psychological experiences. Like learning a new language, mindfulness takes time and patience to master, and ongoing effort to remain fluent.[10]

Living mindfully allows us to stay in the present without worry about the future or regret about the past. It also allows us to relate more skillfully with difficult bodily sensations, feelings, and thoughts without becoming overwhelmed by them. Remember that there are only two days in the year that nothing can be done about. One is called yesterday and the other is called tomorrow. Enjoy this moment because this moment is your life.

Mindfulness meditation
As mentioned above, the primary focus of mindfulness meditation is to observe our thoughts and feelings without judging them good or bad. The intent is to create a sense of stillness or "no thought." Breathing is a primary component of meditation. The goal is maintaining a calm awareness, allowing thoughts and feelings to come and go. Mindfulness meditation can be practiced anywhere, anytime, and for any length of time. Below are a few examples.

Breathing
- Sit or lie in a comfortable position. The object is not to fall asleep, but to "fall awake."[11]
- Focus only on your breath. Breathe in and out without forcing it.
- Observe how air comes into your body and how you release it.
- Observe how your chest or stomach rises and falls.
- If a distracting thought enters your mind that takes you away from your breath, accept it for what it is and let it pass. Put the center of your attention back on your breath.

Continue the process for as long you would like. For beginners, it might be only a couple minutes before your mind becomes too distracted and you lose focus on your breath entering and leaving your body. This is okay. The time you can sit in meditation will increase with practice and also vary depending on the circumstances of that particular day. It is not so much the amount of time you spend meditating, but the effectiveness in which you practice.

You might be wondering, "Is this it; is this all I do?" Yes! You did a great job. The point of mindfulness meditation is to do nothing but focus your attention on one thing by bringing it to the center of your awareness. This might be your breath, a sensation you feel in your body, an object, or a particular intention (or thought) you set for yourself.

Counting
This is a variation of the breathing exercise, but also an exercise in concentration.
- Close your eyes and focus your attention on slowly counting to ten.
- If your concentration wanders to anything but counting, start back at number one.
- When you reach ten, start over and repeat until you get the desired result, whatever that might be for you.

This practice may sound easier than it is. At first, it may go something like this:
"One...two...three...this isn't so hard...oops, I'm thinking. Start over."
"One...two...three...do I have a doctor's appointment tomorrow? Start over."
"One...two...three...four...now I've got it. I'm really concentrating now...oops. I did it again. Start over."

It's okay if your thoughts interfere. Don't beat yourself up. This happens to all of us. That is why meditation is called a practice. Even if you are only able to get to the number three or four before thoughts intrude, you have begun the process and are on your way. In fact, your awareness that this is happening is a practice in mindfulness in and of itself, so be proud of your efforts. Something you can also do is visualize each number to help keep your attention. For example, you can give each number a color, shape, movement, feel, and taste. Use your senses to bring the number to life so you can increase your awareness. You can also choose one number and focus solely on it. Remember that the purpose of these exercises is to clear your mind of clutter and simply be in the moment focused on one thing.

Conscious observation
This technique requires the use of an object. Any random object will do. In Jon Kabat-Zinn's program, "Mindfulness for Beginners", he uses a raisin.
- Sit or lie in a comfortable position.

- Hold the object in your hand.
- Don't study it. Just observe it for what it is.
- Bring to awareness how it looks, feels, smells, and perhaps tastes. Do this without analyzing how it should look, feel, smell, or taste. Allow it to be just as it is and observe all of its unique attributes.
- Continue until you feel a sense of calm come over you.

These are just a few of examples of many mindfulness meditation practices. The interesting thing about them is that they seem so simple, but turn out to be quite challenging at first. Also, many of us incorrectly think that meditation requires lots of time, a special location, and a special pillow to sit on. Meditation can be practiced anywhere, anytime of the day.

Sometimes when I am working at the computer I will sit back for a couple minutes and work on the breathing exercise. If I am waiting in line at the store I might focus my attention for a minute or two on an object, be it something in my cart, a picture or word on a magazine, or a sign on the wall, and practice the observation meditation. The more we practice, the easier it becomes, with the result being more mindfulness (and calmness) as a part of our life. With enough practice, you will do it and not even know it. Instead, you will feel an overall sense of calm in all aspects of your life because mindfulness has become part of your life. This is the purpose.

Letting go
A main component of all meditation is letting go. In other words, let go of the past and the future and just be in the present moment. It is important to remember that at any time we have the power to let go of the things that are bothering us about dystonia or anything else in our life. It is a choice and mindfulness meditation is very helpful in this regard. When we let go, we realize that we can go with the flow and not attach to what we want or push away what we don't want. We can just "be" with whatever is going on. Letting go is different from giving up. When we let go, we are still actively engaged with life, getting up each day and doing the best we can, but we no longer attach to fixing problems. Ironically, it is this letting go of our attachment to a cure for whatever ails us that allows genuine healing to occur.

Let go of what has happened. Let go of what may come.
Let go of what is happening now. Don't try to figure anything out.
Don't try to make anything happen. Relax, right now, and rest.

Someone once asked me a simple yet profound question when I was in the middle of something causing me great stress. "Do you want to be right or do you want to be happy?" I chose to be happy over being right. I was fighting so hard to be understood and to be right that it made me physically sick. Even though I may have been right, it did not matter because the other people saw it a different way so fighting them proved pointless. Their perspective was different and I couldn't do anything to change it.

My anger caused physical and emotional pain. Already living with both, it made no sense for me to keep fighting a battle I couldn't win. In order to heal, I had to let go. I was allowing their actions contribute to my pain. I had to remind myself that I was in control of how I reacted to what others said and did, and that no one can make me feel a certain way unless I give them permission. When I stopped giving them permission my health improved.

When you find yourself in situations such as this, talk to yourself. Ask yourself how relevant something someone says or does is in the grand scheme of things. Is it something that will bother you five or ten years from now? Probably not, so release it now so you can stop needlessly suffering. If you have trouble letting things go, try reciting the Serenity Prayer. If you are uncomfortable with the religious implications, use language that is comfortable to you.

God grant me the serenity to accept the things I cannot change,
The courage to change the things I can,
And the wisdom to know the difference

Prayer

Along with meditation, prayer is an important aspect of self care for me. It helps quiet my mind and bring me closer to a higher power that I believe emanates all of us and all that surrounds us. Connecting to that higher power can be incredibly challenging when we have a health condition because we become so attached to our body and all that it is feeling. We do health checks all the time and we wonder and worry if we will be able to sleep, go to work, take care of the kids, pay the bills, go grocery shopping, etc. Being so body identified can make the remembrance of God/Spirit/Source much more challenging. Prayer and meditation can help keep us balanced so we are not so controlled by our physical symptoms.

The following quote comes from the book, <u>A Course in Miracles</u> (1976) by Helen Schucman, which ties all of this together: "The memory of God comes to the quiet mind. It cannot come where there is conflict. For a mind at war against itself remembers not eternal gentleness. Let all this madness be undone for you, and turn in peace to the remembrance of God, still shining in your quiet mind."

Quiet your mind by turning off the computer, phone, television, and radio. Go outside where you can listen to the sounds of nature or find a quiet place in your home or elsewhere that you feel at peace. Many people are uncomfortable not having "noise" in their lives all the time because it means that they have to deal with themselves and their "problems." Technology is a great escape from reality. However, facing reality is the only way to battle and overcome what ails us. Seek out a quiet mind through prayer, meditation, or whatever brings you inner peace.

Sometimes we get angry when our prayers are not answered. Perhaps they are being answered and we are just looking at it the wrong way. You may recognize the following from the movie, *Evan Almighty* (2007). When we pray for something or ask for something, we may not get exactly what we pray for. Instead, we get the opportunity to be what we pray for. For example, if we pray for courage, we the get the opportunity to be courageous. If we pray for love, we get the opportunity to be loving. If we pray for patience, we get the opportunity to be patient. If we pray for money, we get the opportunity to make money. If we pray for health, we get the opportunity to be healthy. Notice the trend? Opportunity exists everywhere. Sometimes we just need a little more faith that everything is going to work out just fine.

Meaning and purpose

Patanjali, the father of meditation and yoga, said the following: "When you are inspired by some great purpose; some extraordinary project; all your thoughts break their bonds. Your mind transcends limitations, your consciousness expands in every direction, and you find yourself in a new, great, and wonderful world. Dormant forces, faculties and talents become alive, and you discover yourself to be a greater person by far than you ever dreamed yourself to be."

Find enthusiasm in your life. It does wonders for your health. Consider the origin of the word enthusiasm. It comes from the Greek word enthousiasmos, meaning "the God within." Over time the meaning of enthusiasm came to mean "craze, excitement, strong liking for something." One can have enthusiasm for almost anything, from tennis to cooking to reading and writing to teaching...anything. Enthusiasm breeds passion and when we have passion for something, we are inspired to transcend all boundaries. Live passionately and I promise you will find meaning and purpose, and ultimately a much happier life.

In several lectures I heard Dr. Wayne Dyer give, he shared the following story about finding meaning in our lives by being true to ourselves. He talks about happiness, but any feeling or aspiration can be inserted.

There once was a kitten in an alley chasing his tail around. Along comes an old alley cat that stops to watch the show for a while. Finally, the alley cat asks the kitten, "Why is it that you chase your tail?"

Proudly, the kitten states, "I have just returned from Cat Philosophy School where I have learned two things. The first thing I learned is that happiness is the most important thing. The second thing is that happiness is located in my tail. I have determined that if I can just get a grip on my tail, I will have a hold on eternal happiness."

The old alley cat, wise beyond his years, laughs a little, "I am not as fortunate as you have been. I never attended Cat Philosophy School, but I have also learned that happiness is the most important thing and that it is indeed located in my tail. But what I have discovered is that if I chase after it I will never be able to reach it. Rather, if I just go about my business doing what it is I want to do, happiness will follow me everywhere I go."

As Henry David Thoreau said, "If you advance confidently in the direction of your OWN dreams, and endeavor to live the life which YOU have imagined, you will meet with a success unexpected in common hours." This is what the old alley cat was telling the kitten; if you follow your dreams and passions, happiness (his tail) will follow wherever you go.

Just because we have dystonia does not mean our lives lack meaning and purpose. Perhaps having dystonia is to better fulfill our purpose. Be open and honest about this possibility. Look within. Perhaps dystonia was the blessing in disguise to open our eyes to something we have been unable to see. The less we fight and the more we explore, the better our chances that something will be revealed. We are all here for a reason or we wouldn't be here at all. Be good to yourself and be patient with yourself.

Hope

Living with dystonia is sometimes reminiscent of the plight of Sisyphus, a king from Greek mythology. Sisyphus was king of Ephyra who was punished for chronic deceitfulness and condemned to an eternity at hard labor. His punishment was to roll a massive boulder up a hill until he reached the top. However, right before he reached the top the boulder rolled all the way down and he had to repeat the task over and over.

If you have dystonia, this might sound like what you experience on a daily basis. It can be utterly frustrating and exhausting living with chronic pain, shopping for a good doctor, people not understanding, continually fighting to get better and not getting over the hump, trying to find new ways to relieve symptoms, or just getting through the day with as little discomfort as possible.

Although it may often feel like you are rolling a boulder up a hill only to have it roll back down and crush all your efforts, in the face of all your challenges, is it not an accomplishment to even get the ball rolling up the hill? I think so. Dystonia challenges us in ways that we probably never imagined possible. These challenges make each accomplishment more rewarding. With this perspective we realize that dystonia does not diminish our value as a person. In many ways it enhances our value.

Unlike Sisyphus, there is hope for us. We are not alone in our battle and while we have no cure at this point, we do have treatments that can help us manage our symptoms so we can live a productive life. Researchers are working everyday to improve on them, as well as find new treatments. Granted, for many of us life is different than we once knew, but that does not mean it has to be any less enjoyable and fulfilling.

If you have ever seen the movie, *The Shawshank Redemption* (1994), picture the moment when 'Andy Dufresne' (played by Tim Robbins) escaped from prison after crawling through a 500 yard sewage pipe. He came out clean on the other end when he fell into the stream with the rain pouring down on him. He tore off his shirt and raised his arms to the sky as a sign of freedom and triumph after being wrongfully incarcerated for nearly 20 years.

Just like Andy Dufresne, you will have days when you will feel like you are trapped in a prison cell. There will also be days when you feel as he did when he reached the other side and was free. Savor these moments. Remember these feelings. Write about them in your journal. Talk about them. Celebrate them.

Figure out what you did or did not do that made you feel better. Do whatever you can to leave an imprint on your mind about how you felt so you never forget. We have the ability to go back to that place in our minds anytime we choose to get relief and peace of mind.

When you find yourself in the "sewer", remember that hope never dies. You can always get out. You do not have to live in the mental and emotional world of fear and loneliness that is like the prison cell and sewage pipe. When you get knocked down, you can get back up. If you have done it before, you can do it again. It does not matter how many times you get knocked down as long as you keep getting up and keep going. Strength is not defined by how powerful you are but how persistent you are.

Just like Andy Dufresne said in the movie, "There are places in this world that aren't made out of stone. There's something inside that they can't get to, that they can't touch; that's yours; hope. Hope is a good thing, maybe the best of things, and no good thing ever dies." Remember this as you live your life. Just because today may be a challenging day, there is always tomorrow.

Hidden opportunity

Life is ever evolving so it is important to remember that the storms in our lives do not last forever. As previously mentioned, opportunity exists in everything. Granted, the opportunities, or silver lining, can often be hard to find when we are bombarded with dystonia symptoms, but it exists. If we change our thinking around a little, the good fortune will reveal itself.

As Napoleon Hill wrote in Think and Grow Rich (1960), "One of the tricks of opportunity is that it has a sly habit of slipping in by the back door, and often it comes disguised in the form of misfortune, or temporary defeat. Perhaps this is why so many fail to recognize opportunity."

As much as dystonia has taken away parts of our lives and makes us angry, how often do you acknowledge how it has helped you grow as a person? How about the things it has taught you about yourself and others; how you have had doors close and others open that would have never otherwise been opened; met people and grown in ways you never would have otherwise? Instead of focusing on all the things you can no longer do, how often do you take time to appreciate all you can do?

While we most certainly need to vent at times (and I do and it feels good when I need to), we need to spend more time answering these questions and talk more about how dystonia has changed our lives in positive ways. I am not saying, "Oh, just be positive" in a passing, matter of fact kind of way. I am saying it with first hand experience and knowledge about how damn hard it is to live with dystonia and how practicing proactive thinking can make life much easier on ourselves, even if we are in that mindset for just one minute a day. Just one minute a day of being open to the possibility that there is meaning. We can all spend one minute a day in this place and I promise you that the time will increase the more you practice.

A journey of a thousand miles begins with a single step
- Lao Tzu -

Complaining about anything is very easy and actually requires no effort, no matter the issue. We can all very easily go to that well and fill many buckets of things to complain about, but how many buckets can you fill with all the good that has come from dystonia? Not many because we don't do it enough. Plus, it is very hard when we are in the state we are in, so it requires us to truly look deep inside to find those things. This is one of the gifts of dystonia. It forces us to become mentally and physically tough. It forces us to look within and grow.

I have heard so many stories from people who made the effort to find the good fortune and are better people as a result. Some better than they were before dystonia. Many have come from the pits of hell wanting to die, but triumphed by never giving in and finding new ways of living to help them adapt and accept their situation. Their stories teach me, humble me, motivate me, and help me question my perspective so I can live a more productive life.

By no means am I always positive. I do my share of moaning and groaning and yelling at times. Some days are harder than others to cope, but I believe these are the days I am being tested the most, so I view them as an opportunity to learn more about myself. I want to find as much meaning as I can and I want that just as much for you. Changing our inner and outer dialogue about dystonia can do wonders for our emotional well being and helps us remain hopeful in the present moment and about our future.

Some people are not at this point yet, and there was a time I would never have been able to even conceive of anything positive about dystonia. In time, starting with one minute a day, my mindset has changed. While I have lost certain things in my life as a result of dystonia, I have also gained many things. This reminds me of the quote by Robin Williams in the movie *Patch Adams* (1998) where, after losing the love of his life, he said, "I've lost everything. But I've also gained everything." He didn't let the death of his beloved stop him from passionately pursuing his dream to become a doctor. It made him even more passionate. In his loss he learned more about the power of his life and those around him, all of whom made a significant impact on each other.

We are far luckier in so many ways than people who never lived with dystonia or other challenging condition. The things we endure have made us stronger. A reason why you may not see it yet is because you are angry about the symptoms that plague you, as well as the inability to as of yet, appropriately cope with the changes in your life. This is okay and to be expected. It will come if you open yourself up to it. Focusing on how to peacefully cohabitate with dystonia versus angrily listing all the ways it has ruined your life is the way to find happiness. To further illustrate this point, I want to share a poem a friend of mine with dystonia wrote a few years ago:

> *How would you know to experience the true pleasures*
> *of life if you've never experienced the pain?*
> *Sorrow and suffering of any kind, in time, reveals an*
> *exquisite beauty; a secret that is meant to be found.*
> *Life is worth living.*
> *When you learn to embrace the pain and accept what is,*
> *THAT is when life will begin.*
> *Just when you think you can't take it anymore,*
> *When you are ready to give up...don't!*
> *That is when the change is about to arrive.*
> *If you feel your life has fallen apart, rebuild from the ground up.*
> *That is the beauty in being broken.*

I don't think she meant that we are broken, although when she wrote this she may have felt broken, as I am sure many of us have at times. My take is that many of us live life not appreciating our health, among other things, until it is gone. When we feel pain and other noxious symptoms that lessen our ability to do many of the things we once enjoyed, it reminds us how nothing should be taken for granted and to live life to the fullest all the time. When I feel particularly unwell or "broken", the words of this poem help me better enjoy the good days and cope better on the not so good days. Each rough day provides me time to reflect and an opportunity to rise up a stronger person.

The most compelling part of this poem for me is when she says, "When you are ready to give up…don't! That is when the change is about to arrive." This couldn't be truer. The less we fight and embrace what is, opening ourselves up to all possibilities, the better chance our lives will be transformed for the better. We can always rebuild no matter how much things have "fallen apart." The pieces may not go where they once did, but that is okay. You have to know that it is okay. Things may not be how you want them to be, but to be happy you have to make adjustments and find new things in your life that fit in with the new you.

Although your life may have changed dramatically as a result of dystonia and is certainly not what you planned for yourself, you can set a new intention for your life that can be just as joyful and fulfilling. Everything in life is determined by how we think about things so if we change the way we look at things, the things we look at change. As Zig Ziglar said, "You cannot tailor make your situation in life, but you can tailor make your attitudes in those situations."

Are we more or less of a person because of dystonia?
Dystonia reminds me of the bully that picks on kids in the schoolyard every day. Like the bully, dystonia does not follow any rules and after multiple beatings, we can lose our sense of self and feelings of pride. It is not uncommon to then feel weak and not as worthy as others or as worthy as we once were.

In many ways, I think we are stronger than we were before dystonia. Dystonia has probably been one of the greatest challenges of your life, as it has mine. It takes a special person to handle all we do, having to overcome obstacles and persevere every day. If we continue to get up every morning and make a life for ourselves to the best of our ability given our circumstances, we are doing far more than we often give ourselves credit.

People often tell me that they feel that they have not accomplished anything since dystonia started; that they feel like they are "not enough." This is an inaccurate and harmful perspective. Is it not an accomplishment to carry on with life and still seek happiness when dealing with chronic pain and other symptoms? I bet you seek it and value it more now than you once did. The mental strength it takes to persevere in the face of adversity is far more an accomplishment than living a life with few obstacles, or obstacles that are easily overcome, as many were before life with dystonia.

"When the Japanese mend broken objects, they aggrandize the damage by filling the cracks with gold. They believe that when something's suffered damage and has a history, it becomes more beautiful." - Billie Mobayed

The gold is not meant to fix us. It is meant to add a new dimension to our being, much like when we are forced, by change or circumstance, to create a life in the "new normal." By doing so, our understanding is broadened and deepened and we become more beautiful.

It is vital to our mental well being to put in perspective life now versus life before dystonia. With dystonia we have new challenges on top of existing challenges. Being able to endure not only makes us plenty worthy, but an inspiration. Acknowledge your ability to keep living as fulfilling a life as possible. It is an indication of your strong character.

What seems nasty, painful, or evil can become a source of
beauty, joy and strength if faced with an open mind.
Every moment is a golden one for him who has the vision to recognize it as such.
- Henry Miller -

Post Traumatic Growth[12-15]
We often hear the term Post Traumatic Stress Disorder (PTSD), a mental health condition triggered by a traumatic event. PTSD is commonly used in context of military personnel returning from active duty, but it applies to anyone who has faced traumatic events such as sexual or physical assault, an acute or chronic health condition, natural disasters, the unexpected death of a loved one, or an accident. Families of victims can also develop PTSD, as can emergency personnel and rescue workers. Symptoms may include flashbacks, nightmares, and severe anxiety, as well as uncontrollable thoughts about the event.

Most people who experience a traumatic event will have reactions that may include shock, anger, nervousness, fear, and even guilt. These reactions are common and for most people, go away over time. For a person with PTSD, however, feelings of intense fear, helplessness, or horror continue and may even increase, becoming so strong that they keep the person from living a normal life. Some people with dystonia experience PTSD.

A term we hear far less about, if at all, is called Post Traumatic Growth (PTG). PTG refers to people who become stronger and create a more meaningful life in the wake of tragedy or trauma. They don't just bounce back, which is resilience; they bounce higher than they ever did before.

This concept is not new. For centuries people believed that suffering and distress can yield positive changes. It wasn't until 1995 that the term Post Traumatic Growth was coined by Richard Tedeschi, Ph.D., and Lawrence Calhoun, Ph.D., psychologists at the University of North Carolina, Charlotte.

PTG is characterized by people changing their views of themselves, such as an increased sense of strength; "If I lived through that, I can face anything." They tend to show more gratitude and have greater acceptance of their vulnerabilities and limitations, and also develop a sense that new opportunities have emerged from their struggle. Relationships are enhanced; people come to value their friends and family more, feel an increased sense of compassion for others and a longing for more intimate relationships. They can also experience an increased sense of connection to others who suffer. They gain a greater appreciation for life in general, finding a fresh, positive outlook each day; they re-evaluate what really matters in life, become less materialistic, and are better able to live in the present. Another common feature is a change or deepening in spiritual beliefs.

I was never diagnosed with PTSD, but I lived through periods of intense fear, anger, desperation, and hopelessness after experiencing a dramatic shift in my life due to dystonia. Having worked through a lot of these emotions over the years, I have seen a significant amount of growth. For example, I appreciate many things I once took for granted. I realize how fragile life is and how it should be honored by treating ourselves and others with love and respect. I have a much deeper appreciation for people who struggle with life challenges. I have come to better understand the meaning of loss which has increased my ability to live in gratitude. I have also found greater meaning to my life and feel a deeper spiritual connection.

Dystonia and any other life challenge can truly be a source of growth for all of us in ways we probably never imagined, and research has shown that in the face of great challenges, significant human and spiritual growth can occur. In order for it to take place, it is crucial that we are open to the possibilities that lie within our "misfortune." We must abandon hatred and anger, for it will only worsen the pain we feel, preventing us from any kind of growth. Every experience in life is a gift. Something is to be learned from everything to help catapult us to a higher level of being.

You matter!

Most of us our own worst enemy and have a knack for beating ourselves up way too often. We tend to forget or ignore just how much we matter. There are people who think about us every day, often unbeknownst to us. Why? Because we are valuable and have a light inside that touches them. Just like 'Clarence' said to 'George Bailey' in the movie, *It's a Wonderful Life* (1946), "Strange, isn't it? Each man's life touches so many other lives. When he isn't around he leaves an awful hole, doesn't he?" We are no different.

A pencil maker told the pencil five important lessons just before putting it in the box:
1) Everything you do will leave a mark.
2) You can always correct the mistakes you made.
3) What is important is what is inside you.
4) You will undergo painful sharpenings which will only make you better.
5) To be the best pencil, you must allow yourself to be held and guided by the hand that holds you.

This story should remind you that you are a special person with unique talents and abilities. Only you can fulfill the purpose for which you were born. Never allow yourself to think that your life is insignificant and cannot be changed. Like the pencil, always remember that the most important part of who you are is what's inside of you.

The Cracked Pot

A water bearer in China had two large pots, each hung on the ends of a pole which he carried across his neck. One of the pots had a crack in it, while the other pot was perfect and always delivered a full portion of water. At the end of the long walk from the stream to the house, the cracked pot arrived only half full. For a full two years this went on daily, with the bearer delivering only one and a half pots full of water to his house. Of course, the perfect pot was proud of its accomplishments, perfect for which it was made. The cracked pot was ashamed of its imperfection and miserable that it was only able to accomplish half of what it had been made to do. After 2 years of what it perceived to be a bitter failure, it spoke to the water bearer one day by the stream. "I am ashamed of myself because this crack in my side causes water to leak all the way back to your house."

The bearer said to the pot, "Did you notice that there are flowers on your side of the path, but not on the other pot's side? That's because I have always known about your flaw and I planted flower seeds on your side of the path. Every day while we walk back, you've watered them. For two years I have been able to pick these beautiful flowers to decorate the table. Without you being just the way you are, there would not be this beauty to grace the house."

Testimonial

I was diagnosed with cervical dystonia in November 2002 after a lengthy journey of frequenting medical establishments in a vain effort to find "what was really wrong?" My neck, back, and body were very twisted. My fight with dystonia was compounded with the onset of depression which turned my world upside down. Up until 2002, I was a very active person, employed full time, and studying part time pursuing a career as an accountant. I was married and a mother of two robust teenage boys. By all accounts I led a fantastic life of no problems.

My journey was possibly not a lot different from the average person, as I visited every possible person who was prepared to listen to my concerns. I trusted that they had that "quick fix" and I would be well again very soon. I was in denial.

The "hop on and hop off" journey of doctors, specialists, chiropractors, physiotherapists, Botox, Valium, searching the internet for answers, exercise, dietary changes, tears, screams, yells, and pity parties was ongoing for another 5 years. I did really have to reach the bottom of the barrel to really change. Exhausting? You bet!

If somebody could do it, I knew I was that someone. One of my fondest enjoyments is research and study. To find answers I knew that I had to start self educating. Making the decision to change saw me enroll as a student of the Spasmodic Torticollis Recovery Clinic. Upon receiving the literature I knew I was now moving in the right direction. I am a natural girl and personally knew the body does heal when given the right ingredients. I started the program January 4, 2008. True to form, I have not missed a day of using the program since.

If my dystonia was going to change then I had to change. Lifestyle reprogramming for me included exercise, nutrition, massage, acupuncture, and prayer. I love to exercise. I love to nourish my body with whole foods (hunter gatherer nutritional habits- the paleo eating lifestyle). I love my daily massages. I love my regular acupuncture treatments to keep the good energy flowing. I love to pray and through all things give thanks. I totally love that girl I see in the mirror and my body continues to get straighter and straighter second by second.

148

Feeling tremendous, I continued my studies and qualified as a personal trainer and Pilates instructor. Initially this was just to self-educate again. I am now a much stronger person at 53 years. I own a full time health and fitness business. I love life and there is never a day lost that I don't give thanks for my friend "Spasmodic Torticollis." I continue to grow. Every day is a gift. That is why we are blessed by the present.

For me, no one knows why and how this journey began. I was prone to fainting and encountered several falls. I was very insecure and doubted myself. I don't question the why's as I can now say "because..." that was yesterday. Living in the now is me. My advice to others on the journey; never say never. When you truly believe, you will achieve and receive every benefit possible. Impossible actually does say I M Possible.

References
1) www.mercola.com, Retrieved January 30, 2014 from: http://articles.mercola.com/sites/articles/archive/2014/01/30/eft-mapping-emotions.aspx?e_cid=20140130Z1_DNL_art_1&utm_source=dnl&utm_medium=email&utm_content=art1&utm_campaign=20140130Z1&et_cid=66919168&et_rid=413180808
2) Retrieved on February 25, 2014 from: http://www.pnas.org/content/early/2013/12/26/1321664111
3) www.usnews.com, Retrieved January 30, 2014 from: http://www.usnews.com/news/articles/2013/12/30/study-finds-emotions-can-be-mapped-to-the-body
4) Totten, Mindy. 2014. Retrieved on June 17, 2014 from: www.MindyTotten.com
5) Retrieved on February 25, 2014 from: http://www.huffingtonpost.com/dr-carmen-harra/affirmations_b_3527028.html
6) Retrieved on February 25, 2014 from: http://www.vitalaffirmations.com/
7) Retrieved on February 25, 2014 from: http://www.wikihow.com/Use-Affirmations-Effectively
8) Retrieved on February 25, 2014 from: http://www.mindtools.com/pages/article/affirmations.htm
9) Retrieved on February 25, 2014 from: http://www.healyourlifetraining.com/affirmations/positive-affirmations-for-health
10) Quinlan, K. Mindfulness for OCD and Anxiety, Retrieved June 30, 2014 from: http://www.ocdla.com/blog/mindfulness-ocd-anxiety-1920
11) Kabat-Zinn, J. Full Catastrophe Living. (1990). New York, NY: Delta
12) www.ptgi.uncc.edu, Retrieved August 23, 2014 from: https://ptgi.uncc.edu/what-is-ptg/
13) Stephen, J. What Doesn't Kill Us: The new psychology of posttraumatic growth, Retrieved on August 23, 2014 from: http://www.psychologytoday.com/blog/what-doesnt-kill-us/201402/posttraumatic-growth
14) www.livehappy.com, Retrieved August 23, 2014 from: http://www.livehappy.com/science/positive-psychology/science-post-traumatic-growth
15) www.webmd.com, Retrieved August 23, 2014 from: http://www.webmd.com/anxiety-panic/guide/post-traumatic-stress-disorder

Chapter 13
Daily Living

Life with dystonia can be a scary and lonely place. Fitting in, being understood by others, talking about our condition, finding support, doctor visits, and balancing family, work, and social life can be a challenge. The daily grind can be such that we become depressed and isolated, as many of us feel out of place in the world. This chapter provides strategies for how to deal with these challenges. Topics are in no particular order, so jump around to those that interest you.

Staying in the lead

Dystonia is an insidious disorder that can rear its ugly head at any time, day or night. Therefore, it is very helpful to stay one step ahead of our symptoms before they get out of control or further out of control. This is where listening to our body and knowing our triggers becomes so important so we don't shock our already alarmed neurological system. I call it "staying in the lead."

Whenever I have something to do that I know is going to put excess wear and tear on my body, I prepare myself ahead of time so I don't add extra stress prior to the event or activity. For example, when I have to make my three hour trip to the doctor, I will do as much as I can the night before so all I have to do is get up and eat. I will shower, shave, and lay out my clothes, and pack whatever I need for the trip (snacks, paperwork for the doctor, a book to read, trigger point tools, medications).

I wake up at least an hour earlier than normal which allows me time to put heat on my neck and back and do some stretching. It also gives my medication time to kick in so I am at my best once I hit the road. These things may seem minor, but they make a huge difference in how I feel physically. Not having to rush around keeps my body at ease and decreases stress, which helps me better manage my symptoms.

I do similar things to prepare myself for other activities. If I have plans to go to dinner or a ball game, for example, I take time to rest before having to sit in a potentially uncomfortable chair and be in a noisy environment. Before I go I will lie down and do some focused breathing and/or some stretching. Sometimes I will just lay there and read a book or watch television. All of this calms my mind and muscles so when it is time to hop in the car and go, my body is at maximum preparedness for whatever lies ahead of me.

It may sound silly to have to do all this, but this is life with dystonia for lot of us. There are many of you who are unable to go out to dinner, a movie, a concert, a play, etc. I know how frustrating this can be, as there were many years when I was unable to also. Now that I feel better and can do more, I am so grateful that I am more than happy to spend time preparing myself before hand to make it easier on my body. I also factor in recovery time. The mental and physical toll of certain activities sometimes results in more pain, spasms and fatigue, so I plan time to rest afterwards.

Sometimes the increase in symptoms when I do certain things is because I mentally set myself up to expect pain, tightness, spasms, and fatigue because that was my pattern for so many years. Perhaps you do the same. Understanding my pattern, I try to be mindful of my current thoughts and past experiences. I ask myself how true my beliefs really are because there are times when I do certain activities with ease; usually when I don't over think things and let my brain get in the way. One way I make myself more mindful is with an acronym for PAIN: Pay Attention Inward Now. I not only use this for pain, but for any imbalance I might be feeling. It helps me focus on what is bothering me and why I may be apprehensive about doing something. When I can determine what it is, I can let it go and enjoy an activity with more comfort.

Fear
Fear is probably the single most damaging, debilitating, detrimental energy we have. It interferes with our healing process and our well-being in every area of our life. We cannot thrive when we are controlled by fear because fear stresses our immune system and clouds our thinking. Facing fears may feel uncomfortable, but taking action allows the body to release the tension it has built up. Conquering fear could be the saving grace to our mental and physical health. One of my favorite acronyms for FEAR is, "Face Everything and Rise." Sadly, for too long I was afraid to face my dystonia so I followed a different acronym for FEAR; "Forget Everything and Run." This approach didn't help matters at all.

I am reminded of the movie, *We Bought a Zoo* (2011), with Matt Damon. Damon's character, 'Benjamin Mee', is having a conversation with his son about fear and courage. It was in the context of how he first met his wife, but it applies to anything in life where we have fear or apprehension. Damon's character said, "Sometimes all you need is twenty seconds of insane courage. Just literally twenty seconds of just embarrassing bravery, and I promise you, something great will come of it." He's right. Feel the fear, whatever it is, and do it anyway. It will quickly dissipate, allowing us to move forward with confidence. Bravery is not being without fear. Bravery is having fear and walking through it.

A student once asked his old yogi master how he maintained such peace of mind and physical well-being. "Oh, my son", the yogi smiled, "you only see the outside of my life. Inside my mind it is as if two powerful dogs are always waging war with each other." "Wow," said the student. "What do the dogs fight about?" The Yogi answered, "One is always leading me to a better life; good health, strong energy, creativity, wonderful relationships, and constant joy and peace. The other is always leading me away from that wonderful place, to a horrible place that is its opposite. He has only one method, but it is a very powerful one. He leads me to fear. Once I am afraid, I cannot move. I am stuck and I can only spend my energy worrying and being upset, or trying to prevent what I am afraid of. This dog causes me much suffering." "Tell me, Master, which dog most often wins?" The yogi sighed, paused, then smiled and replied, "Whichever one I feed."

Too many of us complicate our lives by feeding the wrong dog, preventing us from living a fulfilling life because we are afraid. Be assertive and push through fear so you live on your terms. If you miss somebody, call; if you want to see somebody, invite; if you want to be understood, explain. If you have questions, ask; if you don't like something, say it; if you like something, state it. If you want something, ask for it. Live your life no matter what obstacles stand in your way.

To show or not to show symptoms

Looking and feeling different is common with dystonia because, quite frankly, many of us do look different. A twisted or turned neck in spasm, as in the case of cervical dystonia, is not a common thing to see in public. Many people go to great lengths to try and hide their symptoms by assuming certain postures or wearing certain clothing to cover it up. This is understandable because it can be embarrassing, but I think it is best to show our symptoms. We have to find comfort in our discomfort and accept ourselves for who we are. When we do that, others will respond in kind. If we embrace who we are no matter our differences, the world will accept us as well. This goes for anything in life.

Also, when we posture to hide our symptoms or when we cover them up with clothing, it tells our brain that something is wrong with us. This may prevent our bodies from healing and learning how to relax.

I think it is more challenging and stressful to hide our symptoms versus just letting our body move the way it wants. You may feel better when you hide your symptoms, but it requires so much effort that it can burden us mentally. Instead of worrying if people can see your dystonia, you might now worry if you are hiding it well enough. Accepting it and letting it be might be a better choice so we can focus our attention on more important things. Also, the more we hide our symptoms, the less likely people will understand what dystonia is all about. Awareness is our ally. On the flip side, since we are all different and have to live the way that suits us best, if hiding your symptoms eases your mind, by all means do what is best for you.

For years there was no way I could hide my symptoms because they were so obvious. People looked at me all the time and I became very self conscious. Many thought I was in a bad car accident. Over time I learned to accept the stares. I had to if I wanted to reduce my social anxiety. I also saw it as opportunity to teach others about dystonia.

Instead of thinking I was a freak, I met all stares with a smile. This made me much more comfortable around others and able to engage the world with less apprehension. It also made others more comfortable because my smile and personality humanized my condition. It also helps to remember that we will never again see most people we encounter on a daily basis, so why care so much in the first place?

For the most part, people are more compassionate than we often give them credit. We just need to do a better job letting them in. Some will judge us no matter who we are or how we look, but the vast majority see past our symptoms and accept us for the person we are inside. We just need to show them that person. Our mental health is greatly improved when we can accept ourselves as we are. Others will follow suit and those who don't are not worth our time. As Dr. Seuss said, "Those who mind don't matter and those who matter don't mind."

Talking about dystonia
Since it is difficult to understand dystonia, I talk about it with as many people as possible. The more people I tell, the more awareness there is and the greater chance I will be better understood. Talking about dystonia also helps eliminate the stigma associated with chronic conditions and it makes me feel less anxious and self conscious, especially in public.

There are times I can sense that someone is uncomfortable and wants to say something, but doesn't know what to say or how to say it. In these cases, I try to break the ice with a brief comment, which is typically a light hearted joke about my particular symptoms at the moment. Whether or not this leads to talking more about dystonia, at the very least it helps reduce the discomfort that I or others might be feeling. Talking about it also provides an opportunity to help someone else with dystonia who may not know they have it. This has happened to me several times. After bringing it up in conversations, some people have literally said, "That sounds like what my friend has! I need to tell him/her about this. Thank you so much for telling me."

This is partly how I found out that I had dystonia. Early on, before I was officially diagnosed, my Mom was talking to her friend about me at a party. She said, "It sounds like he has what my husband Fred has." My Mom called me that night in jubilation. It was the first time we felt any hope. Fred and I spoke on the phone the next day. Having lived with dystonia most of his adult life, he was able to answer many questions no one else was able to, helping to put together puzzle pieces about my condition. Fred provided me with hope and friendship during that very frightening time in my life, a relationship that started from a random conversation where I wasn't even present.

Considering how unaware the public is about dystonia, not to mention the many people who are undiagnosed and misdiagnosed, I see it as a responsibility to tell people about it. How is dystonia going to get more exposure if we who have it remain silent? We live with a condition that is not as well known as conditions that affect fewer people. We need to speak up and play a part in dystonia becoming a household name by telling people about it, both friends and strangers. It matters to those of us living with dystonia to keep talking and answering all the puzzled expressions.

About 10 years ago I walked into a convenience store and the girl behind the counter turned her neck to mimic how mine looked. I was taken aback at first and realized that while it was rude, she didn't mean any harm. She thought I was doing it on purpose. Instead of getting upset, I smiled and told her what was wrong. She apologized for mocking me and we had a nice conversation about dystonia.

This particular encounter made me realize that every situation gives me the opportunity to teach others about dystonia. It also made me realize that everyone responds to us differently and what matters most is how we respond to them. I could have gotten angry, but I looked at it as an opportunity to talk to her. It made me more comfortable, gave me confidence, and better prepared me for future interactions.

Taking advantage of these opportunities helps us educate others and at the same time, reduce our anxiety about dystonia. Give people a chance to show their compassion by letting them in. Smile. Say hello. Engage them in some way. All of this is part of the process of accepting our condition. When we are comfortable looking or feeling different our social phobias diminish.

While I encourage people to talk about dystonia, I understand that there are times when we do not want to talk about it, we can't find the right words, or we simply don't have the energy. This is okay. We all travel this path our own way and need to do what feels right to us.

Testimonial

I used to feel funny around people I know and talking too much about my dystonia because they always told me they never saw any odd movements and I never looked any different to them. I was nervous about them seeing me "posturing" because when I did it was extreme. I've always taken care of the way I dress and look, and being a woman I guess I cared too much about how people viewed me.

I've heard about people who had friends desert them when they got dystonia. Thankfully, the response has been very different for me. People have been very compassionate, loving, and encouraging. I've been even more vocal about it and they want to know about it. I have learned that what really matters is that I am still the same person I always was on the inside and I am loved because I'm me. My friends still want to get together with me and it hasn't made any difference whatsoever. I do not believe I would ever lose a friend because of dystonia. If I did, they would not have been a friend to begin with.

Telling others about dystonia not only breaks the ice, but it helps me see that people really do care and are compassionate. I feel better after telling people what is going on because it makes me more comfortable to just be me. Otherwise, they'd probably look at me funny and it would make me feel worse. The reason people stare is they do not understand what is going on. Once they know about it, most are caring and compassionate. I feel like they understand. Talking about it has helped me to not be as nervous and afraid of being around other people.

It has also given me more confidence and helps me to know it is okay if I posture in front of people. People will often ask me questions which I'm very glad to answer. My friends still want to get together and socialize. That makes me feel good because I know I really mean something to them. I am now able to joke about my dystonia and laugh with friends. It makes them a lot more at ease around me and me around them. It's good to be able to laugh about ourselves and not go around with chips on our shoulders. As I've gotten more used to it, I've actually been less stressed and more relaxed.

Testimonial

I started my journey with cervical dystonia just over 4 years ago when I was 62 years old and planning retirement from my job as a hospital discharge planning nurse. Although my symptoms were fairly mild to begin with, it affected my life in a major way and drastically upended my retirement plans.

When my head first started turning to the left, I could use my other neck muscles to stop it. Now it turns whenever I am doing any kind of activity and I can't stop it. When I am sitting, I can partially stop my head from turning with my hand, which becomes tiring, but helps me concentrate on whatever I'm doing. Friends have asked why I don't just let my head turn. Needless to say, it's very difficult to have a conversation, read the paper, watch TV, attend a concert or play, or do anything for that matter when your head is turning. When I am lying down it is a relief to rest my head, but my head still turns, which makes sleeping a challenge.

From the initial onset, it has affected how I socialize with my family and friends because of the anxiety caused by the fact that I have no control over these muscles contracting and therefore, my head turning. It became increasingly harder to relax and enjoy family and friend's company, with my attention focused on trying to stop my head from turning while trying to be part of a conversation.

Along with the anxiety came an erosion of self-confidence. It is very unnerving to not be able to look at someone when you are talking to them. I have always been a fairly social and active person, and enjoyed doing many activities, such as singing in a choir and belonging to a cycling group. That has now changed. I find it difficult to be around groups of people I don't know.

One of the ironies of dystonia is that I feel like I am fairly physically fit – I can swim 36 lengths at the pool, walk pretty vigorously, and recently dug fence post holes with an auger – yet I am exhausted every day by noon no matter what I have done in the morning. My theory for the cause of the exhaustion is that I am constantly trying to counteract the pulling of my neck muscles. It is exhaustion like nothing I have ever felt.

I am trying to live as normal a life as possible within my limits. All the physical activities that I do are scaled a long way down from what I used to be able to do (except for swimming), but I will keep persevering. I have started to cycle short distances and at times get that wonderful feeling of freedom on my bike again. I am also doing the stretches from the ST Recovery Clinic to keep my muscles strong and supple on both sides of my body.

Although I do get totally frustrated because I'm not able to do all the things I would like, there have been some positives. I have gained some knowledge about how to live my life one day at a time and enjoy the small things that I once took for granted. I appreciate my husband, my family, and friends – time spent with them, appreciating them for who they are, and the support they all give me. My 2 sons, my daughters-in-law, and my 7 grandchildren are all amazing and I love to spend time with them.

Some days I feel like I can conquer this condition and other days it conquers me. So, I will continue on this road, by focusing on the things that are most important to me, being as active as I can and trying to be positive about life!

Being understood

Living with chronic pain and unrelenting muscle spasms is exhausting. Not only are we physically and mentally tired from battling our symptoms all day, we are tired of making excuses and explaining why we cannot join in activities; recreational, social, work, or otherwise. While it is not possible for someone without dystonia to truly understand how we feel, it is nice to know that they have some idea or at least make us feel that they do. They may not understand what it is like, but acknowledging our challenges goes a long way. It makes us feel less alone.

Everyone in my life tries to understand, but no one knows what I really went through when my symptoms were severe or what I still go through today. I believe there is an assumption that because I am much healthier and look much healthier, I am problem free. Some people even think I am cured. For years people saw the pain I was in because of my distorted body postures. Now that it is not as visible, some people think I am free of dystonia. While I am much better, I am not without challenges.

Regardless of the severity of my physical symptoms, the depths of despair and loneliness I experienced, and still sometimes experience, is something most people don't really understand no matter how much I talk about it. These symptoms have been far more significant than anything physical I ever went through. My entire world dramatically changed when dystonia hopped on board, something not often appreciated by others. This is not surprising, nor bothersome to me, as it often takes going through something to understand and be empathetic.

The one thing most people close to me have come to understand over the years is that they don't understand. What they do understand and accept is that I have limitations and there are times when dystonia gets the better of me and I need to take time to care for myself. This understanding helps me tremendously. Being open with them about my symptoms has helped a lot.

What I hope they also understand is how much my limitations upset me because it hurts to not be involved in everything going on, especially when I was able to do anything before dystonia. I have created a new life for myself, but sometimes I really miss parts of the old me. There was a dramatic shift in my life when dystonia arrived, some of which I am still processing. I put on a good face, often not revealing how rough it sometimes is.

I am much better at accepting the fact that life has changed and I may never again be able to do some of the things I used to before dystonia, but the daily grind is what is most difficult. Dystonia itself is utterly exhausting, both physically and mentally, and then certain activities, or sometimes just sleeping wrong or sitting in poor posture for a period of time, can ramp up symptoms even more, putting me out of commission. Many people do not understand this reality. Not knowing from day to day how functional I will be is very distressing. This is my biggest challenge because I am constantly living with symptoms that remind me how much my life has changed.

Even though I have done well to accept the changes, I still get depressed and discouraged from time to time. I also get envious of people who are able bodied and can do whatever they want whenever they want. That used to be me. Learning to live with the new me who no longer plays golf, tennis, baseball, basketball, racquetball, soccer, karate, runs, bikes, swims, boats, hikes, or travels has been quite an adjustment to say the least, even after all these years. Some people become distressed when they have an acute injury or illness that sidelines them from a favorite activity or hobby for only a few days or weeks. Imagine if a few weeks turned into a few years or even a lifetime. This is how it is for many of us with chronic health conditions.

I know that my life with dystonia, particularly the mental side, is very hard to understand, so I don't expect people to get it. I also don't want anyone to feel sorry for me. Everyone has something challenging to deal with in their life. What would be helpful, and this goes for every single person alive today, is if we asked each other more often how we are feeling and how we are managing with everything going on in our lives. This form of acknowledgement reminds us that we are not alone and that we matter.

What saddens me most is that my nieces and nephews never really knew me before dystonia entered my life. They were too young. While we had a lot of fun times that I remember fondly, for them, most of it is overshadowed by years of pain and infirmity. Except for the oldest who remembers a little, none of them knew the fun, happy go lucky Uncle Tom who took an active part in everything they did when I was around. I still have a poem my oldest niece wrote for me when she was 11, a few months after I was diagnosed.

Sugar and spice, my Uncle Tom is nice,
He has a bad neck, but oh what the heck,
It makes me sad to see him feel so bad,
I hope he gets well fast and the pain won't last,
And then we can play with him all day!!

June 2002

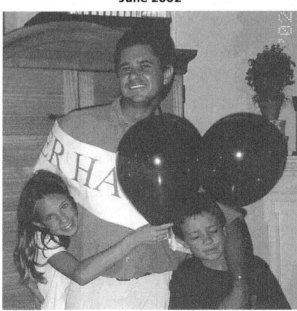

Before dystonia, playing with my nieces and nephews is what I looked forward to most when I visited my family. They would meet me at the door filled with excitement because we had so much fun together. They squeezed me so hard when we hugged. I miss that person and they don't remember that person. They were only 11, 8, 6, and 3 years old when I was diagnosed. My smile in the above picture at my nephew's birthday party very much overshadows my pain, but I still wanted to be involved in things as much as possible. I fought hard to keep up, but not long after this picture was taken, dystonia beat me to the ground. I became isolated with pain and depression for the next five years. I think I had to go through a lot of that to process how significantly dystonia had changed my life. It also taught me how to make better lifestyle choices to help manage my symptoms, both physical and mental.

I once had a conversation with my father about what I can and cannot do (or choose not to do). He invited me to a baseball game at the local college. I told him how much I would like to go, but wasn't feeling up to it. I knew it would be a significant challenge that particular day and my body would pay for it later. Recalling a longer trip I made a month prior to see friends and watch a baseball game, he said, "It seems if you can go that far to see friends and watch a game, you should be able to go to something local." He didn't say it in an accusatory or confrontational manner. He was just making an observation.

Logically speaking, he was absolutely right. However, dystonia is not logical. It brings unexpected challenges every day. I was different the day I went to the other game. I have been different every day since; some good days and some bad days. The day I went to the other game, I was feeling much better and I also did a lot of preparing before going so my body was ready to handle it better. However, it took a few days to recover from everything I did; recover meaning feeling the way I did prior to the trip. My Dad was unaware of all this until I told him. Now that he knows, he understands me better which makes me feel less alone.

Like my father once did, many people don't understand that what may seem easy to do one day may be difficult to do another day. This is simply the nature of dystonia. Pain, fatigue, and spasms all ebb and flow from hour to hour, day to day, and week to week for a lot of us. It is unpredictable, making it very hard to make plans or do things on a whim. Today I may be able to comfortably, or uncomfortably but tolerably, do something like run a few errands, go out to dinner, a show, or a ball game, while the day before or day after, my symptoms are such that I may spend most of my time lying down, not in shape to leave the house. Never really knowing how you will feel is a very frustrating way to live.

Perhaps it would be easier if we change how we think about others and their ability to understand. Dystonia is a mysterious condition so we would do well to embrace the fact that the best understanding we may ever have is that we will never be fully understood. I'm sure you can attest to the fact that not even people with dystonia sometimes understand your specific situation. We can certainly relate much better, but our realities are different. Yes, we understand the pain, the loss of things in our life, emotional issues, anxiety, sorrow, etc., but how we process these things and how they affect our lives and those around us is unique. While we have the same diagnosis, many of our experiences living with dystonia are different.

This is not to say that we are alone. What this means is that there is no way to be fully understood by anyone so we should eliminate this expectation. We only know what we know from what we have experienced, so to expect someone else to "get it" is probably unrealistic. We can get empathy from others, but a complete understanding is out of reach and something we have to live with. This being the case, embrace that you may not get the understanding you desire so you don't beat yourself up over something which you have little to no control.

Describing to others what dystonia feels like
While I would never wish dystonia on anyone, I sometimes wish people could jump into my body for an hour to experience how it feels. It would certainly make explaining it much easier. Since we all experience dystonia in different ways, we have to describe it in different ways.

The best way I found to describe how my neck and back feel is to have people flex their bicep muscle. At the same time they are flexing their bicep, I tell them to try and extend/straighten their arm. Extending your arm while you are flexing/contracting your bicep is impossible to do because it has to relax to let the tricep contract and extend your arm. Opposing muscles, like the bicep and tricep, are not designed to contract at the same time. However, this is what is happening with different muscle groups in dystonia.

People's arms are usually tired and even sore after a short while. I then have them imagine how this would feel in their neck and back (or other body part) all the time. This usually gets their attention because it is hard for them to fathom how it would feel after performing this movement with their arm for less than a minute. I then tell them to imagine having no control over their muscles contracting like this. By now, most people have a better idea for how I feel and are able to relate to me in a different way than before. I also compare dystonia to how a charley horse feels, to which most people can relate.

Your dystonia may not feel like mine so find the best way to describe your unique symptoms. Be creative. Have people perform activities that mimic how your body feels. People relate better to things that they experience, like the charley horse analogy.

Hidden symptoms
I invite you to read a wonderful story called "The Spoon Theory" written by Christine Miserandino, a woman with lupus. Christine's website is called, "But you don't look sick" (www.butyoudontlooksick.com). A friend asked her what it felt like to have Lupus and she described it in a very clever way which is very similar to what we experience with dystonia. We could replace dystonia for lupus in the "The Spoon Theory" story and it would parallel many of our lives.

Although her lupus symptoms are noticeable to others, she also has fibromyalgia, Sjogrens Syndrome, and Reynaud's disease, symptoms of which are pretty much invisible to the naked eye. Being the visual creatures that we are, if we don't see something that looks wrong, we assume a person is healthy.

When my Mom had breast cancer over five years ago, if you didn't know it you wouldn't think anything was wrong with her. She looked just as healthy the day before her diagnosis as she did right after her diagnosis. She just had something inside her that no one could see with the naked eye so she appeared to have nothing wrong. Tests proved otherwise and thankfully she was successfully treated and has been cancer free ever since.

For years my symptoms were such that it was obvious that something was wrong. As I improved, my symptoms were not as evident to where you could barely notice them at all. However, just because my body looks better now does not mean that I am dystonia free. A lot of people seem to think that since I often look fine I must feel fine because it is hard to believe something exists when we can't see it. Just because I often look well doesn't mean I am without pain, muscle contractions, dizziness, headaches, fatigue, or anxiety. Granted, everything is far less severe than it once was, but it still exists to varying degrees. On occasion my symptoms will get bad enough where I have to do nothing all day but rest. Most people don't see me when I am like this so their opinion of me is somewhat skewed. When I am having symptoms in public, most people don't notice. I have become so used to them that I am able to appear quite normal, despite often feeling quite uncomfortable.

Testimonial
It's frustrating to feel that I am atypically atypical. Having dystonia is atypical. My doctors said that I'm not even like the atypical. Unlike most cervical dystonia patients, I don't do typical neck tilting postures. To look at me you see nothing. Only if I close my mouth can one see the involuntary pulling on the left side of my mouth. Yet inside it feels as if Arnold Schwarzenegger is squeezing my neck, shoulders, and side with all his might, all the time. While I am grateful to be spared horrified stares, I long for a clear diagnosis. For with no name, my pain feels invisible. How can I find hope for support and relief for something so invisible no one has a name for? In this day and age, how can I have pain so strong to where I've been suicidal be yet unnamed by the medical profession? I know a cure for "typical" dystonia is a long way off. It feels further off in the distance for what I have.

The opinion of others
While I truly believe that people are well intended, their opinions and comments often miss the mark when it comes to what we are experiencing. Some of the common things many of us hear include:

"It's all in your head."
"You're just having a bad day."
"Everybody gets tired."
"You're just depressed."
"You'll just have to tough it out."
"If you would just get out more."
"There are people worse off than you."
"It can't be that bad."
"If you would just exercise more."

Most of these comments come across to us as indifference, but they are not meant to hurt us. They just do because each statement feels like a judgment not based in reality. While we value the opinions of people in our lives, we have to learn to be independent of the opinion of others. Live your life the best way you know how so you are most comfortable, regardless of what others think. Someone's opinion of you does not have to become your reality.

Whether we like it or not, people will judge and have their opinions about us and how we live our lives no matter what we do or don't do. We are the same way. We all have judgments and opinions about everything. It's the nature of being human. It just tends to hurt more when we are struggling each day with a nagging health condition. Being judged on top of our daily struggle is more than we want to deal with.

When symptoms change and we look better or sound more upbeat because we have come to better accept our situation, there is an assumption by some that we are "healed." We may in fact be better, but maybe not the same as we once were. Those who don't understand this might think we are back to our old selves and can do everything we once did. When this does not happen, people can become frustrated and sometimes even belittle us. This is because they wrongfully assume that by now (whatever time frame it is) we should be better or gotten over it already. Every time this happens I am reminded of a scene from the TV show "Friends."

'Rachel' was nearing the end of her pregnancy and was rushed to the hospital by her friend 'Joey' when she wasn't feeling well. 'Ross', the child's father, arrived from work after the incident was over. 'Ross' was told the following by the doctor, to which 'Rachel' responded with what is not only funny, but similar to what I feel and want to say to people sometimes.

Doctor: She's fine. She was experiencing Braxton-Hicks contractions; mild discomfort caused by contractions in the uterine wall.
Rachel (to the doctor): Hmmm. Mild discomfort? So, I take it you've had one of these Braxton thingies?
Ross: It's no big deal. Most women don't even feel them.
Rachel (to Ross): No uterus, no opinion!

This is how I sometimes feel about dystonia. No dystonia, no opinion; no loss of physical abilities, no opinion; no involuntary pulling, twisting, turning, trouble with balance, walking, writing, seeing, talking, eating, taking a shower, brushing your hair, doing laundry, no opinion; no chronic pain, no opinion; not taking strong medications with bizarre side effects, no opinion; no way of making money because you can't work, no opinion; nothing standing in your way of your plans and dreams that were ripped from under you, no opinion; not able to make plans because you don't know if your symptoms will kick into high gear and knock you to your knees, no opinion. Lack of confidence and self efficacy for fear your body will not be able to withstand the demands of an activity, no opinion.

I know this sounds harsh and a bit melodramatic, but there are times when many of us feel exactly like this. In all honesty, I do value the opinion of others. I do not dismiss what they say because they sometimes have a helpful perspective I may not have thought about. It is important to distinguish between helpful insights and judgmental opinions.

Finding relief should be your number one priority, or at least at the very top of your list; not pleasing others. Family, friends, and co-workers should respect you for this. I doubt any of them would like to be in your shoes. Put yourself in a position of power and don't accept labels that may be put upon you such as lazy, mental, apathetic, sympathy seeking, hypochondriac, or any other thoughtless title sometimes associated with a chronic condition. Be careful to not label yourself either. Wear your challenges as armor. Not as shackles.

Pace yourself and let others know that you might need to take a break once in a while or that it might take a little longer for you to do something. Ask for their patience, but more important, be patient with yourself. Take responsibility for your condition in order to make the best decisions for yourself. This is your life. Own it and live it how you choose, independent of what others think.

Life is deep and simple. What our society gives us is shallow and complicated.
Be a first rate version of yourself. Not a second rate version of someone else.

Suggestions from others

Living with a chronic health condition that dramatically alters one's life can be very confusing, scary, and lonely. I lived in this mental misery for several years when my dystonia was severe. Pretty much everything I did was ripped from my life when dystonia intervened. I went from an active student, businessman, and athlete to a lump of meat on the floor in too much pain to do anything. Adjusting to life with dystonia was very difficult to say the least. It was the biggest mind bender I ever experienced.

Everyone around me wanted to help. They had all sorts of suggestions about treatments, how I should operate in my social life, people I should contact for support, jobs I might do to make some money since I couldn't work a steady job, and activities to do during the day to take my mind off my symptoms. Except for treatment ideas, I didn't want to hear any of it. I was in too much pain and ashamed at how I looked. I was angry and confused. I just wanted the world to stop. Nothing made sense anymore. I was lost and didn't see the point in doing anything. Some days I thought it would be best if life just ended. Many nights I went to bed hoping I wouldn't wake up. This is partly what led me to drink. It was an escape from my misery.

People were well intentioned when they came to me with ideas and suggestions for how to live a better life, but I felt like they were pushing things on me because anything beyond just existing seemed too much to handle. I viewed many suggestions as an insult because it often seemed that my pain and the adjustment to my dramatic life change were being disregarded. People also didn't seem to take my symptoms and range of abilities into account when they made suggestions. This apparent lack of acknowledgment made me feel more alone and misunderstood.

My position at the time was that if someone didn't have what I did or experienced something similar, they were not in a position to tell me what to do or knew what was best for me. I perceived them as arrogant and self righteous because they appeared as though they knew better without understanding the pain and loss I was experiencing. True or not, I felt like no one understood my situation or accepted me as I was, so I either got very angry or refused to listen. I was constantly in fight or flight mode.

As soon as someone suggested something that I felt was out of reach for me at the moment, anger set in and all I could think about was how quickly I could end the conversation. I had a hard time focusing on anything but the pain in my neck and skull which felt like a penetrating drill. No one seemed to get this, no matter what I said, so I just wanted to be left alone. I needed time to sort out the hell I was experiencing.

Some people became so frustrated when I ignored their suggestions that they left my life. I don't blame them because from their perspective I was a fool for not listening to them and doing things that probably would have helped. What they didn't understand was that I needed time to process what happened to me before I was willing to listen. I had to get over the anger. My life was flipped upside down and I needed to find my bearings. The last thing I wanted to hear was people telling me how to live my life. Ironically, it was the main thing I needed help with. I just wasn't ready to listen. People didn't seem to understand that, so they became frustrated and angry when I was dismissive. It was a vicious circle.

A dramatic shift takes place when someone gets sick with a chronic condition. It takes time to accept and get to a place where we are comfortable doing things. We feel like misfits and are learning to acclimate to our new life. Many of us grieve for a long time for the life that was taken away. Thus, the message we hear behind many suggestions is, "Just get over it already." This disregards all that we are experiencing, which goes so much beyond physical symptoms, pushing us further away from people.

Unbeknownst to many and/or not fully appreciated is that we are doing our very best to sometimes just get through the day, let alone do anything more. For many of us it takes time to even find a reason to get on with our lives. We may feel useless and hopeless. We are fighting a body with a life of its own, as well as a mental battle that feels like a war with no end in sight. Everything becomes so "loud" that we tend to shut people off until we can make sense of things and feel like we have gained back some sort of control. Explaining this to people can be very difficult.

My uncle once met a guy on a business trip who had dystonia. He thought it would be good for me to talk to him and get some help. I never called him. I didn't see the point. It hurt too much to talk on the phone and I felt so inadequate that I didn't know what to say to him. I also wasn't in any state of mind to hear how well someone had learned to live with dystonia. I didn't want to learn how to live well with dystonia. I wanted find a way to not live with it at all. I wasn't interested in learning how to cope. I was so angry at dystonia that the thought of learning how to cohabitate with it was out of the question. How dare I give into this beast that took away my life and learn to live with it?!?

While I now understand that this is the only way to live a healthy life with any chronic condition, this thought was preposterous to me at the time. My uncle was unhappy with me for not reaching out, but I didn't know how to explain to him the reasons why I didn't. I tried, but I didn't have the words at the time for him to understand.

On another occasion, my father suggested I contact a guy who helps people with disabilities and other life challenges. After many months, I finally called him and left a message. He called back, but I never returned his call. I wasn't ready to face the world yet, which is what he was going to help me with. I was scared to even make the initial phone call, let alone meet to try and put the pieces of my life back together. My voice was shaking when I left my message.

It was bizarre. It was like an out of body experience. I was afraid of what he might suggest I do because I didn't know if I could handle the pain to endure working, volunteering, meeting other people with challenges, etc. I wasn't even comfortable talking to him, let alone getting involved with anyone else. Like my uncle, my father was disappointed I didn't utilize this resource, but again, I didn't know how to explain the reasons why. It has taken me many years to find the right words and the courage to explain how I felt.

There was another element to my resistance to doing things. After losing control over my body movements, I had little to no self confidence. I felt possessed by some other being. I was living in constant fear and worry. I felt unworthy of anything and anyone. I didn't feel like I could be helped. I was very depressed and wanted to be left completely alone.

It took about 7 years to get my symptoms under better control and into a better frame of mind where I was more open to the suggestions of others; but I was still resistant to a point. Except for the fact that I had prior work and life skills, it was like completely starting over. It was very frightening being involved with other people and doing different activities, and still is at times. So many things were/are brand new to me. I often need to take baby steps and the only suggestions that feel comfortable are the ones where I can take baby steps. Anything more will often put my anxiety into high gear. However, there are times when I take a leap of faith and jump in with both feet. More often than not, I find that I am much more capable than I give myself credit. When I step outside my boundaries and accomplish things I thought were out of reach, it builds my confidence. I bet many of you are very similar in this regard.

I had a lot to process after so many years of living in misery. Hindsight is 20/20, but I probably could have mustered up a little more courage to baby step my way onto a better path than the one I chose. I don't necessarily regret the choices I made because I understand why I made them and had to go through them to get to where I am now. However, I do wish I had been better able to accept things as they were and trust that they would get better with more help from others.

As frustrating as it may be at times, do your best to take steps, no matter the size of the step, toward the helping hands extended to you. We can never do anything in life until we are ready and sometimes we don't know if we are ready until we try. You can always retreat if you find you are not ready. There is no shame in this at all. Take time to decide what you want to do that will bring you joy and then honor what you find by taking a step in that direction.

For our loved ones and caregivers, please understand that we very much appreciate your ideas and suggestions, but we may not be ready to listen. For a while we may be resistant to everything you suggest. Many of us are grieving and need time before we are willing and in some cases, know how to accept help. We will eventually come around once we get a better grasp on what we are dealing with. A big part of our willingness to accept help is to have our situation acknowledged. If you show us that you understand that we are struggling and ensure us that you will hold our hand as we go through certain things, we are much more apt to begin the rebuilding process. When we know we are not alone in our battle, we have much more courage to expand our horizons.

Asking for help
Asking for help and relying on other people when it is necessary does not indicate weakness or failure. It is a sign of strength. One of the emotional barriers to asking for help is feeling guilty for having a condition where we need help. It can cause some to experience negative feelings about themselves; a sense of helplessness and unworthiness, which leads to isolation. Sharing your feelings with others is a way to break isolation. This being the case, open communication about how we feel is vital. Blame and shame must be eradicated.

We can also become negligent in asking for help because we feel we are a burden to others. Put yourself in others' shoes. Like you, other people want to help. They often just don't know how to help us. This is where clear communication on our part is vital by letting others know what we need and also to let them know that we are here for them as well. We are not the only ones who live with dystonia. Our friends and family experience pain as well, as they sit by feeling helpless watching their loved ones suffer. This can put a lot of stress on friendships, marriages, and other relationships to the point that they can be dramatically altered or even end. As much as we want to be understood by others, others want to be understood by us just as much. Please be sure to give your loved ones the opportunity to share what they are experiencing.

While there are relationships that have been ruined because of the life changes associated with dystonia, I have seen many that have become stronger. It is all a matter of how we deal with it individually and collectively. We need to listen just as much as we talk, if not more. An open door policy with any challenge in our lives is the best way for us to help one another and strengthen our relationships.

Be prepared that some people have a strong desire to fix us. When they realize that they are unable to, some will retreat and then less of our needs are met. It is our responsibility to let our spouses, parents, kids, siblings, and friends know that it is okay that they cannot fix us and that we don't expect them to. We sometimes just need to talk. We need to just have people listen to us without trying to fix us or change anything. We need to feel that they are here for us and the best way they can do that is to just listen, open their arms and hearts, and simply acknowledge our feelings. Not change our feelings. Acknowledge our feelings to let us know that we matter and how we feel matters. It is important that they remind us that we are loved and not alone. Sometimes all we need is a hug.

It is important for us to understand that the people we seek all these things from may also need the same things from us. I think it is more difficult to watch a loved one in pain knowing we can't take any of it away than being the one experiencing the pain. Please keep this in mind when you judge how others handle your situation, remembering that it is also very hard on them. Support is a two way street.

If you can't speak with family or friends, there are plenty of support groups where you can talk to others with dystonia. You can also speak with counselors, psychologists, psychiatrists, members of the clergy, and life coaches. Many helping hands are there for us. We just need to reach out. To feel comfortable allowing others to help us, we have to overcome the fact that we sometimes need help. All people do in one way or another.

Support groups – pros and cons

Life with dystonia can get lonely so having a support system to share things with is critical to our mental well being. Thus, it is not surprising that there are a multitude of support groups for practically every health condition and life situation that exists.

Even if you are a very social person, it may often seem that there is no one with whom you can share your daily challenges. It may sometimes feel like you are the only one who lives with pain, fatigue, or debilitating symptoms. This is not true, but it can feel like being stranded on a deserted island. Talking to people with dystonia helps normalize our condition by recognizing that we are not alone. They have great empathy and provide helpful advice and support, especially during tough times. Support groups also help us stay connected to the outside world when don't feel well enough to get out and see people.

While I think support groups where people meet in person are more beneficial because of the social interaction, for those who do not have a group in their area, online support groups, particularly social media, have been a blessing for many people. They offer us the opportunity to speak openly about our lives with dystonia and find common ground. We can say things to members of these groups that we can't say to others because these people "get it." We can share the good, the bad and the ugly without being judged and we can also help others. Helping others is a big part of our healing. We can also build lasting relationships with people who understand us.

A good acronym for how to communicate with one another on forums, and in all of life's situations for that matter, is THINK.

T   Is it **T**rue?
H   Is it **H**elpful?
I   Is it **I**nspiring?
N   Is it **N**ecessary?
K   Is it **K**ind?

While online support groups can be very helpful, you might notice on some of them that the same 10-20 people do most of the talking. The other hundreds of members do not say anything. These people either don't know what to say or ask, they don't feel they have it "bad enough" to offer any advice or ask questions (which isn't true since everyone has something to offer), they get tired of hearing from those who complain about their problems all the time, or they feel that talking about dystonia will make their symptoms worse.

Not to belittle anyone's situation, there is also a lot of melodrama that exists in some online support groups. This gives the appearance that "others have it worse than me", which keeps a lot of members silent because they feel they have nothing to offer; or they don't engage to avoid the drama. Support groups become counterproductive when they turn into soap operas or pity parties.

Most people want and need support when the chips are down, as well as get information when they have a quick question so they can go about their lives.

They don't want to "live" online at the support group as a small minority does, and the biggest complainers tend to be that small minority who dominate many forums. Being realistic and understanding that there is a time and place to vent, most people don't want to hear complaining all the time. It brings them down and squashes their hope. People want to find solutions and ways to be happy; not more reason to be sad or scared.

All that being said, you might be under the impression that I don't think there is any point to a support group if you shouldn't go there to share problems. On the contrary, there is nothing wrong with sharing problems, venting, or complaining. It can be healthy and often when we need support the most. I used to run an online support group so I know how beneficial they are. What needs to be understood is that it is easy to fall into the trap of always thinking we have something wrong with us and we can't help but tell everyone about it. We can become chronic complainers.

In short time you might begin to feel you have nothing at all right with you. Others relate to your situation and they begin to complain as well, creating a pity party rather than a helping support network. Each chronic complainer enables the other by sharing the details of all their trials and tribulations. Rarely are answers, coping tools, or ideas for how to get out of the dark hole provided when this is how the group operates. Complaining incessantly does not help the chronic complainer or the other group members.

This is not to overshadow the many thoughtful people who provide information and genuine support and acknowledgment. The difference between acknowledging others versus complaining with them is that the former provides assurance that they are not alone, that everything will be okay, that they are thought of and cared for, and that there is light at the end of the tunnel. This is a more productive way to support people rather than condone incessant complaining which keeps people stuck where they are with no hope in sight.

If you want to be sad, no one in the world can make you happy. But if you make up your mind to be happy, no one and nothing on earth can take that happiness from you.
- Paramhansa Yogananda -

Forums are also places where certain information should not be shared. Few to none of the people on these forums are doctors, yet it is not uncommon to find people telling others what kind of medication to take or forms of therapy to try. We have to be very careful and responsible about how we communicate this type of information. None of us should be telling others what to do. It is dangerous, particularly given the fact that many people are in a very vulnerable place and are willing to try anything someone suggests or talks about having worked for them.

When communicating with others, add disclaimers. For example, "I am doing A, B, and C for my dystonia and this is what it does to help or hurt me. This is not to say that it will work for others, but this is the recipe I found to be most beneficial for me." Please be sure to emphasize that what helps you may not help others. While we have the same diagnosis, we all respond differently to treatments. Be careful what you say and how you say it.

We need to be particularly careful when sharing what medications we take. Instead of saying, "you should take x, y, z medication," tell people what you take and then leave it up to them and their doctor to decide if it is right for them. Talking about medications is a slippery slope. Be careful how you share this information, if at all. There are some desperate people reading your every word and the medications you take may not be appropriate for them. When you are reading suggestions and recommendations from others, please understand that this is what helps them. It may or may not help you. It is best to discuss all medication use with your doctor, including over the counter medications.

Also keep in mind that it is probably not healthy to spend endless hours on these forums. Human beings require social interaction beyond words on a screen. I think the best way to utilize an online forum is to think of it as a grocery store. Only go when you need something. Log in, get what you need, and log out. While you are there, if you feel you can help someone in need, by all means reach out to that person. Just be careful about online activity dominating your life. Limit your time unless you run a forum and have to be there to moderate conversations. Mutual sharing of health problems can sometimes be system overload and make us feel worse because we tend to focus more on our problems than our successes.

Online support groups can be a wonderful place to learn new information, share your concerns, offer support, make new friends, vent, laugh, cry, and find camaraderie. Please be responsible when making comments and reading comments. Always check with your doctor before trying what someone else is doing or suggesting you do, and most importantly, balance your time spent online with living in the real world.

Comparathon

Theodore Roosevelt said, "Comparison is the thief of joy." What an insightful comment. Anytime we compare our lives with someone else or how our lives were before dystonia, we reject who we are right now which will always leave us feeling empty. We know all the dirty details of our situation and only the surface information about others. It is self punishment to hold ourselves up to some outside vague standard. We should measure the value of our lives by our principles.

Just because someone may be able to do things you can't or find uncomfortable does not make you any better or worse. There may very well be things you can do with ease that others struggle with. Either way, it doesn't matter. You and everyone in your life should focus on the strengths that exist and the accomplishments achieved.

Some people like to compare their dystonia with others. It's almost like a competition, hence the name "comparathon." Have you ever thought or said things such as:

"They don't look as bad as me so I must be in more pain."
"I take more medication so I am in worse shape than them."
"They can work and I am unable to so I must have it worse."
"They are not on disability so money isn't a problem for them. I have to scratch and claw just to get by every month to survive. How dare they complain?"
"They look normal so they clearly don't know what real suffering is like."
"They sure are busy and active. Why don't they get a job?"

I've thought and said some of these things. I don't any longer, but for a while I was very bitter. I compared my dystonia with people all the time. In my mind, if someone didn't look as bad as me then there was no way they could feel as bad as me. How wrong I was. Appearance means nothing. I met people with worse looking symptoms that had little to no pain and some with no visible symptoms with terrible pain. How one looks is not a barometer for how one feels.

I would also hear people say things like, "I can't take it anymore"; "I wish I were dead"; "I wish I were never born"; "The pain is more than I can handle." When I said these things it was usually just a way of describing to others how sick I felt, but there were plenty of times I really meant it and did want to end it all. I could barely function because of the horrible pain.

It was hard to reconcile hearing others use these same words while they were still working, travelling, going to social functions, and living what appeared to be a pretty normal life. I was infuriated. For years, just walking to the bathroom from bed was a major undertaking. I couldn't fathom doing all the other things.

It took me a long time to realize that I was being unfair because we only know what we know. Pain is pain and how it affects our lives is personal to us. Our reality is our reality so for a person who we perceive as having "mild" symptoms, it might be far worse than we think and/or to them it might be the worst thing they ever experienced. People also have different pain thresholds. Thus, their words ring true for them. They can describe it however they want and be involved in whatever activities they choose. We are not in their shoes so we don't know what they are experiencing. Quite frankly, it is none of our business. Focus on getting well instead of comparing your dystonia with others and trying to understand and figure out someone else's life.

Daily routine

Even at my worst when I could barely move because of the unrelenting pain, I got up every day to do something, even it was just to go outside and get the mail. I tried to keep some semblance of a normal routine by waking, showering, and eating breakfast, but this was often asking too much on some days. Most days I didn't want to get out of bed, but I forced myself to do it because I knew if I didn't, I would have been much more depressed than I already was.

Most of the time it was just the innate human desire to survive and feel as though I had accomplished something other than just taking up space, even if my only activity for the day was getting out of bed to walk to the living room floor to watch TV. Some days, this was a big accomplishment given my symptoms, so it was important to acknowledge myself. Acknowledging our accomplishments, however "minor", helps keep us going.

We are all very different when it comes to our daily routine. Being creatures of habit, over the years we have all become accustomed to a certain way of living that is most comfortable to us. Some people are on a very rigid schedule and some are more flexible and just go with the flow; and of course, some fall in the middle. I am a routine oriented person. I like to know what is happening before it happens so I can plan and prepare.

Being routine oriented throughout the day helps me better control my symptoms. The more I know what to expect from hour to hour and day to day, the less stress I have and the better I feel. The majority of people with dystonia that I have been in contact with over the years feel best when they are on a pretty regular daily schedule. The more prepared they are for what is to come, the better they can control their symptoms. For some, the opposite is the case, but the majority of people I know find that a consistent daily schedule helps better manage their stress level and symptoms.

Our brains and bodies quickly adapt to a certain way of being. When we don't shock our brain doing something different all the time, it pretty much knows what to expect so stress levels remain lower. The more wrinkles thrown into our lives, the more our brain becomes stimulated, which then alters how we feel physically. Since many of us have sensitive nervous systems, the less unexpected events in our lives, the more calm our mind and body. Being on a schedule is also important for people who take medication on a daily basis.

However, there is a downside to too much structure. Sometimes we can become so routine oriented that the routine runs our life. In other words, when we have too rigid a routine, we become slaves to that routine and anything unplanned or unexpected can make us very uncomfortable. Having structure in our lives can be good, but too much structure can be crippling. Sometimes we just have to go with the flow and have enough faith in ourselves that we will manage things just fine.

Since we have to handle curve balls that inevitably come our way, having some variation in our days to keep our brains from becoming too programmed is helpful. Sometimes if we have a very rigid routine our bodies feel better and worse at certain times of the day to the point that we begin to expect to feel well or unwell at certain times of the day. This is when our dystonia really starts to control us. We can become so locked into a regimen that we can almost predict how we will feel at certain times of the day or even in certain locations of our house or wherever we spend most of our time. Rigid routines can also become just plain boring.

Our environment

It can also be beneficial to change things in our immediate environment. Add some plants or rearrange a room. Change the towel color in your bathroom or get rid of something you are not using. Just a minor change to your immediate environment can do wonders for getting out of the doldrums of expectation living. What I mean by expectation living is that when we spend a lot of time in the same place that never changes appearance, our dystonia symptoms also never change. They too become part of the environment. Getting away, whatever that means to you, can bring great peace of mind.

Think of a time in your life when you went on vacation. More than likely you did not have the same worries and stressors that you do on a daily basis in your regular environment. You were probably able to leave much of it behind and be more at peace. There was less to worry about because you weren't caught in the daily grind.

When we remove ourselves from our environment, even if it's only for an hour or two at the park, library, a friend's house, church, or a movie, it can give us greater peace of mind. Another way to relax is to turn your phone off so you are not constantly distracted by calls, texts, tweets, etc. Take a break from everything so your mind can rest and recharge.

I have the luxury of living about 15 minutes from the beach. There are times when I grab a book, music, beach chair, and towel, and away I go for a couple hours or however much time I have. Just that small change in scenery and new environment clears my mind and rejuvenates me. I feel the same when I go to the park or sit by the river. Being out in nature is very soothing for me. I also find peace of mind when I involve myself with people and activities I enjoy. It helps take my mind off my "problems."

There was a period of about six years when I didn't even want to hear people talk about the beach because I was too sick with dystonia to drive there and too symptomatic to be there if someone else drove me. It sounds so silly thinking about it now since it is only about ten miles away. To me it seemed like 100 miles. The pain of being in a car was often unbearable. Even if I were to get a ride, I couldn't walk on the sand or lie down comfortably. Thus, to keep from getting more depressed, I put it in my mind that I didn't live near the beach.

When my symptoms began to get better, I mustered up the courage to drive there one day. I was also dealing with high anxiety at the time from the symptoms of benzodiazepine withdrawal (see chapter 15), so that made it even more challenging. Driving was also one of my triggers for panic attacks. When I got there I was so excited that I didn't know what to with myself. All that mattered to me was that I had done it! I was finally at the beach after six years of painful avoidance. I was not in the kind of physical shape to enjoy the beach the way I wanted, but I was there! For me, the beach is a place to swim in the water, take long walks, go for a run, hunt for shells, throw a Frisbee, and ride waves. My body was not and is still not in the kind of shape to do most of these things, so now I enjoy it for other reasons.

As time went on and I went more frequently, I was better able to enjoy what I could comfortably do and accept the things that were out of reach. I love the beach, so for me to enjoy it I had to change the way I looked at my experience there. Having done that, I enjoy every moment. Thinking about how far I came in those six years is the most rewarding part of all. Back in the days of those debilitating symptoms, I truly never thought I would ever go to the beach again. Never say never.

It has been seven years since that first trip to the beach. I have been back many times since and I am able to walk a little on the shoreline and even swim a little if the water is calm. I find bobbing around in the salt water to be very soothing. Before I leave, I always put a shell in my pocket to take home as a reminder of my progress. Doing little things like this mean so much to my healing.

If we continue to think and act the same way, we will continue to get the same results. We must be willing to think and act differently if we want to change.

Social life
One of the biggest changes when dystonia hit was in my social life. I was in so much pain that just getting through the most mundane tasks took the wind of me, let alone anything beyond that. I became very isolated. I was also depressed about my dramatic life change and embarrassed about how I looked. At first it wasn't so much embarrassment as it was the pain. The less I did and the less going on around me the better I felt.

I tried to maintain relationships with family and friends, but it became too much for me to handle. Driving was dangerous because I could not see the road well or turn my head because it was in a locked position, and talking on the phone was very uncomfortable. People stopped visiting and calling me. The novelty of my health condition with which people originally expressed interest soon waned. I also changed so I was not the most pleasant person in the world to be around. I was frequently complaining. Granted, I was miserable, but no one wanted to hear about it all the time.

Before too long, I lost almost all connection with people. Some left me, but I also removed myself from some people's lives. I was very isolated and felt truly lonely for the first time in my life. When I began to get my symptoms under better control and decided to re-engage the world, at first my anxiety skyrocketed. I felt like a fish out of water and still do at times. The more persistent I was and understanding that it was a transition after years of isolation, the easier it was to feel more comfortable engaged in the world again.

I urge all of you to maintain connections with people as much as possible in any way you can. Even when I was in bad shape, I could have done a better job keeping some connections alive which might have helped prevent my downward spiral. For those who have a hard time being mobile, there are many forms of technology at your disposal to communicate with people. Use it. For those who can be more active, BE more active. Stay involved with the world. We are social beings and little else provides us with all the feel good hormones as much as human interaction. It also helps us forget the pain, even if for just a little while, when we are engaged in meaningful activities. Also, the more we engage the world, the less social stigma we create about life with a chronic health condition.

Doctor visits

Be prepared for your doctor visits. I can't stress this enough. Dystonia is complex and our symptoms are very specific to us. Doctors need to know as much unique information about us as possible. Be sure to provide them with your medical history, all of your symptoms (even those that seem minor), medications you are taking, nutritional supplements you are taking, and the things that exacerbate and calm your symptoms. Also be specific about how your symptoms fluctuate throughout the entire day.

If it is your first visit with your doctor, add as much additional information as possible to supplement the paperwork they ask you to fill out. If you know you have dystonia prior to your first visit, get as educated as possible about it. Be familiar with the different kinds of dystonia and the various treatment protocols. We need to keep our doctors on their toes and sometimes educate them. It does not matter how many patients they have seen. They have never seen you. You are different than every other person who walks through their door even if you share the same diagnosis.

The more you know about dystonia and how it affects you, the more effective your doctor will be in treating you. You will be working more as a team versus you being a lab rat. When your doctor suggests something, go home and learn more about it to decide if it is right for you. The wrong treatment at the wrong time can do harm. Do your homework. We have to be our own best health advocates with our doctor working as a partner in our treatments. Ask questions, no matter how many you have.

Many find it helpful to keep an ongoing journal of their symptoms so they can share it with their doctor. It's hard to remember all the little nuances we experience which may be more important than we think when it comes to our treatment. Keeping a journal or a checklist of symptoms is especially helpful if you are getting botulinum toxin or taking medications. It helps doctors modify your treatments as needed.

I suggest keeping a symptom journal that highlights the problems you are having AND a wellness journal so you don't lose focus on the positive things in your life. Your wellness journal should include your physical health as well as your mental, social, and spiritual health. Unless it is a routine check-up, we rarely go to the doctor because we feel well. We go to the doctor when we are sick. Thus, our journals tend to focus on how sick we feel, which can make us feel even worse if we are committed to only talking about negative things.

Remember that when you see your doctor, this is your time and your money. Spend as much time as you need to have all your questions answered and health concerns addressed. People with dystonia tend to be people pleasers who don't want to ruffle any feathers, but this is your life and your health. It is vital that you take as much time as you need with your doctor. If you leave a visit and have something you forgot to address, do not be afraid to call the office. Our doctors are there to help us better manage our health and it is our responsibility to make sure they do their job. I am not suggesting that we be difficult patients, but sometimes we have to be pushy if we feel we are not being given the time we require (and paying for) to have our needs met. Many doctors appreciate patients who are diligent about their health because they know it is conducive to better treatment outcomes.

Medical Folder

I've been to so many doctors that I feel like a broken record telling my story over and over. Plus, my symptoms have changed over the years. To make visits easier, I created a personal medical folder to bring to the doctor so I can share as much pertinent information about myself as possible so they have a clear picture into my life.

My medical folder includes pictures of me showing how my dystonia has changed over the years, all medical treatments I currently receive or have received, medications I am taking and have taken in the past (prescription and over the counter), nutritional supplements I take, allergies, and results from various tests (blood work, MRI, CT, x-rays). I also include a journal of my symptoms and any changes I have had, as well as all other relevant information a doctor might need to better treat me.

It is important to go a step further by letting a family member and/or friend have access to your medical folder in case of an emergency. If you become incapacitated and someone needs to speak on your behalf, they can simply grab the folder and present it to the attending nurse or doctor. It is also helpful if you educate your family and friends about you and your condition beyond what is in your folder so they can be even more thorough when discussing your health details if you are unable. Also get a medical ID card for your wallet or purse (and/or bracelet) to put your illness, emergency contacts, medications, allergies, and other pertinent information in case of an emergency.

Taking a little time to get your medical information organized can pay dividends. It can make doctor visits far less laborious and it can help you in case of an emergency where this information could prove vital to doctors in order to treat you most effectively.

Your health specialist
My overall experience with doctors leaves a lot to be desired. I have heard the same thing from countless others when it comes to the diagnosis and treatment of dystonia. There are some great doctors out there and then some who do us more harm than good or make no difference at all. Find the one who is best for you and your unique needs, and hold them to a high standard.

It does not matter if your doctor is considered the best in the world or an "expert" in the field. The notion that a particular doctor is an expert is only relevant to the results we receive from their care. Others may not fare well with your doctor who may be hailed as one of the best, just as you may not fare well with their doctor who might be completely unknown. Either one can be of help to us depending on how we mesh. Thus, we have to find the "expert" that is best for us.

Remember that doctors work for us. We can hire and fire them at our discretion. I had one doctor tell me this on my first visit. He viewed himself as a part of my health care team with me as the manager of that team who could hire and fire whoever wasn't carrying their weight. This mindset made him work hard to constantly learn more and stay up to date with the literature about my condition and related issues.

Doctors may know more about the pathology of dystonia and treatment protocols, but they don't know what it's like to live with it every day. I am no expert on dystonia, but I am the expert on my dystonia. No one knows more about me than me. The same goes for you. There is so much that doctors do not see or know about because they are not with us all day long. They don't know how our symptoms fluctuate unless we tell them. They have a small window into our lives and do their best with the information they have. This is why keeping a journal is so important. We need to tell them what they can't see.

The main problem I have with doctors is that they don't often think enough outside their scope of treatment. Very few of my medical doctors have suggested things such as proper nutrition, exercise, therapy (physical and otherwise), or stress management techniques. Doctors should be discussing these things with us because they can have a profound affect on our well being. They can also enhance/complement the treatments they are providing. By the same token, doctors who don't fall under the category of "traditional medicine" should acknowledge what is offered by mainstream medicine, which does have a good track record. Both parties have a lot to offer so they should work together more so we get the best care possible.

The people I know who do best in managing their symptoms are those who utilize a comprehensive approach to their care using a variety of protocols. To this end, it is important to remember the definition of health: "A state of optimal physical, mental, and social well being and not merely the absence of disease or infirmity."[1] If your doctor only addresses one aspect of this triangle, it is your responsibility to address the others.

Do your best to seek out a healthy balance of outside care and self care. This includes medical, spiritual, emotional, social, psychological, and physical health. In addition, seek out joy, peace, love, and laughter. Although dystonia may affect many aspects of your life, it does not have to control your life.

Testimonial

My story with dystonia appears to be one of a sudden twist of fate, so to speak. One day I was fine and the next day my life was irreversibly changed. A whiff of a formaldehyde based substance was the catalyst to my life slipping away like sands through the fingers of a child innocently playing on a beach. Although I do believe the severe blow to my head during a car accident in the 1980's is what started me on this journey, I know odors are a trigger for me. I've heard some doctors say toxic odors shouldn't cause such a reaction, while other doctors say it may for some and not for others. Quite honestly, that is a debate that feels a long way off from being rectified. In the meantime, what I do care about is how this debate negatively impacts the well being of the patient.

I remember when I first started seeing my movement disorder specialist. Whenever I would attempt to get a better grasp of the treatment method he was planning, he would reassure me that I just needed to think more positively. As if to say, "If you were more positive about this experience and less concerned about what may happen; you'd be fine." It is experiences with medical professionals like this that can overshadow the day to day challenges of living with dystonia because of the mental and emotional torment those situations cause within me. I sometimes feel like a fraud.

The very nature of dystonia, being that it is different for each individual, I think lends itself to being a thing that is easily dismissed by others. It's our nature as humans to look to others for similarities; that 'where do I fit in' quality of our existence. It has taken me a few years to reconcile that need to 'dystonically' fit in, believing my symptoms had to be to a certain threshold before I am not an impostor and to realize that one of the gifts of the disorder is that it truly is uniquely my own. I am ok with this realization, and even find greater comfort in it than I expected; that is until I have my yearly check up with my doctor.

His comments about my movements not being of a progressive nature, said with a slight hint in his voice of, "there is nothing wrong with you", can put me back months emotionally while I try to regain my resolve. His two minute comment said at the end of a 10 minute consult is like a tentacle spreading out; reaching deeply into areas of my life that I believed I had long ago found peace and it ultimately puts me into a tailspin. It is at that moment that I begin to doubt my body. Doubt my mental state. There seems to be a schizophrenic type by-product built into the typical medical journey patients must trudge through in an effort to get relief from the actual malady for which they are being treated.

Starting life over at the age of 45 was disheartening enough. I tried to find the positives in the experience, since regardless of what reality I wanted my life to be, I would still have my home, I would still be employed doing the job I excelled at, and I would still be hitting the open road in the car that felt like an extension of myself. When dystonia came knocking, all of that was now my past. But none of that dealt as severe a blow as when I left my doctor appointment and realized that if what I felt he was implying was true, in essence, he was saying I caused myself to lose almost everything that mattered to me.

The fact that Gabapentin is keeping my movements to an almost unnoticeable state is good and encouraging to me. In a typical day, when I am experiencing my new level of independence, I am able to function at such a level that many would never know that just a mere 5 years ago I resembled someone who had survived a stroke. I am abundantly blessed by the opportunities that have unfolded for me in this time and I am eternally grateful for the successes in my new life.

Ironically though, in light of the growth and my positive attitude, it is the self doubt imprinted upon me by the responses of some of the medical personnel that has been far more debilitating than the actual disorder. That isn't to say the physical pain or the sometimes awkward postures haven't caused me to question if I have what it takes to endure the challenges they present. That is always ever present in my mind, but it's the lurking, more debilitating mental chastising that resides in the back of my mind that causes far more discomfort for me. It's an odd line I feel I walk when I allow myself to actually think about it. On the surface I appear to be without any true effects of dystonia, to the point that I too at times believe I am without the disabling responses of having muscles spasm against one another, and it is in that blindness that I have had momentary lapses of respect for what the disorder will do if it feels slighted.

I still need to remain mindful that my body requires more time to perform mundane tasks; that at the most inopportune time the facial tics that I've grown accustomed to and think little of will become more pronounced, deceiving my facade. It's during those times of the rare flare up, especially immediately afterwards, that I realize how much I have learned to adapt my day to day routine. I know this isn't uniquely my own response to dystonia. It's not what the doctors say I do or don't have and it's not the comparison of symptoms with others living with the disorder. People living with dystonia learn to adapt to their unique symptoms in a way that suits their day to day life. I now recognize that to some degree, the ability to adapt is what provides me the reference to answer the question, "Where do I fit in?"

The life I was planning and working towards prior to 5 years ago has no resemblance to the life I am living now. I still mourn the profound loss, but it no longer defines who I am today. I was slow to accept my new reality, but have since embraced that what does define me is my desire to continue to live my life to the fullest.

References

1) www.who.int, Retrieved on July 14, 2014 from: www.who.int/about/definition/en/print.html

Chapter 14
Dystonia Speaks

Understanding dystonia is difficult for all of us. We do our best to remember that having dystonia does not mean we are no longer a worthwhile human being. We desire to do what we used to but we feel stuck inside a body over which we have little or no control. We still want to enjoy work, family, friends, and leisure activities, however much dystonia puts that enjoyment out of reach.

Despite our condition, we are still very much alive. We just have to adjust how we live. We can still laugh, love, and enjoy good times. For some of us, symptoms are mild enough where we can involve ourselves in many things. For the rest of us, we have a hard time doing a lot of the things we used to do. Making plans is often uncomfortable for us because we may not be feeling up to following through. Some of us have trouble driving. We have also become overly sensitive to certain stimuli, such as bright lights, certain noises, colors, crowds, smells, and tastes, so we carefully pick and choose our activities.

Many of us depend on people who are well to support us at home or visit us when we feel too crummy to go out. Sometimes we need help with shopping, cooking, cleaning, a ride to the doctor, or help with the kids. People who are well can be our link to normalcy. They help keep us in touch with parts of life that we enjoy that we are not as involved with as we once were.

Daily dystonia living is very inconsistent. We may not know how well we will feel each day, let alone hour to hour some days. There are days when we can do more than other days, but just because we did something one day doesn't mean we can do it again the next. Maybe we can or maybe we have to wait for another day or time of day. Patience is one of our greatest challenges living in a body that does not cooperate. Doctor appointments, treatments, medications, the rest needed to function, anger, worry, frustration, and fear are all part of our every day life.

Since our symptoms are so varied, we ask that others be patient with us. We sometimes feel that people expect us to get better faster, get over it already, and act as though we are cured when our physical symptoms are unseen or after we get a treatment, most of which just mask our symptoms at best.

At times we may talk differently from people free of constant pain. Just because we say we are fine does not mean we are not experiencing pain or discomfort.

Sometimes words are not adequate to describe how we are feeling. We attempt to hide our symptoms to not be a bother and to try and forget. We desperately want to feel "normal."

The pain some of us feel is like the pain one experiences at the moment of an injury, but never goes away. Recall a time when you hurt yourself, such as a broken bone, a stubbed toe, or a paper cut. The feeling you had right when it happened is the kind of pain many of us deal with non stop. This kind of pain has forced us to adopt coping mechanisms that don't necessarily reflect our real level of discomfort. When we say we are in pain it is usually worse than usual; much of the time we are just coping, trying to sound happy and look normal.

For many of us, our body does not allow us to do what our mind wants it to do. Being able to stand for ten minutes doesn't necessarily mean that we can stand for twenty minutes, or an hour, or give a repeat performance tomorrow. Just because we managed to go for a walk, out to lunch, or grocery shopping yesterday doesn't mean that we will be able to today. We want to do all of these things and more, but our body often tells us we can't. We often don't listen and push past our limits because we want to live beyond merely existing.

Some people like to give us pep talks. While this is well intentioned, it can be demoralizing because our symptoms are so variable. As mentioned, there are days we can do more than others. It's quite possible that one day we are able to go out to lunch or for a walk in park, while the next day we have trouble getting to the next room. When people say things like, "But you did it before" or "Oh, come on, I know you can do this", we feel pressured and misunderstood.

For many of us, "getting out and doing things" does not make the pain vanish and can often exacerbate our symptoms. If we were capable of "getting on with things" we would, and those who can do. All of us are constantly striving to improve and do the right things to manage our symptoms so we can "get out and do things" more.

Sometimes we hear others say, "You just need to push yourself more; try harder." It may be hard to read how we feel on our face or in our body language, but we push ourselves all the time. Sometimes too much and we pay for it later with worse symptoms. Finding balance is one of our greatest challenges. For some of us, every day we do nothing but push just to get through the day.

Each day has to be taken as it comes. We have to mentally prepare and carefully consider if an activity is going to cause more symptoms. This is one of the hardest and most frustrating traits of dystonia. It can lead to a great deal of fear and anxiety because we never really know how much our bodies are going to cooperate.

Many of us very much miss our social life. When we tell people that we can't come over or go out to lunch or dinner or to the movies, it's not because we don't want to, but that we are having a difficult time at the moment. Moving too much or sitting too long might wreak havoc on our body. Sometimes we will have spasms and spill food when we eat. It can be embarrassing and cause anxiety. Just the thought of what might happen is scary for some of us. Going on day long trips or walking through the mall may be out of the question for us. We tend to need frequent rest breaks so "making a day of things" means something different to us than it once did.

Sometimes we sense that we are unwanted and unwelcome. This is logical since it probably feels like a slap in the face getting rejected most every time people ask us to do something. Even if we say "no" most of the time when we are asked to do things, we still want to be asked. It means more to us than we can put to words. It's important to know that we have not been forgotten and are still valued. Just because "no" is a common response, there are times when we will say "yes." It's hard for us to sit on the sidelines and we feel deprived when people stop asking us to join in activities. When we are physically and mentally able, we will always say "yes", so please give us that opportunity. It also makes it easier for us to join in activities when we are given lead time to help us plan and prepare our mind and body.

We understand that communication is often difficult. We don't always know what to say to one another. People often hear us complain about our dystonia, which we know can be a burden. Likewise, we hear comments that burden us. For example, we hear statements such as, "Oh well, that's life, you'll just have to deal with it", or "You'll get over it eventually. Until then, you'll just have to do your best", or, "Well, you look well enough." These comments are true to a certain degree, but often distance us from people because they don't address what we are really experiencing.

It helps more when people engage us with questions such as, "What does it feel like?", "How have you been able to manage?", and "How can I help?" Being inquisitive about what we go through versus telling us how to go through it is more helpful. It shows interest which helps us open up and feel more comfortable about something that is often hard to talk about. It may also reduce our complaining. Sometimes we talk so much about our symptoms because we feel alone. We want to be heard so we are better understood and feel accepted.

When we talk about dystonia, one of the worst things people can do is respond with silence. Our days are hard and tiring, and living with the knowledge that our symptoms may never leave us weighs heavily on our mind. When you thoughtfully respond to the things we share and ask us questions with vested interest, it gives us a chance to lighten our load. If listening to the details of our condition makes you uncomfortable for a short while, consider this: what is your short term discomfort of lending an ear compared to the long term discomfort of your friend or loved one?

Talking about dystonia is one of our most important coping tools. Denying one of our best survival mechanisms makes a hard day even harder. We rarely tire of answering questions about our condition. Many of us love it when someone takes the time to ask us about it. Efforts to understand help us feel valued.

If asking questions is too difficult, hearing things such as, "I really appreciate you coming along when you're not feeling well. It's good to have you here" or, "I know you're not feeling well, so thank you for making the effort", mean so much to us. I can remember almost every single time someone said this to me because it made me feel understood and appreciated. While I also remember moments of ridicule and avoidance, the times I have been positively acknowledged stay much closer to me.

Sometimes we can be testy and short fused. It's not how we try to be or want to be. No one wants to be this way whether they have dystonia or not. We all go through difficult times making it hard to always be level headed. When we have something unpleasant going on that we feel we can't escape, it can cause fireworks. Our behavior towards others is not personal in most cases. We are just trying to find our way as we learn to accept our new reality.

Don't be surprised if we cancel a meeting, don't answer the phone, walk out in the middle of a gathering, it seems like we are not listening or appear disinterested, or we suddenly sit or lay down. We still love being with you, but sometimes dystonia prevents us from doing certain things.

Common misperceptions and things we often hear

"Just get on with it." This undermines our determination to cope. We are making great effort to get on with life the very best we can. It just might not seem that way sometimes because it takes more effort to do things that once came easily to us. "Just get on with it" ignores all our efforts.

"There are so many people worse off than you." We can only feel what we are experiencing so this discounts everything we are experiencing. Knowing there are people with worse symptoms or a worse condition (not that there is any real way to measure "worse") doesn't make our situation any less difficult. We only live in our bodies and when something is wrong with it, it stinks, which is all that matters. We know there will always be someone with worse symptoms, but we can only relate to how we feel.

"You always feel bad." In some cases this is true. Then there are times when our symptoms are at a low level where we are more comfortable. This can last for varying amounts of time. We also sometimes get in the habit of saying we feel bad all the time because we are inundated with symptoms that can often overwhelm us. This is our fault for always saying we feel bad and something we all need to work on, but it is often the truth.

"No one can be as bad as you say you are." It might seem out of the ordinary, but many of us do feel as bad as we say and sometimes worse than we let on.

"You should look worse so people know you're in pain." Many of us are able to hide our pain and other symptoms. We have also learned over time how to live with it so it doesn't appear as bad as it is. We also want to look as normal and as good as we can, just like everyone else does. Furthermore, what does someone look and sound like that has a disabling condition? Are there certain criteria we should be aware of? Of course not. Disabling conditions come in all shapes and sizes, some of which are obvious and some which are invisible.

"How come you don't laugh anymore?" We can laugh. We love to laugh. It just gets more difficult sometimes when the pleasure centers of our brain are shut down from pain and medications. While we still laugh, for many of us it has become more difficult. Many of us are sad and angry about a life so dramatically altered.

"You look fine. How can you have chronic pain?" The simple answer is that you can't see pain so how we look doesn't always reflect how we feel.

"You can't hurt that bad. You need to push through the pain." This reminds me of some former coaches and personal trainers. Chronic pain from dystonia and pain from exercise are very different. When we "push through the pain" it can make it worse.

"You can't do that. You're hurt." Actually, we can do a lot of things. We just choose not to most of the time because of the pain it causes or how it will make us feel later on or the next day. Our recovery time is not what it used to be or that of a "normal" person. As much as we appreciate other's concern, none of us likes being told we can't do something. It reduces our feeling of self worth more than it may already be. Give us a chance to try something. If we can't do it we will let you know.

"Why don't you get a job?" Some people have symptoms mild enough where they are able to work. Others are not so fortunate. For the latter group, on good days some could probably work a job, but many have pain and other symptoms that kick in, making them unable to function for a day or a week or more. No employer would keep them on the job. Some days we are well enough to do some things like everyone else. Unfortunately, these moments are few and far between for many people and often last only a short while. We also take more time to recover from some of the most seemingly innocuous things so it is actually irresponsible for us to take a job when we may not be able to consistently perform. This puts an employer and business in an awkward position because it may affect their productivity.

"You must enjoy having an everlasting vacation from work." We would like nothing more than to be physically well enough to work. Many people take for granted how lucky they are to be able to work. If we could work, we would. I miss working more than people can imagine; more than I ever imagined I would. Be grateful if you are well enough to work. We envy you. Our life is not a vacation. We are on indefinite sick leave.

"You must be earning a gold mine from your disability payments." Disability payments keep people below poverty level.

"Since you don't work anymore you must have a lot of spare time." This can be true for some of us, but it is far from fun as this comment is often implied. Much of our spare time is spent dealing with very uncomfortable symptoms.

When my dystonia was more severe, I mentioned to someone that I felt lost without my watch. She responded by saying, "What do you need a watch for? You don't do anything or have any responsibilities." Unbeknownst to this person, who only saw me about an hour every few weeks and therefore had a very small window into my world, I did have responsibilities of which she was unaware. Many were related to managing my symptoms so I could have some level of function during the day, which was the hardest job I ever had in my life. In addition to that "job", I was spending time finding ways to get my life back on track, make money with some small at home businesses, and learn to live a more productive life given an obstacle greater than she could fathom. I also needed to know the time so I could make it to doctor appointments and take my medication on schedule. Instead of an obnoxious comment, she could have just accepted that I liked wearing a watch, regardless of the reason.

Many of the comments above come from people closest to us; those we rely on the most for support. As well intentioned as these comments may be, when we hear them it distances us from people and makes us feel more isolated.

Even though we may at times complain and sound needy and demanding of your rapt attention, we want you to maintain balance in your life. If you don't take care of your own needs, health, and work-life balance, it can bring you down. We understand that life with dystonia is not easy on anyone. Just as we want you to show us compassion, patience, and understanding, we want to give the same to you.

Just as we have had to make adjustments to our lives and our relationships with others, we know you have to do the same. If you ever have a question, please ask. We are open to speaking with you about anything. Everyone is fighting a battle we know little to nothing about. The more we talk about our personal challenges, the better off we will all be.

There comes a time in your life when you walk away from all
the drama and people who create it. You surround yourself with
people who make you laugh. Forget the bad and focus on the good.
Love the people who treat you right. Pray for the ones who don't.
Life is too short to be anything but happy.
Falling down is a part of life.
Getting back up is living.
- Unknown -

Chapter 15
Treatment Options and Therapies

Introduction

There is currently no cure for dystonia so treatments are focused on reducing symptoms. A treatment that helps one may not help another, or help as much, so there is no cookie cutter approach. Thus, finding the right treatment/symptom management program can take some trial and error. I have explored a variety of treatments, some being more helpful than others.

Whatever your treatment of choice, it is important to know beforehand how you will evaluate its usefulness; in other words, your expectations. When discussing a particular treatment I often hear people ask, "Does it work?" This is a vague question. "Work" in what way? Reduce symptoms, reduce pain, reduce spasms, eliminate dystonia altogether? Anything might "work" so we need to be more specific to satisfy our personal definition of the word "work." Plus, what works for one may not work for someone else so we have to experiment to find what is best for us based on our desired outcome.

Perhaps a better question is, "Does it help?" Every treatment and symptom management protocol available to us has the potential of helping so it is best to be open-minded to every possibility. If we get 20% help from one treatment, 10% from another, and 15% from another, it starts to add up. Use anything and everything that helps.

Also keep in mind that just because something has not been approved as a treatment for dystonia does not mean it is ineffective for dystonia. There are plenty of FDA approved treatments that are ineffective for some of us so this standard is not absolute. Further, there are no medications for dystonia, but medications used off label have proven effective. This being the case, especially with a complex disorder like dystonia with so many symptom variations from person to person, every single thing that may help manage our particular symptoms deserves our attention.

No matter which symptom management approach you use, one of the most important things is to establish is a good working relationship with those who treat you. As with any condition, the more your health care team knows about you and your body, the better they can identify what is and is not working. When you have a close relationship with your team, they can follow patterns and determine what changes need to be made, if any. In addition, the more informed you are about your treatment plan and goals, the more likely your chance for success. Educated patients are more prone to better treatment results.

One of the most important aspects to any treatment is how much we believe it is going to help. Our dedication to a treatment and belief in its efficacy is just as important as the treatment itself. Trust is a big factor in our body's ability to positively respond to a particular treatment.

Treating dystonia is not a sprint. It is usually a meandering journey on a trail with many side paths. Close monitoring by you and your health care team is paramount to best managing your symptoms. Having people on your side that you can talk to and count on in times of need is priceless. When you have the added comfort that you are truly being cared for by those who treat you, it has a profoundly positive effect on your overall well being.

The length of benefit for all treatments should be noted because every day our bodies endure new stresses and strains. We are different every day in terms of how our body is functioning and how we respond to treatments. When we go for any kind of treatment, we can't expect that we will get the same results each time. Our mind and body are always changing so "who" the doctor/therapist worked on during the last visit is different this visit. Thus, the doctor/therapist has to adjust their approach to meet the needs of you that day and not the you they saw at a previous visit.

When I was grappling with expecting to get the same results after every treatment, one of my doctors shared the following quote by the Dalai Lama: "I am open to the guidance of synchronicity and do not let expectations hinder my path." I recite this at every visit, regardless of what kind of doctor or therapist I am seeing. It helps me let go and allow the treatment to do its job.

It would be impossible to cover every treatment option for dystonia, so this chapter focuses on those most commonly used by patients.

Botulinum neurotoxin (chemodenervation)
One of the most well known and popular treatments for dystonia is botulinum neurotoxin (Botox, Xeomin, Dysport, Myobloc). Botulinum toxin is a protein and neurotoxin derived from bacterium clostridium botulinum. When it is injected into muscles, it blocks signals from the brain that tells a muscle to contract, helping to reduce or eliminate pain and spasms. It results in decreased

muscle activity by blocking the release of acetylcholine, the neurotransmitter believed to be most involved in dystonia.

Neurotoxin therapy does not work on everyone the same way and it may take a few treatments to find the correct muscles to inject to achieve the desired result. It does not have a long lasting or curative affect, as it only lasts for roughly 3 months (less for some and longer for others) so you need to get it done on a routine basis. This 3 month standard has been in place since Botox first became available. It is used to guard against immunity to the toxin where you would no longer benefit from the treatment. Many insurance companies also use this 3 month standard for reimbursement purposes. In recent years, companies have improved their formulas to reduce the chance of immunity and new neurotoxins have become available. Researchers are also exploring shorter injection schedules, as there tends to be a 1-2 week period of increased symptoms pre and post "injection day" for some people. Efficacy varies between individuals.

Botox is probably the most well known brand of botulinum toxin and a lot of people think that the other neurotoxins (Xeomin, Dysport, Myobloc) are the same as Botox and call them Botox. Their intended uses are the same, but there are some differences in how they are made, stored, and administered which can be nominal to substantial depending on the individual. They are not interchangeable, as they each have their own characteristics and preparations. Sometimes doctors switch brands if they feel another one may be more effective. It is also possible to develop antibodies to a particular brand which would also be cause to switch.

It is usually best to have your neurotoxin administered by a neurologist who specializes in movement disorders (Movement Disorder Specialist or MDS). There are other doctors who can effectively administer your injections, but an MDS is usually the most skilled and knowledgeable in this area.

Toxins are usually administered using an Electromyography (EMG). An EMG is a machine that measures muscle activity by inserting needles into muscles. Some doctors do not use an EMG. They will instead use ultrasound or palpate the muscles and look at movement patterns to determine which muscles to inject. Most people I know prefer doctors who use an EMG or ultrasound machine because they are typically more accurate in identifying which muscles are most active. It is also easier to help determine what part of the muscle to inject. There are certainly some doctors who do very well without an EMG or

194

ultrasound, but it seems most patients prefer one that uses a machine as a guide.

During your visit, the doctor will assess your muscle activity with their hands, eyes, and EMG machine (if they use one). They will determine which muscles are most active and actively involved in your dystonic movements. These muscles will be injected with the neurotoxin using a hypodermic needle. Sometimes the same muscle will be injected more than once at different parts of the muscle. For example, you may get injections in more than one spot along your trapezius or sternocleidomastoid (SCM) muscle.

More than one muscle is typically injected during a visit and the number of injections and the amount of neurotoxin delivered varies depending on your symptoms. I've had treatments where I received as few as four injections and as many as twenty injections, ranging in amounts from 75 units to 400 units. If you have consistent movement patterns and positive results from your neurotoxin therapy, you will more than likely receive similar treatments each visit. However, since symptoms can be variable, it is not always known how many shots you will receive and how much neurotoxin. Some doctors only do injections one or two days a week, so getting an appointment, especially your first, may take a few weeks to a few months.

As with all treatments we all respond differently. Be prepared that your first or first few treatments may not be effective or as effective as you had hoped. For some there is relief after the first set of injections, but in a lot of cases the first few times may be trial and error or exploratory. Try to not get discouraged. There is an art and science to neurotoxin therapy, so it may take time for a doctor to pinpoint the exact muscles that need to be injected and with how much toxin.

I have never done well with neurotoxin therapy. This puts me in the minority since most derive at least some benefit. I have been to several doctors and the results have always been the same regardless of the amount given and muscles injected. I have been to local doctors with limited experience and seasoned doctors at major universities. After all my treatments, I have either had no change or I have had an exacerbation of symptoms.

I have a theory as to why I have poor results. In cervical dystonia, many muscles appear involved, yet they are not all primarily affected by dystonia. Some of the cervical muscles are overactive due to secondary compensation. In other words, there are non-dystonic muscles that are active because they are working to try and balance the neck (compensatory muscles). They may look, feel, and test as being dystonic, but they are not. Doctors will sometimes inject these muscles because they have yet to determine the primary dystonic muscles. This weakens compensatory muscles, causing them to become more tense and painful because they have to work even harder to compensate for the true dystonic muscle activity that was not addressed. This does two things: 1) the dystonic muscles continue to contract and 2) it forces other muscles (primarily the upper back for me) to get involved to help out the weakened compensatory muscles, causing more pain and exhaustion.

After a treatment I have to work much harder to maintain good posture. Just standing sometimes becomes a chore. My head feels much heavier and I get sluggish from so many compensatory muscles being overworked. I can feel my back and shoulders working much harder in order for me to move around. I also have to do what I call "pre-movements" with other parts of my body before I begin to walk or do some other activity. For example, if I have to lift or turn my head, I might consciously engage my shoulders first. It makes the other movements easier. Since I have not had positive results with neurotoxin therapy, I no longer get it done.

Injection day
The injection day is different depending on who you are. Some are in and out with no problem whatsoever. Some will not experience pain or any of the common side effects, while there are others who always do. The stress of getting shots can exacerbate symptoms and/or bring on other unwanted symptoms. It varies depending on the person. The first time I got shots was the most painful. I didn't know what to expect so I was anxious and tensed up the entire time which made it worse. I had minimal pain in all of my subsequent treatments. Knowing what to expect was very helpful.

Many people look forward to "injection day" because the toxin gives them so much relief. People don't necessarily look forward to the procedure itself because it can be painful and an inconvenience, but more what the toxin does to relieve their symptoms. If you have never gone for injections, learn as much about it as possible so you know what to expect. This will decrease any anxiety you may be experiencing.

Unfortunately, there is no specific way to approach "injection day" or know how you will respond to the injections in terms of efficacy and side effects.

Results are so varied that I do not want you to think that you will get great results after one treatment or that it will take 3-4 treatments before you get the results you are looking for. This is all unknown. It is best if you can remove all expectations and simply allow the process to unfold. You do yourself no good expecting that on a certain day after the injections and for so many weeks thereafter, you will feel a certain way. Until you know what neurotoxin therapy does for you, it is best to have few to no expectations, but to be positive and set your prayers and intentions that you will get the best results possible. The same applies to oral medications, which are discussed further in the chapter.

Neurotoxin side effects
There are many possible side effects from botulinum neurotoxin injections. The most common reported include bruising, pain, redness, or swelling at the injection site, difficulty swallowing, headache, fatigue, body aches and/or joint pain, muscle weakness and stiffness, dizziness, drowsiness, dry mouth, and flu like symptoms.

Not everyone experiences side effects. For those that do, they usually go away as your body adjusts to the medicine. Your doctor may also be able to tell you ways to prevent or reduce some of these side effects. Most side effects do not need medical attention, but always check with your doctor if any side effects continue or are bothersome.

A common side effect is pain and inflammation around the injection site, as well as overall body pain for a couple days up to a couple weeks for some people. A few of the things that have helped me with these symptoms include ibuprofen (or other over the counter pain medication of your choice), ginger root capsules (a great natural alternative for pain), topical lotions with different minerals, such as magnesium for example (magnesium in supplement form also helps me), Epsom salt baths, ice, drinking lots of water, and rest.

Another common side effect you may experience and hear others talk about, and one that is at the top of the list of potential side effects for all neurotoxins, is dysphagia. Dysphagia is the medical term for difficulty swallowing. The sensation is usually described as food stuck in the throat or tightness from the neck down to just above the abdomen. This symptom can last for several days to a couple of weeks or more. It varies from person to person. While dysphagia is typically talked about in dystonia circles as it relates to side effects of neurotoxins, it can also occur from dystonia itself where the muscles required for swallowing may become compromised.[1-4]

When my dystonia was severe, and even at times now when I have significant tightness in my neck, shoulders, and upper torso, swallowing was/is difficult. In order for me to eat, I had to push as hard as I could in the other direction my head turned so I could put food in my mouth and be able to swallow. I did the same thing when swallowing liquids, but they were easier to get down. I also had to push my head in order to speak clearly. My voice had become muffled and my breathing was labored because my air passage was constricted.

Dysphagia is not to be confused with Dysphonia (a.k.a. Spasmodic Dysphonia). Dysphonia is a generic term for any issue with one's voice. Spasmodic Dysphonia (SD) differs in that it is a neurological disorder in the same family as dystonia. SD is task specific, meaning that the muscles spasm only when they are used for particular actions and not when they are at rest. When a person with SD attempts to speak, involuntary spasms in the muscles of the larynx cause the voice to break up or sound strained, tight, strangled, breathy, or whispery. The spasms often interrupt sound, squeezing the voice to nothing in the middle of a sentence, or dropping it to a whisper. However, during other activities, such as breathing and swallowing, the larynx functions normally.

According to the National Spasmodic Dysphonia Association, SD is estimated to affect approximately 50,000 people in North America, but this number may be inaccurate due to ongoing misdiagnosis or undiagnosed cases of the disorder. One of my friends has both cervical dystonia and spasmodic dysphonia. Both his CD and SD fluctuate in terms of severity, but he has found treatments that help (intrathecal Baclofen pump, Botox, and oral medications) to where he is easily 75% more clear sounding than he once was. His CD has also been well managed. His testimonial can be found in chapter 15.

Testimonial
I decided to get Botox about 3 months ago and it has helped me a good 70%. When I'm around large crowds my neck still wants to act up though. But man, I'm pretty happy with the results. It gives me more freedom and I look normal again!! It's not the best scenario but much better than it has been in years. I'm still hoping that with gentle stretching I can keep it at bay. My specialist says Botox can wear off in about 2-3 months. I was actually really scared to have the shots done. I cried after receiving the injections (after I left the office) because my reaction to the Botox was now out of my control. After 4 days, when I realized I wasn't going to choke to death or suddenly stop breathing, I calmed down. It took a little over a month to see its full effect.

198

Testimonial

I was nearly 60 when I developed stiffness in my neck before I realized it was dystonia. By that age, I was already generally less supple than when I was younger. I turned to Botox shots and the ST Recovery Clinic program for relief. I found that I could not do many of the ST Clinic exercises so I eventually stuck to about six I could do and left it at that. It worked for me, although I still get Botox every 3 months.

For those who are on Botox, my experience is that for at least 2 weeks after the injections, one should exercise very gently. The injections kick in at different rates; some in a few days and others in ten days or more. In that time, the dynamics of the neck are changed and doing the same exercises to the same extent as previously may result in injury (I have made this mistake many times). Then one has to rest the neck completely for a couple of weeks which is obviously counter-productive.

The first two neurologists I consulted over a period of 12 years would assess my neck on each visit and change the 'recipe' claiming that different muscles were affected since my last visit. My head has always tilted towards the right shoulder and rotated to the left. Two movements are more difficult to treat than a single one. In the last 5 years I have a new neurologist who got the injections pretty well right from the first visit and, while he does assess my neck on each visit, he has never changed the recipe. I have done so much better under this regimen. I no longer have a good set of injections followed by a bad set of injections.

Testimonial

My cervical dystonia symptoms started in the fall of 1990 at the age of 48. My symptoms started just after I had inguinal hernia surgery. I believe the anesthetic may have triggered the symptoms. I don't have anything to back this up, but it is believed that some anesthetics may trigger dystonic reactions. My first line of attack was to see a chiropractor. I went to him for a few weeks and his diagnosis was wry neck. I wasn't getting better under his care and he had no idea what he was dealing with so he referred me to a more experienced chiropractor. After a couple of visits it was obvious that this doctor also had no idea what my problem was.

I then went to my family doctor who also had no idea what was wrong. He referred me to a neurologist who finally diagnosed it as dystonia and prescribed an oral medication, the name of which I do not remember. He then referred me to Dr. Joseph Jankovic at Baylor College of Medicine, Movement Disorders Department, one of the most respected doctors in the country on dystonia. His recommendation was to start on Botox. I waited four months before starting Botox. The two main reasons were because I didn't like the idea of injecting poison into my body, even if it was diluted many times, and I was torn because my theology stressed a strong belief in God's healing powers.

In the meantime, I took the oral medication first prescribed to me. I also learned that if I put my left hand against my neck it would loosen me up. It was a sensory trick that gave me a little relief before I knew there was such a thing as a sensory trick.

It was getting difficult to do my work so I began taking more medication. The regular dosage wasn't helping much. Unfortunately, I began having side effects from the larger dosage such as sleep walking, dry stools, and a very dry nasal area. The worst was that I would lose my train of thought in mid-sentence.

Everything came to a head in an important meeting for a job I was managing. I lost my train of thought in the middle of a sentence and changed to another topic. I'm not sure what the others thought about the kinds of drugs I might be taking, but they knew I was having difficulty with my neck. I was fortunate that they assumed the best and told me to go home until I was better. This led to a two year disability. I never thought it would take so long to get better.

I didn't want to get Botox so I stayed home and tried to deal with the symptoms the best I could. In the beginning I had some tremors which made it difficult to go to sleep. I would lie awake in bed for hours. The muscle tightness in my neck was so bad that I could barely be on my feet long enough to take a shower. After a shower I would run to bed to get comfortable. I spent my days lying in bed or in a sleeping bag on the floor.

It wasn't long before I couldn't sit up to do normal paperwork for the family banking or anything unless I was leaned over to support my neck. It is pretty unhandy to do many things from that position. I didn't drive for more than a year.

One of the unfortunate results of not getting Botox soon after having the symptoms was that the muscles and tendons shortened and I lost range of motion because of the delay in starting treatment. When I decided it was time to get Botox, they started me on a low dosage at first and built it up over the next 6 months which brought me back to somewhat normal, but I have never recovered full range of motion.

I went back to work part time after being off for two years. I was still uncomfortable, but I could get by. After a couple of months I started working full time. I continued to improve. I started playing tennis and getting into some sort of shape. It was so great to be back to almost normal. Then around December of 2000 I had Botox injections that didn't seem to work. I had a test for antibodies to Botox which was inconclusive. My doctor tried Myobloc. It didn't help much, but I stayed with it. I soon found it was not fun playing tennis anymore so I gave it up.

In 2005, I went to Baylor for my regular Myobloc shots. Dr. Jankovic was unavailable so I saw another doctor. She mistakenly ordered Botox rather than Myobloc and was almost done with my injections before I remarked that the syringes looked smaller. It turned out to be Botox, not Myobloc. She was embarrassed, but it couldn't be undone so we decided to see if I still had a resistance to Botox. To my delight, Botox worked so I switched back.

To further help me manage my symptoms, I take Klonopin (clonazepam), and Artane (trihexyphenidyl). Something I feel has hurt me is that I have gotten out of the habit of exercising. I am in poor physical condition so I am considering getting back into tennis and/or joining a gym, but overall I am doing very well.

Testimonial

When my condition first manifested, my head would pull severely to the left so I was looking over my left shoulder and in quite a lot of pain. After searching the internet for ideas on the best ways to get relief from my symptoms, I decided to get the Long Distance Recovery Program put together by Abbie Brown at the ST Recovery Clinic. I dedicated myself to the exercise program hoping that the more effort I put in, the more relief I would get. Wanting instant results, I overdid it and paid the price. My condition became worse than it was before I started and the pain was increasing. My muscles were being aggravated even further and began to fight back.

About 3 months after starting the program, I had my first appointment for Botox treatment. I had hoped to be able to do without the treatment, but I was in pain and fed up so I decide to go for it. My wife drove me to the appointment while I lay flat in the back seat of the car to get some relief from the pain. About a week later the pulling to the left began to ease and it has never been as bad since. The Botox enabled me to be more aggressive with my exercises and by the time the next appointment came round, I was feeling good enough to pass up on further treatment. It didn't mean that I was back to normal but my condition became a lot easier to live with than before.

After the pulling to the left eased, I started to find it more difficult to turn to the right. This has continued to the present day in some respects, but at the beginning I had to turn my whole trunk if I needed to look to the right. Driving became difficult any time I had to look over my right shoulder and I can remember giving way on filter lanes, not being able to turn to see what was coming.

My condition was always better when I wasn't working and at home on weekends. I could have a weekend barely noticing I had dystonia and then return to work on Monday and stiffen up again, but it's something I learned to live with.

As I began the Christmas holidays in 2011, my symptoms went from pulling to the left and not being able to turn to the right, to my head pulling left and down. It was like starting over again and caused me quite a bit of stress. I was convinced as I went into the new year that I wouldn't be able to go back to work, but I started on a strict regime of exercises from the ST Clinic Program again and it wasn't long before things started to improve. I went back to work again and also booked myself for Botox to see if it could also help.

This time around, Botox had a big effect on me. I've had it four times since, each treatment 4 months apart. It's helped me become better every time to the point that now sometimes I forget that there's anything wrong with me. The whole experience of going backwards and developing new symptoms scared me enough to never relax my routine again. I now know what it takes for me to keep the more serious symptoms away and I'm prepared to put the work in. I've seen the alternative.

Testimonial
My dystonia began in 2003, but years before I had a very sore neck and shoulders. I also had some trouble with my right ear; ringing, dizziness, and slight loss of hearing. I was a school teacher and during the summer I noticed my head starting to pull to the right. I wasn't too concerned until October. It was getting worse so I went to see my doctor. He first took me off two medications I was taking, Lipitor and Reglan, because he though they might be causing it. He then sent me for x-rays. Of course nothing showed up and it kept getting worse so I went back fairly quickly to see him. Thankfully, he figured out what I had and sent me to a neurologist. Unfortunately, it took about 3 years to find a good neurologist who really knew what he was doing.

In November of 2003 I had to quit working. It was just too painful. The only relief I got was when I was lying down, so that's what I did almost all the time. I started to get depressed. I went from a pretty active life to doing nothing.

I couldn't take it anymore so I made the choice to get up and start moving a little at a time. I knew lying there getting depressed wasn't good for me. I was going to do what I could. My head was pretty much stuck to my right shoulder so I wasn't able to drive. Losing my independence was very difficult, but I learned to accept help from others and trusted that God had me in this place for a reason.

In 2006, I began seeing a doctor at USC that specializes in movement disorders. I had been seeing another doctor there who was injecting me with Myobloc. It wasn't helping. He kept upping the dose each visit, but still no relief. When I finally got to see the doctor that I'm seeing now, he first injected me with Myobloc and still nothing. The next time, Botox was "accidentally" ordered, but I don't believe in accidents. I believe God sent it. It was the first time I ever got relief!! Each time after that it seemed to get a little better. Then my head started to pull backwards! I couldn't believe it! It took quite a few trips for my doctor to really see it but when he did, I finally started getting relief for that also. During all this time I was also trying physical therapy and massage. Both seemed to help some, but it didn't last. Although, I did learn some things in physical therapy that helped me cope with daily living.

In 2010, I heard about Dr. Demerjian who specializes in TMJ treatment for people with movement disorders. One time he showed up at a support group meeting because he wanted to learn more about dystonia. Another time he came to speak and test people for TMJ disorder using popsicle sticks. When he stuck them in my mouth (on my back teeth) and I bit down, I could feel some instant relief in my neck and shoulders. In September 2010, I decided to go see him to get fitted for an oral orthotic. It hasn't given me as much relief from my symptoms as I would like, but it has definitely helped. It helps take some of the pressure off my neck and shoulders, and relieve some of the pain I am experiencing. I still get Botox every 3 months and find the two together give me great improvement.

I still continue to see a chiropractor, a PT periodically, and a massage therapist. Since I'm unable to work, I spend as much time as I can volunteering. I spend 2-3 afternoons a week helping kids with their homework. I help one of my friends, a Kindergarten teacher, in her classroom for a couple of hours each week. I help with the children's ministry at my church. I am also co-leader of a dystonia support group in the LA area and attend a support group in the Orange County area.

I believe God brought this into my life for a reason, so I try to help as many people as I can with this disorder. I think it's good to share stories to let others know what works for us. This disorder is always changing and different for every person so I encourage people to find doctors who specialize in movement disorders to get the best help they can. I'm also very open to non-traditional treatments. Whatever works!

Phenol therapy

Phenol, also known as carbolic acid, is an anesthetic drug given by injection. This drug is used in patients with spasticity where the muscles are overactive. Phenol acts as a chemical neurolytic agent, which means that it works as a nerve block by temporarily destroying nerve pathways to prevent over-activity in specific muscles. These nerve pathways eventually grow back.

Phenol therapy is done by attaching small electrodes to the skin over the muscle and nerve areas that will be injected. The electrodes are attached to an Electromyography machine (EMG). The EMG is used to be sure the needle is in the right place before the phenol injection, similar to how neurotoxins are administered. The amount of phenol you receive depends on the degree of spasticity and groups of muscles involved. The phenol is injected around the nerve using a small needle attached to the EMG.

The physician may inject small amounts of phenol into several locations along the nerve or within several muscle or nerve groups to get the most benefit. The advantage of using phenol is that you see the effect immediately after the treatment and it may last for six months. Because every patient is different, the degree of relief will vary from person to person. Patients should resume activity slowly and carefully following the administration of phenol.

The most common side effects are pain during injection, dysethesia (a burning, tingling sensation), and swelling where the phenol was injected. Less common side effects include skin sloughing (rubbing off), motor weakness, sensory loss, and injection site infection. Serious side effects such as tremors, convulsions, slow breathing, fatigue, drowsiness, shortness of breath, and chest pain are very rare. Like botulinum toxin, phenol is an ongoing treatment for the relief of symptoms only. It is not a cure.[5]

Oral medications

There are no drugs specifically for dystonia, but several classes of drugs have been found effective for various forms of dystonia. These medications are used "off-label", meaning they are approved to treat conditions other than dystonia but have been found effective for easing dystonia symptoms. Please note that the response to medications varies among individuals and even in the same person over time. Pain medications are not discussed, as the list is too long and varied from over the counter NSAIDS -Nonsteroidal anti-inflammatory drugs- (acetaminophen, ibuprofen, naproxen, etc.) to prescription narcotics.

Anticholinergic agents block the effects of the neurotransmitter acetylcholine, which is involved in controlling a number of involuntary functions in the body. Drugs in this group include Artane (trihexyphenidyl) and Cogentin (benztropine).

Dopaminergic agents act on the dopamine system and the neurotransmitter dopamine, which helps control muscle movement, among many other things. When there is a deficiency in dopamine in the brain, movements may become delayed and uncoordinated. An example is dopamine-responsive dystonia, or dopa-responsive dystonia (DRD), also known as Segawa's disease, which most commonly affects children. It is sometimes referred to as DYT5 dystonia which is a dominantly inherited condition. When this gene is impaired and cannot fully accomplish the task of producing dopamine, the levels of dopamine in the body are compromised and a person will have problems with movement. It is often managed with Levodopa (L-dopa). Levodopa is often combined with Carbidopa (Sinemet and Atamet) to reduce nausea.

If there is an excess of dopamine, the brain causes the body to make unnecessary repetitive movements. In this case, people may benefit from drugs that block the effects of dopamine, such as Xenazine (tetrabenazine).

Antispasticity medications include Zanaflex (tizanidine), Catapress (clonidine), Dantrium (dantrolene), and Baclofen, also known as Chlorophenibut (brand names Beklo, Baclosan, Gablofen, Kemstro, Lioresal, Liofen, and Lyflex).

Antidepressants are used in the pharmaceutical treatment of dystonia if it is accompanied with depression. However, there is a dilemma with antidepressants because some are thought to contribute to the onset and/or exacerbation of dystonia symptoms. This varies from person to person, but something to keep in mind. Some of the more common antidepressants are Elavil (amitripyline), Tofranil (imipramine) Pamelor (nortriptyline), Zoloft (sertralene), Paxil (paroxetine), Effexor (venlafaxine), Wellbutrin (bupropion), Lexapro (escitalopram), and Cymbalta (duloxetine).[6]

GABAergic agents are drugs that regulate the neurotransmitter GABA (gamma-aminobutyric acid). GABA is the chief inhibitory neurotransmitter in the central nervous system and is responsible for the regulation of muscle tone. It is known as the brain's calming neurotransmitter.

Benzodiazepines are probably the most well known GABAergic drugs and also the class of drugs most commonly prescribed for dystonia. They include Ativan (lorazepam), Klonopin (clonazepam), Xanax (alprazolam), Valium (diazepam), Restoril (temazepam), and many others (see Table 1 below).[7, 8]

Some people are prescribed more than one benzodiazepine at a time, such as Klonopin and Valium, which may also be prescribed with other medications, such as Baclofen. Baclofen is a skeletal muscle relaxant and anti-spastic medication that is closely linked to GABA.

A large number of benzodiazepines are available to us (see Table 1) and there are significant differences in potency. Equivalent doses vary as much as 20-fold. For example, 0.5mg of Klonopin (clonazepam) is approximately equivalent to 10mg of Valium (diazepam). Thus, a person on only 1mg of Klonopin daily is taking the equivalent in strength of about 20mg of Valium.

These differences in strength have not always been fully appreciated by doctors. Thus, people on potent benzodiazepines such as Xanax, Ativan, or Klonopin tend to be using relatively large doses. This has implications on effectiveness, side effects, tolerance, tapering, and withdrawal.

Benzodiazepines also differ in the speed at which they are metabolized in the liver and eliminated from the body in the urine. For example, the half-life (time taken for the blood concentration to fall to half its initial value after a single dose) for Halcyon (triazolam) is only 2-5 hours, while the half-life of Valium is 20-100 hours with active metabolites from 36-200 hours. This means that half the active products of Valium are still in the bloodstream up to 200 hours after a single dose. With repeated daily dosing, accumulation occurs and high concentrations can build up in the body.[9]

Table 1: BENZODIAZEPINES AND SIMILAR DRUGS[5]

Benzodiazepines[5]	Half-life (hrs) [active metabolite][1]	Market Aim[2]	Approximately Equivalent Oral dosages (mg)[3]
Alprazolam (Xanax)	6-12	a	0.5
Bromazepam (Lexotan, Lexomil)	10-20	a	5-6
Chlordiazepoxide (Librium)	5-30 [36-200]	a	25
Clobazam (Frisium)	12-60	a, e	20
Clonazepam (Klonopin, Rivotril)	18-50	a, e	0.5
Clorazepate (Tranxene)	[36-200]	a	15

Diazepam (Valium)	20-100 [36-200]	a	10
Estazolam (ProSom)	10-24	h	1-2
Flunitrazepam (Rohypnol)	18-26 [36-200]	h	1
Flurazepam (Dalmane)	[40-250]	h	15-30
Halazepam (Paxipam)	[30-100]	h	20
Ketazolam (Anxon)	30-100 [36-200]	a	15-30
Loprazolam (Dormonoct)	6-12	h	1-2
Lorazepam (Ativan)	10-20	a	1
Lormetazepam (Noctamid)	10-12	h	1-2
Medazepam (Nobrium)	36-200	a	10
Nitrazepam (Mogadon)	15-38	h	10
Nordazepam (Nordaz, Calmday)	36-200	a	10
Oxazepam (Serax, Serenid, Serepax)	4-15	a	20
Prazepam (Centrax)	[36-200]	a	10-20
Quazepam (Doral)	25-100	h	20
Temazepam (Restoril, Normison, Euhypnos)	8-22	h	20
Triazolam (Halcion)	2	h	0.5
Non-benzodiazepines with similar effects [4,5]			
Zaleplon (Sonata)	2	h	20
Zolpidem (Ambien, Stilnoct)	2	h	20
Zopiclone (Zimovane, Imovane)	5-6	h	15
Eszopiclone (Lunesta)	6 (9 in elderly)	h	3

Reprinted with permission from Dr. Heather Ashton: *Benzodiazepines and Similar Drugs, Table 1, Benzodiazepines: How They Work & How to Withdraw*, Professor C H Ashton DM, FRCP. www.benzo.org.uk/manual/

1. Half-life: time taken for blood concentration to fall to half its peak value after a single dose. Half-life of active metabolite shown in square brackets. This time may vary considerably between individuals.

2. Market aim: although all benzodiazepines have similar actions, they are usually marketed as anxiolytics (a), hypnotics (h) or anticonvulsants (e).

3. These equivalents do not agree with those used by some authors. They are firmly based on clinical experience but may vary between individuals.

4. These drugs are chemically different from benzodiazepines but have the same effects on the body and act by the same mechanisms.

5. All these drugs are recommended for short-term use only (2-4 weeks maximum).

My experience with benzodiazepines

In April 2002, roughly 8 months after my symptoms began and about 3 months after they became severe, I couldn't take the pain, spasms, and muscle pulling any longer. I didn't want to take any medication, but I had to do something to get some relief. I researched the most common medications for dystonia and found Klonopin (clonazepam), a benzodiazepine, which seemed to be effective and widely used. My doctor agreed that it would be good for me to take.

I began with .5mg of Klonopin three times a day. It helped a lot. In a couple weeks my pain went down and my spasms were not as severe. My mood improved as well. However, I was still not sleeping well so I was prescribed 30mg of Restoril (temazepam), a benzodiazepine used for insomnia.

Within a couple of years, the medications were not helping as much so my doctor increased Klonopin to 3mg/day (as much as 6-8mg for a short period of time) and Restoril to 60mg/night. He also decided it would be good if I went on Baclofen to help with spasticity. I started at 30mg/day which was eventually increased to 60mg/day. By 2004, I was taking 3mg of Klonopin, 60mg of Restoril, and 60mg of Baclofen; quite a potent cocktail of medications.

Using Table 1 above, 3mg of Klonopin is equivalent in strength to 60mg of Valium and 60mg of Restoril is equivalent in strength to 30mg of Valium. I was taking the equivalent of 90mg of Valium a day. I didn't think twice about it because 3mg of Klonopin sounded like a small amount and I was led to believe that 60mg of Restoril was also a small dose. However, if I were prescribed 90mg of Valium (the equivalent strength to what I was taking), red flags would have been flying around like crazy. Add in 60mg of Baclofen and I was pretty heavily drugged.

In September 2007, my doctor and I decided that I should start going off my medications since I was doing much better physically. My diligent efforts following a customized exercise routine, healthy eating, at home therapies, massage, and stress management (things I neglected for the previous 5 years) significantly reduced my dystonia symptoms. He also wanted me to go off my medications because I was experiencing what seemed like side effects. Little did we know, I was actually in benzodiazepine withdrawal.

He reduced Klonopin from 3mg to 2mg, Restoril from 60mg to 30mg, and Baclofen from 60mg to 30mg. Within two weeks I began to experience very bizarre symptoms. Still thinking it was side effects, my doctor tapered me even more! This of course made everything worse. Below is a partial list of my symptoms and the severity varied throughout the day:

- My body felt like it was swaying back and forth; like I was stuck in cement and my body was heaving in a strong wind.
- I felt like I was on a boat bobbing up and down in the ocean, especially when standing.
- When standing and walking it felt like I was on an unstable surface, like slippery rocks or a sheet of ice.
- The floor felt soft as if I was sinking into it with each step. I often had to stand on tip toes to reduce this feeling.
- The floor and walls looked like they were moving.
- My head did not feel attached to my body. It felt like it was floating or being pulled off.
- My skin felt like it was dripping off my bones and I was invisible.
- Anxiety and depersonalization.
- Severe muscle weakness; my arms and legs felt like telephone poles.
- Vertigo and tinnitus.
- High sensitivity to visual and auditory stimuli.

These symptoms lasted for nearly two years. In that time I went to neurologists, an internist, a physiatrist, general medical doctors, chiropractors, physical therapists, ENT's, and eye doctors. I also had blood tests, an MRI, and cat scans. Everything was normal. No one knew what was wrong with me and not a single person ever mentioned the possibility of benzodiazepine withdrawal.

Since none of these symptoms manifested in my physical appearance, convincing doctors and others how sick I felt was very difficult and frustrating. Plus, during this time my dystonia, miraculously, pretty much disappeared which added to the difficulty in diagnosis.

My symptoms were so severe at times that I literally thought I was dying. It was like I was not in my body. I was so weak that lifting a glass of water to my mouth felt like a 10 pound weight. There were numerous times when I was standing and wondering how I could possibly remain upright because I was so weak and dizzy. I couldn't feel my arms or legs sometimes and any tiny visual or auditory stimuli would shock my system to such an extent that I would have to lie down because of how exhausted it made me. At times, benzodiazepine withdrawal was worse than some of my dystonia symptoms at their most severe. It was very scary, to put it mildly.

Unlike some people who go through benzodiazepine withdrawal, my cognitive abilities remained intact. In some ways they were actually heightened and my memory was clearer than it had ever been. Being so lucid baffled doctors. I looked healthy and came across as an intelligent, able-bodied person, making the benzodiazepine withdrawal diagnosis even more difficult. I eventually diagnosed myself.

I clearly didn't do my homework before I started taking Klonopin and Restoril because I had no idea that they are addictive and should be taken with great caution. Plus, no doctor ever told me about the potential problems of long term use. It wasn't until I began having bizarre symptoms five years later that I began to learn about benzodiazepines.

It is unfortunate how little many of us know about the affects of benzodiazepines. Even more unfortunate and surprising is how little some doctors seem to understand the true nature of these drugs. Many people I know who have taken them for any length of time have been affected in some way. While some experience uncomfortable side effects, withdrawal is also a problem because of their addictive quality. Some have compared the potency of benzodiazepines to heroin.

Withdrawal not only affects those who are tapering off benzodiazepines. It can also affect those who are taking their prescribed dose. The reason is because chronic exposure to benzodiazepines causes physical adaptations in the brain to counteract the drug's effects, which is known as tolerance. When the body builds up tolerance it needs more of the drug to maintain equilibrium. When more of the drug is not taken, numerous physical and psychological symptoms often occur. This is exactly what happened to me. I was taking the prescribed dose and had become tolerant without knowing it.

By incorrectly thinking my symptoms were medication side effects, I started to taper off them. Since it was withdrawal I was experiencing, what I should have done instead was increase my dose until I reached a comfortable level (comfortable meaning a reduction in symptoms) and then begin tapering slowly under close supervision; not the cavalier approach taken by my doctor. The reason for starting a taper from a comfortable level is to try and minimize withdrawal symptoms as the brain adjusts throughout the taper process.

As a result of my doctor's negligence and my lack of knowledge about what I was taking, I spent a year trying to get off my medications thinking they were causing my symptoms, but I was instead going through withdrawal and making things worse by continuing a rapid taper. When I figured out I was in withdrawal, I left my doctor to work with an addiction medicine specialist.

The first thing we did was increase Klonopin to reduce my symptoms. I then followed a taper plan designed by Dr. Heather Ashton, one of the leading experts on benzodiazepines. Please see her online manual called, *Benzodiazepines: How they work and how to withdraw*. It has some of the most comprehensive information I have found on the subject. Ashton's approach requires taking Valium and then tapering off Valium and the other benzodiazepines you are taking, all at the same time. The reason for adding Valium is because it has a very long half life so it is supposed to help reduce withdrawal symptoms as you taper, with the ultimate goal of being off all medications around the same time with little to no withdrawal symptoms.

Unfortunately, I ran into trouble with my dystonia and instead of tapering off all my medications, I used Valium to help me taper completely off Klonopin and Restoril, and reduce Baclofen from 60mg to 30mg. Although I am off Klonopin and Restoril, and taking less Baclofen, I am still taking Valium. Had I to do it all over again, I would have been sure to taper off Valium along with the other medications as suggested, and deal with my dystonia some other way; or I never would have introduced Valium in the first place.

Dr. Ashton's approach is successful for some and not for others, which is par for the course with pretty much all medications and treatments. To date, my dystonia and benzodiazepine withdrawal symptoms are pretty stable, but not where I would like to be. I still have work to do to get longer periods of relief. However, my life now is a stark contrast to the hell it once was.

As frustrating as it was, had I not seen numerous doctors, gotten extensive testing, and spent thousands of dollars looking for answers, I never would have narrowed my search and been able to diagnose myself. It was similar to what I went through before I self diagnosed dystonia.

With this in mind, please become as educated as you can and be your own best health advocate. Find a doctor who will be your partner in your health care, rather than one who follows their own agenda without your input. In the very beginning when you are still finding your treatment protocol, use as little medication as possible in its weakest form possible. It is much easier to move up the ladder than it is to come back down. Do not let your doctors over-drug you and before taking anything, research the drug itself (uses, side effects, how it is typically prescribed, addictive qualities, etc.) and then decide if it is right for you. It is always wise to err on the side of caution.

While it may appear that I have completely condemned benzodiazepines, I want to make it clear that I believe these medications can be very helpful, as they were for me, but to be very cautious regarding dosage and long term use. Each of us is different so not everyone who takes benzodiazepines experience or will experience what I did, but it is best to become as educated as possible. If you do experience withdrawal, please find a doctor who understands how to modify your intake or safely get you off the medication. If need be, please also get involved with the many online benzodiazepine support groups for help.

Testimonial

My first memory of feeling something was wrong was around 3 years ago. I felt this internal trembling that was not apparent to others. I just knew I didn't feel right. So I began the search to feel better. I went to my doctor who said it was anxiety, and I agreed. I've always been kind of an anxious person who worried a lot about illness. I figured I was making a mountain out of a molehill once again. I tried two different antidepressants which didn't work and she referred me to a psychologist. To rule out tumors or lesions in the brain, I was sent for an MRI, which was normal. I had more blood work done than ever, and other than low vitamin D and a few other minor things, all was okay. I saw 2-3 chiropractors, who ordered more X-rays, a naturopath, a life coach, had acupuncture, my eyes read (iridology), and made every adjustment I was told to do. I went gluten, dairy, red meat and soy free, and lost 15 pounds, of which I did not need to lose. Still, I could not shake the mild spasms and tremors.

Somewhere in the midst of that, I took my first Klonopin (clonazepam). I still recall how much it impacted me. God, it was good. I felt like myself again, actually better than my usual self. That started a whole new battle. In time, I realized my body had become addicted to Klonopin and I was in what they call "tolerance withdrawal." I thought my blood sugar had plummeted. My tongue was tight, pulse racing, and the trembling was worse. I searched the internet for "tight tongue" and the first hit was "benzodiazepine withdrawal." I couldn't believe it. I found a wonderful website for benzodiazepine withdrawal and learned how to properly wean off Klonopin, which took over a year.

Meanwhile, this other goofy thing was happening. When I bent over, my head would turn to the left. With everything else going on, I tried to put it out of my mind. Plus, I felt it might have been due to the Klonopin withdrawal. I was hoping it was. As I weaned further and further, it became more and more apparent it was not going away. In fact, it was getting worse and I began more internet searches. They say one can find things that really are not the actual diagnosis, but I was right. I knew I had cervical dystonia long before I was diagnosed. To top it off, I had my 2nd spot of skin cancer removed from my nose. A week later, I was done with work as a school teacher and I completely plummeted into pretty severe depression.

I was officially diagnosed with dystonia in June of 2012. I was numb. I set up my first Botox (Xeomin) appt in July and could not wait for the turning to feel better. But it didn't. It took 3 visits, 3 months apart each, to finally feel relief. By then, my head was turning to the left when I walked and I was having more pain. But I had started the ST Clinic program, so I thought maybe the seemingly sudden turn for the worse was due to the exercises. The jury is still out on that one. I went down to only working half days and felt the sadness creeping back in. But still, I had hope. I knew the ST Clinic program took time. I knew it would get worse before it got better, so I kept at it. A week after my January appointment, relief finally came. It wasn't perfect, but it was a glimpse of what I'd been praying for. A month later, I went back to work full time and was able to finish the school year in far better condition than my fears had me believing.

Thinking back to the fear, guilt, and anger I was gripping onto, I'm so thankful to be here right now. I was convinced my life was over; that I was headed for a life filled with pain and disfigurement. I won't claim that I've completely changed my ways and that I'm a new person. I still have a semi short temper, I get moody, and like things to be just so. BUT, it's on a different level. Things are let go much more easily now. I shift out of my "moods" and try to love more openly. I try to not act out of fear, but out of love and knowing we are all in this together. If dystonia brought me that, then I'm truly thankful.

I can honestly say that I try to appreciate everything, and not out of fear that some day I'll be in too much pain or too shaky to do what I can do today. But because now is all we have. To live in the future is to live in fear. To live in the past is to live in regret. I know my story has only begun, but it will be a fantastic one. I'll make sure of it! There is always a blessing in the midst of a storm.

Medications to avoid[10-12]

Below is a list of medications that are thought to possibly cause and/or exacerbate dystonia symptoms. This is not a complete list and the medications included may not cause a reaction in some. However, whenever possible, dystonia patients should probably avoid these medications, except at the recommendation of a physician knowledgeable in the treatment of dystonia.

When I was in college, I was put on one of the medications on this list (Dilantin/phenytoin) for a "seizure disorder." I had a total of four idiopathic tonic-clonic (grand mal) seizures over a three year period. To try and figure out the source of my seizures, I had an MRI, CAT scan, x-rays, blood work, and an EEG. Everything was normal and I had no signs of epilepsy. It was concluded that they were caused by stress. Instead of being taught stress management techniques, I was told to just stay on Dilantin. Since my seizures were so intense and scary, I decided to take it, not really sure what it was doing for me (I had two seizures while on it) or what it might be doing to me long term. Even though I had two seizures while taking it, I still believed that it provided me some level of protection. I was afraid, and told by doctors, that I might have more if I stopped taking it.

All of the seizures took place in my sleep, so it took me a while before I was able to go to bed without worrying about a seizure. When I finally got over the fear and learned some stress management techniques, I eventually stopped taking Dilantin. About 2-3 years later I noticed my first dystonia symptoms.

I do not know if taking Dilantin or going off Dilantin caused dystonia, but having been on it for 8+ years makes me wonder how much it may have played a role. I mention all this as a reminder to always check and then check again when given any recommendation about your health, no matter the source.

Medications to avoid[10-12]

Generic Name	Trade Name	Classification
Alprazolam	Xanax	Anti-anxiety
Amitriptyline	Elavil, Endep	Antidepressant
Amoxapine	Asendin	Antidepressant
Aripiprazole	Abilify	Neuroleptic

Benzquinamide	Emete-Con	Anti-nausea/vomiting
Bupropion	Wellbutrin	Antidepressant
Buspirone	Buspar	Anti-anxiety
Citalopram	Celexa	Antidepressant
Carbamazepine	Tegretol	Anticonvulsant
Chlorprothizene	Taractan	Neuroleptic
Chlorpromazine	Thorazine	Neuroleptic
Cimetidine	Tagamet	Gastrointestinal
Comipramine	Anafranil	Antidepressant
Clozapine	Clozaril	Neuroleptic
Desipramine	Norpramin	Antidepressant
Desvenlafaxine	Pristiq	Antidepressant
Diphenhydramine	Benadryl	Antihistamine
Doxepin	Adapin, Sinequan	Antidepressant
Droperidol	Inapsine	Neuroleptic
Duloxetine	Cymbalta	Antidepressant
Ergotamine	Cafergot	Antidepressant (MAOI)
Erythromycin	many brands	Antibiotic
Escitalopram	Lexapro	Antidepressant
Fluvoxamine	Luvox	Antidepressant
Fluoxetine	Prozac	Antidepressant
Fluphenazine	Prolixin	Neuroleptic
Gabapentin	Neurontin	Anticonvulsant
Haloperidol	Haldol	Neuroleptic
Imipramine	Tofranil	Antidepressant
Isocarboxazid	Marplan	Antidepressant (MAOI)
Levomilnacipran	Fetzima	Antidepressant
Linezolid	Zyvox	Antidepressant (MAOI)
Lithium	Eskalith, Lithobid	Anti-manic
Loxapine	Loxitane	Neuroleptic
Mesoridazine	Serentil	Neuroleptic
Metoclopramide	Reglan	Anti-nausea/vomiting

Midazolam	Versed	Induction anesthetic
Milnacipran	Ixel, Savella	Antidepressant
Molindone	Moban	Neuroleptic
Nortripyline	Aventyl, Pamelor	Antidepressant
Olanzapine	Zyrexa	Neuroleptic
Perhenazine	Trilafon	Neuroleptic
Paroxetine	Paxil	Antidepressant
Phenelzine	Nardil	Antidepressant (MAOI)
Luminal	Phenobarbital	Anticonvulsant
Phenytoin	Dilantin	Anticonvulsant
Pimozide	Orap	Neuroleptic
Prochlorperazine	Compazine	Anti-nausea/vomiting
Promazine	Sparine	Neuroleptic
Promethazine	Phenergan	Antihistamine
Protriptyline	Vivactil	Antidepressant
Quetiapine	Seroquel	Neuroleptic
Ranitidine	Ranitidine	Gastrointestinal
Risperidone	Risperdal	Neuroleptic
Sertraline	Zoloft	Antidepressant
Thiethylperazine	Torecan	Anti-nausea/vomiting
Thiothixene	Navane	Neuroleptic
Trifluoperazine	Stelazine	Neuroleptic
Triflupromazine	Vesprin	Neuroleptic
Thioridazine	Mellaril	Neuroleptic
Tiagabine	Gabitril	Anticonvulsant
Trazadone	Desyrel	Antidepressant
Trifluoperazine	Stelazine	Neuroleptic
Trimipramine	Surmontil	Antidepressant
Verapamil	Calan, Isoptin	Antianginal, Antihypertensive
Venlafaxine	Effexor	Antidepressant
Ziprasidone	Geodon	Neuroleptic

Surgical procedures for dystonia

Surgery for dystonia was first performed in 1641 by the German surgeon, Isaac Minnius. It involved cutting the muscles in the neck that were involved in torticollis. During the 19th century, a better understanding of the regions of the brain involved in movement helped surgeons address movement disorders through brain operations. The earliest surgeries for movement disorders involved removing these surface areas of the brain.

Victor Horsley, a British surgeon, was the first to describe a procedure where the primary motor cortex was removed to treat tremor. An American named A. Earl Walker later described a less invasive procedure in which the nerve fibers of primary motor cortex cells, connecting the brain to the spinal cord, were partially cut to produce weakness and relief of tremor. This procedure, called pediculectomy, remained popular until the 1950's.

In 1942, Russel Meyers first reported the effects of surgery on the basal ganglia for Parkinson's disease. He removed the caudate nucleus (a part of the basal ganglia) and found that tremor and rigidity improved without creation of weakness.

Later surgeons improved upon this technique, introducing heat or cold to create a permanent lesion in the brain. Once doctors realized that lesions of specific structures deep within the brain could treat individuals safely and effectively, surgery for movement disorders began in earnest. Over time, surgeons became more precise with what brain structures to treat.

Understanding that the brain is an organ where cells communicate with each other through chemical and electrical signals, in 1973, Yoshibo Hosobuchi was the first to perform chronic deep brain stimulation using implanted electrodes for the treatment of pain. This technology was adapted from the heart pacemaker, which was introduced in 1958.

In 1987, Alim Louis Benabid, a French neurosurgeon, found that chronic stimulation of the thalamus resulted in disappearance of tremor. He later reported successful long term stimulation of the pallidal (a major component of the basal ganglia) in the treatment of Parkinson's disease.

These discoveries are among the most significant in the field of modern brain surgery for the treatment of movement disorders, as well as other neurological and psychiatric disorders.[13]

Deep Brain Stimulation (DBS)

Deep Brain Stimulation (DBS) is a technology using an implanted device to deliver electrical stimulation to the brain to help alleviate symptoms associated with movement disorders. The US Food and Drug Administration (FDA) approved DBS as a treatment for essential tremor in 1997, Parkinson's disease in 2002, and dystonia in 2003.

The idea of this surgery being a "last resort" is an evolving concept. Around 10 years ago, doctors were operating on only the most severely disabled patients. Now they are operating on patients with moderate-to-severe cases of Parkinson's, essential tremor, and dystonia. The thought is that this trend will continue. Instead of saying, "wait another five to ten years until you become more disabled," doctors are realizing that the earlier they use DBS, the more they can improve the quality of life of their patients. That being said, and although it is no longer considered experimental, DBS is still used as a second or third-line treatment. It is typically for patients with more advanced cases of their respective disease and those for whom medication alone is inadequate or cannot be adjusted precisely enough to keep their symptoms under control.

DBS surgery procedure

DBS surgery involves implanting stimulating electrodes into selected targets in the brain in order to mimic the effects of lesioning (removal of an injured or diseased area on or in the body). The procedure is performed with the patient awake, using only local anesthetic and occasional sedation. The basic surgical method is called stereotaxis, a method useful for approaching deep brain targets through a small skull opening about the size of a nickel.

To maximize the precision of the surgery, a brain mapping procedure is employed. Microelectrodes are used to record brain cell activity in the region of the intended target to confirm that it is correct. Brain mapping produces no sensation for the patient. The brain's electrical signals are played on an audio monitor so the surgical team can hear the signals and assess their pattern. Since each person's brain is different, the time it takes for mapping varies.

Once the brain target is mapped and identified, instead of creating a lesion, the surgeon places the DBS electrode into the target. The electrode is then tested. The testing does not focus on relief of dystonia, but rather on unwanted stimulation-induced side effects. This is because the beneficial effects of stimulation may take hours or days to develop, whereas any unwanted effects will be present immediately.

DBS surgery does not cure dystonia. When the stimulator is turned off or if it malfunctions, symptoms return. DBS can decrease the abnormal movements and postures of dystonia, but usually does not totally eliminate them. The degree of benefit appears to vary with both the type of dystonia and the duration of symptoms.[14]

The complete DBS apparatus includes the DBS electrode, a connecting wire, and a pulse generator/stimulator that contains a battery. All parts of the device are internal so there are no wires sticking out. The wire and pulse generator may be implanted at the same time as the electrode or at a later date. The generator is implanted under the collarbone and the wire is tunneled up the neck and behind the ear to the site of the electrode.

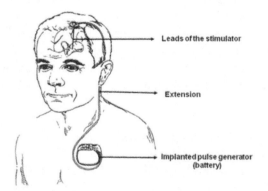

Reprinted with the permission of Medtronic, Inc. © 2005

Once the generator is implanted, the patient must wait a week or two before the batteries are activated. This waiting period is necessary to allow the swelling that normally occurs with surgery to diminish. The DBS electrode conveys electrical pulses into the brain using power produced by the battery in the generator. A series of visits to the doctor are required to adjust the voltage settings to the needs of the individual. It may take several weeks or months to achieve the correct settings. The patient can check the status of the generator using a handheld device that resembles a remote control. Using this device, the patient can determine if the generator is on or off, and can turn it back on in the event that it shuts down unexpectedly. Certain phenomenon such as magnetic fields caused by medical testing devices and security devices may cause the battery to temporarily stop working.

The expected life span of a battery at a typical voltage is about four years. At a very high voltage, the battery may need to be replaced after a year; at a very low voltage, perhaps up to seven years. There is now a rechargeable battery available which has an expected life span twice that of a standard DBS battery. Replacing a battery can be done under general or local anesthesia as an outpatient procedure.

Dystonia does not respond to DBS the same way as other movement disorders. For example, persons treated for tremor will generally improve within seconds of turning the generator on. In patients with dystonia, improvement may be delayed for days and weeks, or months may pass before full benefit is reached. DBS does not necessarily eliminate the possibility of subsequent drug or botulinum toxin treatments.

As previously mentioned, although no longer considered investigational, DBS is in its relatively early stages as a treatment for dystonia. The preliminary results are quite positive and the procedure is expected to evolve over time as more patients are treated and more data is collected.[15]

Testimonial

I woke up one morning in the early 1990's with a stiff or "wry neck." It was as though some invisible force was pulling my neck and I was resisting. The more I tried to resist the greater the pulling sensation became. I quickly developed spatial disorientation, began having falls, and developed an intoxicated gait, yet I continued working as a nurse in one of the busiest medical centers in the U.S.

Within months my neck was not getting any better and my head hung to one side weighing like a two ton rock. It was frozen in position, locked and causing intense discomfort. Life was getting difficult, almost unbearable. Not a single physician was able to diagnose my symptoms. Eventually, I self diagnosed by finding a picture of a woman with a similar condition in a neurology textbook.

By now my hands were gripping my hair in an effort to stop the violent twisting and turning of my neck. While this had the effect of stopping my head from flailing around, it was only a very short term solution to what was to become a lifelong problem.

When I walked, I looked like someone who had too much to drink. When using public transport I learned to run past people so I could get an unoccupied seat while at the same time avoiding those seats reserved on the public transit system for "the disabled" - after all I wasn't one of them! I tried wearing a soft cervical collar at work to control the twisting and spasms.

I hated looking in a mirror or at a photograph. I was distressed and upset at the person looking back at me. I didn't like that person. There were moments when I felt caged in by dystonia. I was lonely, isolated, and embarrassed in social settings. In public I began wearing a variety of scarves and sweaters that had collars to hide the physical distortion I saw in the mirror each day. I stopped wearing dresses. The mental anguish persisted, often in silence unbeknownst to family, friends, and colleagues.

Next began a long, tedious 13 year ordeal of being fed oral medications. Driving became impossible and I relocated to Manhattan where Botox was available to patients. It worked for a short while, but I soon became immune to its effects. I began getting Myobloc and derived benefits from this toxin for 8 years, even being able to ride my bicycle again.

Immunity to Myobloc eventually developed. The toxins were no longer working for me and oral medications were losing their effectiveness. I began investigating Deep Brain Stimulation (DBS). I didn't want to live in darkness when there was light. I was also tired of alternative or complementary care. I wanted a treatment that was more permanent and for me. DBS was it. I knew the procedure would help correct and diminish many of my dystonic symptoms. I wanted to live; to simply "be still ", yet live a life in motion.

I embarked on the meticulous journey into deep brain stimulation in December 2004. The operating room was filled with anesthesiologists, nurses, doctors, and electrophysiologists. I was surrounded by a staff of 15 people at all times. I felt no pain during the procedure except for a vibratory effect as my skull was drilled open. The operation began at 5:45am and was completed by 6pm. Within 24 hours of the operation, I was walking back to my apartment from the hospital eating and laughing. I was out on Fifth Avenue buying a new wardrobe that Sunday and attending mass at St. Patrick's Cathedral within 48 hours of undergoing brain surgery. I had not experienced any of the risks: seizures, stroke, hemorrhage, or frontal lobe headaches.

I returned for programming of my pacemaker in January 2005 with a new outlook on life. DBS had proven to be my ticket out of the realms of a devastating, debilitating disorder called dystonia. No longer must I plan every aspect of my life; no longer am I surrounded by dystonia or the despair of depression and pain. I was free to return to a life that had begun 15 plus years ago- a life filled with promise and hope. It was all rather amazing to me. The entire world seemed new to me. It was like I woke up from a bad dream and that the 15 plus years with dystonia didn't exist. I spent days just looking at things and commenting to myself how different things looked because I was not twisting, posturing, or in constant pain. Even colors looked different. I could wear high heels! It might sound ridiculous, but DBS had given me the start of a new life; one that I left so long ago and couldn't remember at that point. It was all about relearning life now.

First of all, let me make it absolutely clear that DBS is not a cure for any type of dystonia. Second, each type of dystonia responds differently to DBS settings. Third, don't assume that what another person experiences with DBS is what you will experience with your own settings, programming etc. Fourth, there are no set guidelines for DBS and selection of patient criteria.

In February 2005, I returned to work which proved to be immensely tiring. Assignments were heavier than before during those 12 hour shifts. By March I felt like a sinking ship. My gait became weaving in nature again, and I couldn't keep my hands out of my hair to hold my neck in place. I was leaning against walls again. I no longer felt fluid in my movements. They had no beginning, middle, or end. Was this the way it was with programming? Was this so-called DBS a success? Adjusting to DBS was not just adjusting to new settings, but it also involved adjusting to a new set of life circumstances. I began recognizing that DBS was a life-changing event emotionally, physically, socially, and mentally. I am not too sure if I was as well prepared as I should have been at the start of DBS. There was so much to learn.

I still did not understand how frequently adjustments or reprogramming were in order for me. I felt lost about programming. Voltages, amplitudes, pulse rates and widths. It all seemed like a foreign language in me. I was frustrated and distressed. I also began noticing a pattern. My settings were clearly lasting only 6 to 7 weeks at a time. 20% of my battery had already been used up. What was it about my dystonia that was making it so hard to ensure success? Was this happening to others with dystonia as well? Was I emotionally undone at this point? What was my programmer going to think of me? What about my neurosurgeon? I wasn't in the mood to see him anyway. I didn't give a hoot about programming, my neurosurgical team, voltages, DBS, dystonia, or pretty much anything at this point. I wasn't as tough as I was always being portrayed. I was on a new journey. I wasn't on top of society life either. Life was new and right now I was a real human being with too many chaotic-like emotions. Least of all, I didn't know what was coming next for me.

Labor Day was nearing and my body began feeling the effects of dystonia again. I wanted to punch a wall. I solicited some of my other DBS friends for their suggestions and sent a letter to my neurosurgeon about device improvements. We all wanted a rechargeable battery. The current design felt too clumsy and bulky. I was still afraid to use it. My symptoms steadily, but menacingly, returned over an 11 day period while I was on vacation with my family.

While visiting the new Super Walmart on vacation, for some unknown reason I decided to check my IPG (Implantable Pulse Generator) battery, to see if things were working properly. A yellow light appeared indicating that my IPG was in the OFF mode. I became frantic. I turned myself back on and needless to say, ended up with a power surge erupting in my head followed by my usual over-stimulation side effects of headaches and nausea. At one point I thought I had gone into a cardiac arrhythmia. That was the last thing I needed. My neurosurgeon concluded that the store's anti-theft detectors had most likely turned me off.

My symptoms felt 10 times worse than they did before DBS. What had I gotten myself into? Was this the right decision? DBS was only a band-aid. This I clearly understood. Yet frustration levels soared. I didn't know what to believe; who to believe, least of all myself. Did I truly have the finesse to be able to live with the hardware, its pitfalls and successes on a continuous basis? I wanted to, but was unsure of how to do so. I also felt at a loss for how to troubleshoot the system independently without the help of anyone.

As an ICU nurse, I learned the skills to problem solve patient issues and equipment failures in a matter of minutes. Now I couldn't even problem solve my own device. However, I was beginning to understand that stress, lack of sleep, and fatigue played a role in how well I coped with the hardware. These were 3 factors that I dealt with rather confidently over the years. Having them chopped like fine tuna was scary, demoralizing, and unsettling.

I arrived at my one year post DBS anniversary filled with too many expectations that were not explained to me prior to the procedure. I felt raw, awkward, and misplaced. I felt dreadfully lonely; like I was the only person on the planet with the device.

A year came and went and I was still learning about the DBS system. It had its successes, but pitfalls and failures also existed. One of the most important points to make is those considering DBS should examine themselves as individuals, persons with dystonia, their emotional levels, DBS expectations, and coping mechanisms. It is also essential that those considering DBS become as well-informed as they can and find qualified physicians who perform the procedure.

I think Roberta Rubin-Greenberg, a skilled programmer in California, said it best, "The thing to emphasize is that even though the surgery is the big dramatic moment, it is only the first step in the DBS journey. Once one is implanted, one is far from being *done. Sadly, patients give little thought to how and where they will receive this care, even though, really, it requires equal or even greater consideration than the implanting decision. Patients need to place thought into what they're going to do when they get home after traveling thousands of miles for the implant. But regardless, they are still traveling miles and searching with little educational back-up. Good programmers are few and far between. A great additional need is to bring programming up in its stature and recognizing it for the special talents that it requires. However, basic scopes of practice need to be conveyed with patients being educated on these guidelines and individual DBS expectations."*

No one could tell that I had a movement disorder at times with proper programming. Yet, as time went by, programming became more difficult and time-consuming. Finding those optimal settings was tricky and would cause many side-effects including leg dragging, loss of speech, hoarseness, loss of verbal understanding (expressive aphasia that is seen in stroke patients), gait difficulties, and tingling of the limbs during the sessions. My neurosurgeon, Dr. Mike, and I continued to try and find the right settings. With time we eventually did, but it was an exhausting, strenuous, laborious, and arduous time. Anyone not expecting this during programming is being unrealistic about this process. Worrying about the Halo Frame and loss of hair is meager compared to the aftermath of DBS surgery and long term effects.

Feelings of darkness, hopelessness, doom, gloom, and despair continued with my mother calling me practically every day for months. I felt disappointed that programming was now an ongoing issue. Then BOOM! We found the right settings and for 9 months I was able to work solely in the Open Heart Unit without any programming at all. Life was good again. My mood improved as I worked and traveled.

By September 2007, I really had no complaints. It had been a long, rocky, and winding road. However, from nursing colleagues I began hearing comments that DBS had changed me, tweaked my brain in the process, altering my personality. What could I do? Had I changed personality wise? I really couldn't tell you if this is true or not. Physically, the feelings of doom had left me with immense weight loss- 110 pounds, Height 5'8. Some said that I was now perfect for running down a fashion runway as a model. Foolish!

The Effexor XL I was taking was slowly tapered which led to an increase in dystonia symptoms, pain, and DBS headaches. Klonopin became the drug of choice for me. Difficulty walking again became routine. Planning life became a routine again. Sleeping on ice packs to diminish the pain became a norm. Heat did nothing for me. I was wearing a soft cervical collar again. In reality, dystonia had been waxing and waning for the past year, yet everyone else with dystonia desperately wanted to know "how well DBS was working for me?" I would really limit my answers. I desperately wanted DBS to last. I tried to ignore the return of symptoms.

After all, I had not experienced any lead breakages, wire breaks, lead migration, infections, or battery changes. Yet, with each programming session, we noticed that I required less and less voltages to obtain sensitization to the settings. Scientific papers were now describing the loss of optimal DBS effects occurring between years 3 and 5 for all 3 disorders – Parkinson's, Tremor, and Dystonia. This was utterly disappointing; a loss, defeat, failure; 100% unexpected. Twisting returned along with a diagnosis of thoracic 6 thru 10 disc degeneration and fractures. Back pain!

As I read the "Neurotic Adventures of a Law Student", I was forced to face that there was a very good possibility that DBS might not last as long as my battery would. I had faced the Neurotic Adventures of DBS, but failure had never been in the picture. Nor had I even been told that was a possibility. So, what now? My last programming session resulted in two high jolt-like electrical shocks. I thought I had been electrocuted. I recall leaving the office, finding myself in the cereal isle of a local bodega, then crawling into bed and not waking up for 36 hours. I suspected I had experienced a sub-clinical seizure of some sort as I had no recall of being in the supermarket. Generally, brain fatigue and fog is not an uncommon experience after a programming session.

There was something else Dr. Mike and I observed over that year. It had to do with electromagnetic forces or EMI. I worked in settings that contained an immense amount of electrical equipment, especially the Open Heart Unit. Physical electrical forces in each of the 4 ICUs I worked in were completely different. Each affected me and altered my settings, thus bringing about a return of symptoms. This phenomenon was unexpected. Taking notice of your employment setting is critical when you have DBS.

I've now passed my 8th year anniversary, 2013, years filled with chaotic, chilling and unexpected, but indecisive emotions along with social and physical changes. There are no guarantees or set rules and outcomes to the procedure. There have been ups and downs, and successes and setbacks filled with emotions and coping challenges that were unexpected.

As I finish this portion of my journey, I want to note that each person's journey with DBS is different. What I have experienced is not what you may experience. There is no-cookie cutter recipe for DBS or dystonia today. Yet, you need to be aware that programming is the greatest problematic issue that goes along with the procedure. Anyone telling you otherwise is minimizing this problem.

DBS is not a cure for your dystonia. You will have highs and lows. Also, be aware that you may require medications to manage certain physical, cognitive, and emotional effects. Socially, life can improve to a certain extent, but over-expectations can be detrimental, especially since dystonic symptom breakthroughs can occur at anytime. Physical adjustments include simply feeling comfortable and an inner sense of peace with an implantable device.

It took about 3 years for me to feel safe with the device and hardware in my brain that could go array at anytime. I have also learned what to avoid and the strength of electromagnetic fields on individual settings. What lies ahead I'm not so sure. I went for the rechargeable battery in May 2013...

Testimonial

My dystonia symptoms started in 1984 while I was going through a divorce. I had slight movement and pain in my neck, but dystonia wasn't diagnosed until 1990 when my neck locked to the right. It also started to move all the time and it was very painful. After a couple of years, the dystonia spread to my back causing me to lean over to the right quite badly. This started to affect my mobility.

In 2001, I heard about Deep Brain Stimulation surgery (DBS) while I was on holiday. As soon as I got home I went to see a neurologist at the Hallamshire Hospital where I was informed that there was no funding for this operation in the area where I lived. This news hit me hard, but after talking to family and friends I decided to try and raise the money myself. I also got my local MP (Member of Parliament) involved and she helped a lot.

I wrote to all major soccer and cricket clubs, as well as supermarkets and department stores. I was inundated with gifts to auction and raffle off. We held a disco/auction night at the company's sports club and raised over £5000 for the night. The company I worked for also informed me that they would donate two thirds of the cost of the operation. After another couple of functions we had raised enough money to pay for the operation. All I needed now was a surgeon to perform the operation.

I was referred to Professor Aziz at the Radcliffe Infirmary in Oxford. After a couple of visits he decided I was a good candidate for DBS. In June 2002, I went to Oxford where I spent 12 days in hospital undergoing two operations; one to put the electrodes in my brain and one to fit the neuro stimulator (battery). After the electrodes were fitted I was pain free for the first time in years! I'd say I was around 75% better than before the surgery.

The next few months were a bit up and down. I was still relatively pain free but still leaning over quite a bit. I was back at work now doing the planning for the shop floor. I managed to bang my head while at work, so in May 2003 I had to have an electrode replaced at the Charring Cross hospital in London.

In early 2005, I had to have the battery changed. In October 2006, things took a turn for the worse and on inspection, my consultant, Mr. Rowe, decided that he would have to replace a broken electrode. This took longer than anticipated as scar tissue had formed around the broken electrode. Mr. Rowe also noticed the other electrode was also broken so it meant another operation just before Christmas 2006. All was okay, but I had to have another battery fitted in August 2008. By this time, I had retired from work due to the company closing down.

In 2010, I was really struggling with my mobility so Mr. Rowe decided to fit an extra set of electrodes in my brain. I also had a rechargeable battery fitted (this should last 9 years). After this operation I could stand up straight for the first time in years.

I am currently struggling with my mobility again and my voice is very weak. The doctors think that DBS may give symptoms of Parkinson's disease, which may be causing my mobility problems, so I am currently undergoing tests for Parkinson's. My dystonia may be the cause of this, but it is still unknown.

Despite some of the challenges that come with the DBS, I am very satisfied and would definitely choose this treatment again. It has helped me in so many ways. I will not let this dystonia get me down and plan to keep on smiling.

Selective Peripheral Denervation (The Bertrand Procedure)

In severe cases of disabling cervical dystonia when oral medications and neurotoxins have failed or the side effects are too severe, selective peripheral denervation may offer relief of symptoms. Selective peripheral denervation began in the 1970's. It is a procedure in which nerves are removed at the point where they enter the selected hyperactive muscles, while innervation to uninvolved muscles is maintained. Studies have indicated that this procedure is useful in selected patients. Positive response to prior botulinum toxin therapy appears to be a good indicator of outcome following selective peripheral denervation.

The term 'selective' refers to the care taken to identify the muscles of the neck affected by dystonia. The term 'denervation' refers to cutting the nerves that supply those muscles. The purpose of the Bertrand procedure is to reduce abnormal contractions in the affected muscles by severing the nerves to these muscles. The goal of the procedure is to leave intact the supply of nerves to unaffected or less-affected muscles.[16]

Myectomy

Selective myectomy or myotomy is a surgical procedure where a portion of an overactive muscle is removed in the eyelid or brow squeezing muscles. This procedure was a common treatment for blepharospasm; however, with the advent of botulinum toxin treatment, selective myectomies are rarely performed.[17]

Ablation surgery

Ablation (or ablative) brain surgery, also known as brain lesioning where certain nerves are severed, is a procedure for severe dystonia. The procedure locates, targets, and destroys (ablates) the clearly defined area of the brain that produces chemical or electrical impulses that cause abnormal movements (i.e. the thalamus, which is responsible for sensory perception and regulation of motor functions).

A heated probe or electrode is inserted into the targeted area. A local anesthetic is used to dull the outer part of the brain and skull. In some cases, it may be difficult to estimate how much tissue to destroy and the amount of heat to use. It is safer to treat a small area and risk the symptoms returning or not being eliminated than to treat a larger region and risk serious complications, such as paralysis or stroke.

The patient remains awake during the procedure to determine if the symptoms have been eliminated. A related procedure, called cryothalamotomy, uses a very cold probe that is inserted into the thalamus to freeze and destroy areas that produce tremors.[18]

Ablative surgery carries risks. The thalamus is very close to another part of the brain used for speech and if that area is disturbed, the patient may experience speech impediments following the procedure. Adverse effects of surgery often cannot be reversed and may result in permanent disfigurement.

Types of ablative surgery include thalamotomy and pallidotomy. During a thalamotomy, a selected portion of the thalamus is surgically destroyed. A pallidotomy involves destruction of part of the globus pallidus. The goal of surgery for individuals with dystonia is to attempt to "rebalance" movement and posture control by destroying one of these regions deep within the brain. These procedures have been performed in relatively few patients with dystonia as compared to those with Parkinson's disease.[19, 20]

Baclofen pump

Baclofen is a medication that was introduced in the 1960's as a treatment for spasticity and to ease muscle movement. It helps to supplement the body's supply of the chemical neurotransmitter called gamma-aminobutyric acid (GABA). GABA is the chief inhibitory neurotransmitter in the central nervous system and is responsible for the regulation of muscle tone.

For some people it takes a high dose of oral Baclofen to have a therapeutic benefit, which may cause intolerable side effects such as drowsiness, sleepiness, weakness, and fatigue. As an alternative, an Intrathecal Baclofen Pump delivers Baclofen directly into the cerebral spinal fluid (intrathecal means 'in the spinal fluid') and only small doses are needed which reduces these side effects. Other medications may also be delivered in this manner to minimize side effects often associated with higher oral doses.

A battery-operated pump (about the size of a hockey puck) is surgically implanted under the skin on the person's upper trunk, usually to the left or right of the belly button. The pump is connected to a small tube that delivers Baclofen directly to the spinal fluid. The pump works by use of a small computer that is programmed by the doctor to deliver the amount of medication appropriate for the individual at any point throughout the day. This way of delivering Baclofen decreases spasticity without drowsiness. Intrathecal Baclofen therapy is an adjustable and reversible treatment.

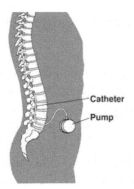

Retrieved on March 17, 2015 from: http://multiple-sclerosis-research.blogspot.com/2013/08/complications-of-baclofen-pumps.html

Regular maintenance is a key component of this therapy. The pump needs to be refilled every one to six months, depending on the dose. This is done by inserting a thin needle through the skin into the pump. This is a straightforward, outpatient procedure. How often the pump is refilled depends on the dose. The pump battery needs to be replaced about every seven years.

To determine if you are eligible for a Baclofen pump, you will undergo a screening to observe your body's response to Baclofen. You will receive an injection of Baclofen using a standard lumbar puncture. Relaxation of the muscles (which is temporary and should only last several hours) indicates that an intrathecal Baclofen pump may likely be effective. If you do not respond to the screening test, a second test using the same procedure may be tried the next day or at a later date. Some physicians use a continuous intrathecal infusion of Baclofen as a screening method. In this technique, a small catheter is inserted into the spinal fluid and is connected to an external pump that infuses Baclofen in increasing doses over two to three days.

Studies have shown that intrathecal Baclofen can dramatically improve symptoms and quality of life. Some centers have reported significant improvement in as much as 85% of patients. However, like any surgery, the procedure is not without risks. Hardware complications may arise including infection and catheter breakage and disconnection. In a small percentage of cases, patients may lose effect within the first year of therapy or experience a worsening of symptoms. The most common side effects are constipation, decreased muscle control, and drowsiness.[21]

Testimonial
I was diagnosed with cervical dystonia in 2003 at age 39. I was already living with spasmodic dysphonia (SD), which I had since I was 11 years old, but it got much worse when dystonia started. Spasmodic Dysphonia is a disorder that involves spasms of the vocal cords, causing interruptions of speech and affecting voice quality. It can cause the voice to break up or to have a tight, strained, or strangled quality. My voice was such that it was hard for others to understand me. I am a well educated professional with a PhD, but I sounded intellectually disabled because it was difficult to speak smoothly and enunciate my words. My dystonic movements added to my awkward appearance and presentation.

I started receiving Botox shots in Spring 2003. It took time to find the right muscles and amount to inject, so unfortunately my condition continued to worsen. I could not move without severe pain and straining. My face was turned upwards making it extremely difficult to walk, shower, or do anything on my feet. I was drinking large amounts of alcohol to try and minimize my pain and depression. I was also on many medications (benzodiazepines and muscle relaxants) to try and help me stay functional, but they made me very sleepy. I would sometimes fall sleep in mid sentence. I eventually lost my job and had to move in with my parents.

On occasion I would take more medication than was prescribed to try and get relief, but it just made me more loopy. Driving was extremely painful and difficult. Worse yet, on three occasions I fell asleep at the wheel, totaling three different vehicles. I almost lost my life after one of the accidents. Thank God I never hurt anyone else.

At the end of 2005, I spoke to my doctor about my deep frustration with dystonia, my lack of progress with the treatments we had been using, and my deliberations about having deep brain stimulation surgery (DBS). He had been having similar thoughts. However, he suggested an alternative that was not so brain invasive; a Baclofen pump.

Surgery would be required to implant a medication pump in my stomach along with a tube (catheter) that runs from the base of my spine into my brain stem. It is a delicate procedure, as the placement of the catheter providing the medicine (Baclofen) comes perilously close to the medulla oblongata; the small structure at the base of the brain that controls vital body functions such as breathing, swallowing, digestion, and heart and blood vessel function. The idea was that the pump would continually bathe the neurons in my spinal cord and brain with Baclofen to reduce the pulling in my neck.

I was desperate and liked the idea of trying the slightly less invasive Baclofen pump procedure, with DBS still available as an option. To determine if the procedure might work, I had to go through a trial that simulated the effect of the pump. Simply, they injected a trial of Baclofen directly into my spinal cord.

The effect was magical, amazing, exhilarating. No pain! The pain from the continuous pulling and red-hot poker disappeared. Relief! I knew then that I wanted to have the pump. I was warned, however, that the effect of the trial was quite different from the actual pump.

When the pump is installed, you receive a very small dose of the medication to start. Just like Botox, it can take up to a year (perhaps two) of trial and error before getting the dosage right. My wait would be even longer. During the trial procedure, I contracted spinal meningitis, a serious illness that could be deadly if it migrated to my brain. I had to go on intravenous vancomycin for the infection. It was nine months before I could have the pump implant surgery; nine long, agonizing months before the infection would clear.

On September 17, 2007 I had the pump implanted. At first, the change in my dystonia was minimal, as I had been given a low dose of the medication as promised. I continued getting Botox injections and continued taking oral medications. Botox soon became more effective since the pump provided enough muscle tension relief to allow Botox to better do its job.

Gradually, I started to feel better. At first, it became slightly easier to walk and take the bus to travel. In two months I was able to join a gym. In the beginning, the only aerobic activity I could do was the recumbent bike. In order to use the machine, I had to have a high back support (obusforme) placed between me and the back of the bike to keep my neck somewhat straight as I exercised. I could only do some of the Nautilus machines for weight training, whereas now I use free weights, Hammer weights, and Nautilus to vary my strength building routine.

Exercising gradually became easier, both on my body and my neck. This was fortunate because my previous sedentary lifestyle, accompanied by depression, led me to overeat. I gained 90 pounds since being diagnosed with dystonia. I started exercising at a robust 310 pounds. Currently my weight varies between 220 and 230.

Since the pump was first implanted, I have continued improving in many ways, small and large. I became more active and functionally less impaired. Over a period of two years, I made slow but measurable progress that continues to this day. My spasmodic dysphonia has also improved. I have to exert less effort to enunciate my words and find speaking much easier most of the time. My friends tell me that there are times that they can't even tell I have dysphonia.

I was able to taper down my oral medications which made me more alert and less sleepy. I am no longer provided driving oversight by the DMV medical board. I have had no accidents since getting the pump (other than bumping into someone in a parking lot when I wasn't paying attention); I am taking on leadership roles in volunteer projects and starting to work again. I also began dating again and got married just over two years ago. In fact, we just had a baby! I've come a very long way.

All is not perfect of course. I know that cervical dystonia is a disorder that I will need to manage for the rest of my life, just as if I had Parkinson's, diabetes, and less severe forms of muscular sclerosis or muscular dystrophy. I manage my dystonia by getting my pump filled with Baclofen every 2 months, Botox shots every 3 months, and oral medications when my neck starts to tighten up. I also go to the gym up to four times a week.

My regimented gym workout includes neck stretches and exercises to improve flexibility and increase muscle strength to compensate for the pulling sensations I often feel. I also speed walk for 40 minutes. This is not only good for the waist line, but it allows me to practice relaxing my neck to compensate for the pulling to the right I feel under extreme conditions. I also exercise my biceps, triceps, back, shoulders, abdominals, shoulders, and chest. I find it important to have a strong upper body to help me compensate for the dystonia symptoms. I was never able to exercise like this with dystonia before the pump. My current abilities are a stark contrast to the life I used to live where I essentially resided in my recliner all day watching TV or on my computer, and ate things like pizza and other unhealthy foods I would have delivered.

I still have periods when I get tired and have to nap. I still need to take oral medications (Klonopin, Baclofen, and Flexeril) when my neck starts to tighten and spasm. Because of these medications, I am likely not as sharp or efficient as I once was. Still, utilizing the Baclofen pump along with Botox has greatly reduced my reliance on these medications.

I have also had Baclofen overdoses when the wrong amount of medication was administered through the pump (as we were adjusting my dose), causing side effects such as extreme nausea, vomiting, dizziness, and stupor. If the pump somehow malfunctioned and stopped delivering Baclofen, it could be a life-threatening event. Without this medication bathing my spinal cord, I would likely have a dystonic storm and require emergency attention. My muscles would tense and become extremely rigid, so much so that I might suffer convulsions and be unable to breathe.

Finally, there are financial considerations. Medicaid in my state does not cover the Baclofen pump procedure or refills. Medicare does. However, there is a coinsurance fee which varies depending on how much medication you receive. For me it costs about $350 every two months. However, there is some relief from these expenditures. One is that if your income is low, many hospitals and health care facilities will forgive or write off these coinsurances through "charity care." Also, if you have private insurance, many have caps on out of pocket expenses, particularly if the care is in network.

As you can see, the Baclofen pump can present significant challenges, but it can make a tremendous difference in one's life. The pump not only reduced my dystonia symptoms enough so that Botox is more effective, the synergy created by these treatments has allowed me to greatly reduce my reliance on oral medications to control my symptoms.

My doctor would say that I owe the improvements to my hard work at the gym and my ability to stay calm and effectively manage stress (especially when I start experiencing dystonic symptoms). He gives me too much credit. What allows me to function as well as I do are the conditions created by my amazing and caring health care providers, Botox, and the Baclofen pump. However, I do give myself some credit because I have worked hard and taken risks. I choose to live my life to the fullest without letting dystonia stand in my way. Having this type of attitude is probably one of the most important factors in me being able to live a fulfilling life. I know that I can do whatever I put my mind to, no matter the obstacle.

Medical marijuana

Medical marijuana is a popular, albeit controversial, topic for many people with and without a health condition. Medical marijuana refers to the use of cannabis and its constituent cannabinoids, such as tetrahydrocannabinol (THC) and cannabidiol (CBD). Cannabis has been effectively used with some people to reduce nausea and vomiting from chemotherapy, AIDS patients, and for pain and muscle spasticity. Researchers are actively investigating the possible therapeutic uses of cannabis for a multitude of other health conditions.

Proponents argue that it is a safe and effective treatment for the symptoms of cancer, AIDS, multiple sclerosis, pain, glaucoma, epilepsy, and other conditions. Opponents of medical marijuana argue that legal drugs make marijuana use unnecessary, it lacks FDA approval, is addictive, leads to harder drug use, interferes with fertility, impairs driving ability, and injures the lungs, immune system, and brain. Clearly, there are strong opposing viewpoints.

Marijuana is illegal under federal law, but states can decriminalize it if they choose and also allow exemptions for medical use. There are currently 20 states (and Washington, DC) where marijuana is legal for medical use. "Medical use" means the acquisition, possession, cultivation, manufacture, use, internal possession, delivery, transfer, or transportation of marijuana or paraphernalia relating to the administration of marijuana to treat or alleviate a registered qualifying patient's debilitating medical condition or symptoms associated with the debilitating medical condition.[22]

Each state has a list of conditions that are approved for the use of medical marijuana. If your condition is not on the list, you can submit a request to the health department for an exception. If you qualify, you can obtain a medical marijuana ID card, which is required to purchase medical marijuana.

Since marijuana can't be obtained at a conventional pharmacy and insurance won't cover it, qualified patients purchase their marijuana from either a caregiver or a dispensary. A caregiver is a person whom the state deems qualified to grow or acquire marijuana, sell it to the patient, and help the patient use it. However, the caregiver is not required to have medical or health care qualifications.

Dispensaries are formal business entities licensed by the state to sell medical marijuana. Medical marijuana can also be purchased in vending machines in some states. They are operated by dispensaries and strictly controlled, requiring a fingerprint scan and the insertion of an ID card provided by the dispensary. There is no standard dosage for marijuana so patients are left to regulate their own intake of medication, but each state sets limits for how much marijuana a qualified individual or caregiver can possess or grow.

Medical cannabis can be taken using a variety of methods, including vaporizing or smoking dried buds, eating marijuana-based products and prepared foods (chocolate, smoothies, cakes, cookies, etc.), and taking capsules. Synthetic cannabinoids are available as prescription drugs in some countries. There are also products made from the marijuana plant that are legal to purchase without an ID card. They come in the form of sublingual preparations (dissolve under your tongue), tablets/capsules, sprays, and topical lotions. Speak to your doctor and research the internet for all options if this form of treatment is of interest.[22-27]

I do not use marijuana, but I know people with dystonia who benefit from it. I've also heard stories about people with other health conditions who benefit from medical marijuana. Medical marijuana is not an approved treatment for dystonia, but there are many treatments for dystonia not recognized and/or endorsed by doctors, or officially or specifically approved for dystonia, that people find helpful to treat their symptoms. For some people, medical marijuana is the only medicine that relieves their pain and suffering and/or treats symptoms without debilitating side effects.

The use of marijuana for the treatment of dystonia and other health condition comes down to legality and personal choice. Like any other treatment protocol, it may or may not be effective for you. If this is a route you would like to pursue, please consult your doctor to see if it would be appropriate in your case. Ideally, find an open minded doctor who will give you the pros and cons of this type of treatment so you can make an informed decision. It is also important to know the steps to gaining access to medical marijuana, with which your doctor should be able to help you. Lastly, keep an eye on the laws in your state as they are frequently changing.

Physical Therapy/Physiotherapy

Physical therapists/Physiotherapists (PT's) work with patients who have impairments, limitations, disabilities or changes in physical function and health status resulting from injury, disease or other causes. Their role includes examination, evaluation, diagnosis, prognosis, and interventions toward achieving the highest functional outcomes for each patient. They provide services that help restore function, improve mobility, relieve pain, and prevent or limit permanent physical disabilities. They restore, maintain and promote overall health, wellness and fitness.

Therapists examine medical history, as well as test and measure strength, range of motion, balance and coordination, posture, muscle performance, respiration, and motor function. They develop treatment plans that describe the treatment strategy, as well as its purpose and anticipated outcome.

Treatment often includes exercises for patients who lack flexibility, strength or endurance. PT's encourage patients to use their muscles to further increase flexibility and range of motion before advancing to exercises that improve strength, balance, coordination, and endurance.

PT's also use electrical stimulation, hot packs or cold compresses, and ultrasound to relieve pain. They may also use traction or deep-tissue massage. Therapists also teach patients exercises to do at home to address their issue. As treatment continues, therapists document progress, conduct periodic examinations and modify treatments when necessary.

Some PT's treat all physical problems, while others specialize in areas such as pediatrics, geriatrics, orthopedics, sports medicine, neurology, vestibular (balance), and cardiopulmonary physical therapy. PT's will often consult and practice with a variety of other professionals, including physicians, nurses, educators, social workers, occupational therapists, and speech and language pathologists.[28]

Physical therapy/physiotherapy can be helpful to people with certain forms of dystonia. While dystonia is not necessarily a progressive disorder, over time the integrity of our muscles and joints, as well as our strength and balance, can become compromised. To offset the negative effects of sedentary living and chronic muscle imbalances, physical therapy can be excellent for keeping your body in better shape, as well as treat specific symptoms.

As with all treatments/therapies, it is very important that the therapist has some knowledge about dystonia and how your dystonia manifests. Even if they treated dystonia patients in the past, it does not follow that you are the same and should be treated the same way. Be careful about what they suggest. Do your homework and make sure they are doing what seems best for you and your specific needs.

I have been to several physical therapists, none of whom were able to help me. Most of them were baffled by my symptoms and did not know what to do. PT has helped me with other problems, but never with dystonia. However, this is not to say that PT is not a useful modality for dystonia. I know plenty of people who have derived great benefit working with the right PT. As with anyone you see or any therapy you try, it has to be the right fit for you.

Massage Therapy

The human touch can be very therapeutic, especially for dystonia if the right therapist is working on you. Massage increases circulation, reduces tightness in muscles, stimulates the release of pain relieving endorphins, and lowers stress hormone levels. When I began having dystonia symptoms (before my diagnosis), I thought massage would help, but I had no idea what would be a good type of massage to get. I just assumed a massage was a massage. Boy was I wrong.

About two months before my symptoms went from mild to severe, I saw a massage therapist a couple times a week for about a month. While I think she was a good therapist, she was not good for me. She worked heavily on my overactive muscles which irritated them, resulting in more pain and spasms. She told me this was normal for people who were as tight as me and after a few more visits, it should resolve itself. The opposite happened. To be fair, I still had no diagnosis at this point so both she and I were approaching my treatments somewhat blindly. My symptoms at the time mimicked that of a person with moderate to severe muscle tightness and rigidity, so the approach taken was targeted at that body type.

What she did that was most problematic was heavy duty trigger point work on my dystonic muscles. She also pinched muscles to try and break up knots. This put my symptoms over the moon so I stopped seeing her. I didn't stop sooner because I had massages like this for other conditions and it always helped.

Since learning more about dystonia and massage, and what works best for me, I find it to be a great form of therapy and a complement to everything else I do to manage my symptoms. The most effective massage for me is one that elongates my muscles with deep, long strokes along the length of my back, the sides of my neck, and across my shoulders. Trigger point work on my back and at the ridge where my neck and skull meets is also very helpful. This area is called the external occipital protuberance (EOP) and is often very tight in people with cervical dystonia.

Along with helping some people with dystonia, massage can be helpful for a variety of other conditions, some of which may or may not be associated with dystonia. These include pain, stress, anxiety, flexibility and range of motion, muscle relaxation, soft tissue strains or injuries, temporomandibular joint pain, posture, circulation, digestive disorders, headaches, immune system health, joint flexibility, spasms and cramping. Massage therapy is also really good for releasing endorphins. Endorphins are neurotransmitters that can block pain, relieve stress, and enhance feelings of pleasure, among other things. They are often referred to as the body's natural opiates.

If you choose to explore massage, there is a book available that is specifically written for spasmodic torticollis/cervical dystonia called, Spasmodic Torticollis Massage Guidebook, by Myra Murphy. It can be found at www.torticollismassage.com. If you are unable to get a massage from a therapist or loved one, there are massage machines available. The one that I use is called Kneading Fingers and can be purchased from Clark Enterprises at www.clarkenterprises2000.com. You can also find the same or similar massage machines from other stores. I use the kneading fingers machine on a daily basis and find that it really helps restore mobility and reduce pain.

Massage may or may not be of help. For me it is great tool. There are many types of massage so choose what you think is best. You may also find massage combined with other therapies to be helpful.

Cranial Sacral Therapy

Cranial Sacral Therapy (CST) is a gentle, non-invasive form of bodywork that addresses the bones of the head (including the face and mouth), spinal column, and sacrum to release tension and improve body movement. It was pioneered and developed by Osteopathic Physician John E. Upledger after years of clinical testing and research at Michigan State University where he served as professor of biomechanics.

CST practitioners palpate soft tissues that surround the central nervous system to evaluate the cranio-sacral system. They gently feel various locations of the body to test motion and rhythm of the cerebrospinal fluid around the brain and spinal cord. Soft-touch techniques are then used to release restrictions in any tissues influencing the cranio-sacral system.

By normalizing the environment around the brain and spinal cord, CST is used for a wide range of medical problems associated with pain and dysfunction, and for its ability to help bolster resistance to disease.

I have had a few CST sessions with good results. They were not long lasting, but I was able to achieve greater relaxation and balance, allowing me the opportunity to function better for a period of time, anywhere from a few hours to a few days.

Reflexology

Reflexology is the application of pressure to specific points and areas on the feet, hands, or ears. Reflexology practitioners believe that these areas correspond to different body organs and systems, and pressing them has a beneficial effect on those body organs and systems, improving a person's overall health. It is called a "reflex therapy" because practitioners work with points on one part of the body to affect other parts of the body.

Reflexology may reduce pain and psychological symptoms, such as anxiety and depression, and enhance relaxation and sleep. Practitioners claim that reflexology can also treat a wide variety of medical conditions, such as asthma, diabetes, and cancer. However, scientific evidence is lacking to support these claims. Reflexology is generally considered safe, although very vigorous pressure may cause discomfort for some people.

On occasion I do foot reflexology on myself, with varying degrees of pressure depending on what I can tolerate. At times it definitely relaxes my body and reduces tension in my neck (it also makes my feet feel good). I really don't know what I'm doing since I was never trained, but by following the guidelines in a book called, Healing Yourself with Foot Reflexology (2002) by Mildred Carter, I am able to achieve some benefit.

After a reflexology session, drink plenty of water to flush out the toxins that were released during the treatment. The same should be done after massage and cranial sacral therapy.

ST Recovery Clinic

The ST Recovery Clinic (STRC) provides natural, non-medical, individualized education and therapy for people living with Spasmodic Torticollis/Cervical Dystonia (ST/CD). The STRC offers clients a clear, structured program, empowering them to achieve a state of ongoing recovery from the symptoms of ST/CD. While there is currently no cure for this disorder, via this program it is possible to drive the symptoms into dormancy and live a normal life again. This is achieved with daily reinforcement of stretching, exercising, and massage to help lengthen muscles, break up scar tissue, detoxify muscles, and bring circulation back into the musculature. Over time, new muscle memory is established for normal movements because new neural pathways are created; the same thing that happens when you learn a foreign language or musical instrument.

The program is tailored to each client's individual needs. It involves a combination of specific exercises, stretches, massage, daily habit patterning (posture work and ST/CD friendly ways of doing daily activities), nutritional guidelines, and emotional/attitudinal work. Psychoneuroimmunology (the mind-body-emotion connection) is at the center of this program.

This clinic provides people with options beyond medications and surgery. However, there are some who use the STRC program in conjunction with other symptoms management protocols, such as oral medications and/or botulinum toxin. It all depends on the individual. You can attend the clinic in person or purchase the long distance program, which includes a workbook and 2 DVD's. The second option allows you to stay in the comfort of your own home, but does not mean it is best for everyone. Attending the clinic has the added benefit of one on one education that you do not receive at home.

Clients experience a professional, knowledgeable staff that has the empathy, compassion, and true understanding of dystonia and what it takes to address physical, emotional, and spiritual needs. They provide ongoing support, staying in contact via phone and email for as long as clients require help.

My visit to the STRC
I had the pleasure of attending the clinic in March 2002. It was shortly after being diagnosed with dystonia. Not being one who likes medication, surgery, and at the time was opposed to Botox injections, I chose to attend the clinic. Also, after spending so much time with doctors with no success, I felt it was the best next step. Despite the pain, I was determined to put my body through the rigors of travelling across the country. I felt it was my only hope, and in some ways it turned out to be.

Back then, attending the clinic was my only option because the long distance program was not yet available. However, knowing what I do now, I still would have attended versus getting the long distance program by mail. Hands down, aside from the brutal pain of travelling to New Mexico from North Carolina, it was the best experience to date with anything related to my dystonia.

I recall the absolute horror I was living at the time. I was rolling around on the floor most of the day because I had so much pain in my head, neck, and back. When I called the clinic to register, I was literally face down on the floor as I was giving them my information. Pressure on my forehead slightly helped reduce the pain which made it easier to speak. It was often hard for me to breathe because of the pain, making my voice sound labored.

The trip from North Carolina to New Mexico is etched perfectly in my memory. My father accompanied me because I was unable to travel on my own. To give you an idea for where my ego was at the time, my parents wanted to get me a wheelchair to get around the airport; I refused because I did not want any special treatment. I was in denial that I was so sick and I was embarrassed to look so different. I wanted to try and be as normal as possible. That was a big mistake. I needed the wheelchair, if not additional help. Every chance I had between flights I laid down on the floor. People stared at me as I writhed in pain. When it was time to check in and board, I could barely stand. To make matters worse, this was shortly after the World Trade Center in New York City was attacked, so security had been beefed up making for longer waits.

After a layover and what seemed like hours waiting for a rental car once we landed in NM, we were finally there. It was the worst experience of my life. I got there on sheer will power. I checked into my hotel and I literally dropped onto the bed face down when I got to the room. My Dad got ice bags and draped them over my body. It was then time for dinner so my Dad ordered in because I was in too much pain to get out of bed.

He was amazing the whole trip. I had never before seen my Dad so attentive and caring to my needs. He is a very attentive and caring father, but taking care of the kids when we were sick was always Mom's forte so I never saw him in this role. It was like he had been doing it for years. He took such great care of me that trip for which I am so grateful.

Since I couldn't sit up to eat, I laid in the hotel bed on my side sliding food into my mouth. This was nothing new since I did this all the time on my floor back in my apartment. I probably got about 3 hours of sleep. I then went to the clinic with my Dad in the car we rented. I went with another person who was also attending the clinic that week. He was from Norway. The clinic only allows for one or two people a week so they can give individualized attention. He was not nearly as severe as I was. He was still able to work and support his family, but was not getting enough relief from Botox so he wanted to try the ST Clinic. I was very envious of him. He was almost pain free and able to work. He could walk around. He went sight seeing and shopping after we were done at the clinic, while I stayed in bed on ice. He was able to sit in a chair to eat, watch TV, have a conversation, etc. He also flew all the way from Norway! I barely made it across the country and he made it halfway across the world.

When I first entered the clinic and met the director, Abigail Brown, I instantly felt like I was in the presence of someone who knew exactly what I was going through and how to help me. To this day, I have yet to meet anyone with as much knowledge and compassion for people with ST/CD. I tried to sit in the chair as we went through orientation. After about an hour, Abbie saw the pain I was in and said it was okay if I wanted to lay down on the floor. Some of her clients opt to do this. I was trying to be macho and act like I was able to handle sitting. Thinking back, it was so silly of me to try and play it off like I was not in pain. Not just there, but anywhere I went.

During the four days I spent with Abbie and her staff, I learned so much about dystonia and how I could utilize the program to reduce the pain, pulling, and spasms. I knew that it would require months to years of dedication and I am happy to say that my symptoms have improved at least 75% since the day I walked into the clinic.

When I left to travel back home, I was in tears as I said goodbye to Abbie. My Dad was as well. We had finally found someone who could relate to my pain and misery; someone who showed me that there was a light at the end of the tunnel and that I could get better. No one prior to that week or since then has provided me with the same hope, motivation, and tools for getting better as much as Abbie.

Much of what I learned has become part of my lifestyle. It is to the point now that I don't think too much about what I have to do each day to manage my symptoms. It is all part of my daily routine. As you read in my personal story in chapter 2 and saw from my pictures, you get a good idea for how bad things were. If I can come from where I once was to where I am now, so can you. It just takes grit and determination.

The STRC has had great results with their clients with all degrees of severity, but every situation is different. Some use it as their sole means for managing symptoms, while others use it as a complement to other treatments. I think most everyone with ST/CD would benefit from this program and urge you to call and speak with the director to learn more.

Abigail Brown
S.T.R.C., Inc.
5 Bisbee Ct. 109-238
Santa Fe, NM 87508
(505) 473-0556
Email: stclinic.info@gmail.com
Website: www.stclinic.com

Testimonial
I am a true believer and an example of how the ST Recovery Clinic changed my life after Botox did little to help. I started the program in October 2000. I was fortunate to get this addressed early on because I was walking straight by my February 2001 birthday, which I set as a goal after going to the clinic. I am blessed that my ST/CD is now in remission.

Testimonial
I'm doing well. Between the ST Clinic program and Dysport injections, I am rarely turning at all. Better and better everyday. So much better! I don't know how much is due to the ST Clinic program, as I started doing better before I had the injections, or how much I'm doing better because of Dysport. Sometimes I wonder if Dysport is even working. It seems if the muscles were paralyzed they would act the same every day. Whatever the case, I'm thrilled.

Testimonial

The onset of my ST/CD started when I was 45 years old, which I suspect was brought on by stress. My symptoms started a few minutes after I got out of bed and continued until I fell asleep. Severe pulling to the right caused back spasms that caused me to miss work for the first time in my 23 year career.

My doctor prescribed muscle relaxers, pain killers, and physical therapy. Along the way I also went to a chiropractor. None of this stopped my neck from involuntarily pulling to the right. Most of it made it worse, but I still didn't know at the time what was wrong with me. I was finally referred to a neurologist and he diagnosed dystonia within two minutes and recommended Botox treatments. The first set of shots were right before the Christmas holiday; no improvement. I felt like a freak in front of my kids. A week later, another set of Botox shots and still no improvement. It was time to check out the STRC and see if this would straighten me out.

My wife joined me when I visited the clinic and I was encouraged as soon as Abbie answered the door. Her history with dystonia was dreadful and she was able to overcome it. What a comforting feeling. I made it a point to follow her routine when I got back home and that I did. A complete detox for one straight week, stretching exercises every day, daily prayer and relaxation, lots of reading and relaxation, I cut back on caffeine and sugar, and got a daily massage, all of which was identical to Abbie's routine. Within six weeks of returning home, I was beginning to straighten out and never looked back. The STRC was the answer to my prayers.

I have been working and traveling extensively for the past 12 years and have managed to stay straight. My personal down pillow comes with me on all trips and I try to do a 3-day detox at least 3-4 times a year to cleanse my body from the toxins it accumulates. ST/CD can be put into remission following the STRC program, but it takes a lot of discipline and patience. It is not going to happen overnight. If you have the persistence and confidence to stick with the program you can overcome this dreadful disorder. Never Give Up!

Author's note ~ Consult with a doctor before doing a detoxification program, especially if you are taking medications.

Testimonial

When I first started the ST Clinic program I was also getting Botox. I felt great and thought it was just the stretching that accounted for that in the beginning. So, I stopped getting Botox and spent six months barely able to move (once the Botox wore off). My husband and mother-in-law finally convinced me to get more Botox and probably within six months of getting it again (in combination with stretching and massage) I was able to return to a "normal" life again. I guess my point is that for me it was definitely a combination that helped.

Don't be afraid to use whatever works to help you get to the point where the muscles can relax and actually stretch!! I am now in recovery and haven't had Botox for 3 years. I do the stretches every day, get a massage every six weeks (that is what works for me - won't be enough for everyone), and I take a fish oil supplement daily which seems to help me with stiffness.

Testimonial
It all started in 2003, several days before I went to Kuala Lumpur, Malaysia to cover a news story. I am a news anchor for one of Indonesia's biggest private television stations. I felt something wrong with my neck. Every time I prayed (Muslim people pray 5 times a day) I couldn't look down properly. My head was dragging to the right. Since everything was set for the conference, I decided to go to Malaysia, cover the stories, and get back home.

The day after I got back from Malaysia, I fell down. This had never happened before. I felt something different with my balance. The next day I went to my doctor who referred me to a neurologist who diagnosed me with spasmodic torticollis/cervical dystonia. I was given a narcotic for my pain. I don't remember the name. My doctor also suggested I get Botox in my neck to reduce the severe spasms.

After a few months doing Botox therapy and taking medications, it didn't make my neck better. My parents insisted I use traditional medicine, but some were more like 'black magic'. The worst was when I went to a witchdoctor in Central Java who gave me baby turtle ointment. To make the ointment, she killed a baby turtle and burned one of its veins mixed with oil. I was so sad thinking about that poor baby turtle. It also did not do anything to help me.

I was so tired of all the medications the neurologist and witchdoctor told me to take. I prayed to God to help my condition go away so I could get back to normal without any chemicals or medications. God answered my prayers. I found a website for the ST Recovery Clinic. I sent an email and explained my condition. A few days later, Abigail Brown (the clinic director) replied to my email. She explained many things about dystonia and suggested I order her program.

Around 4-6 months of doing the program, I felt better. After one year, I was almost back to normal, but still had to do the program to maintain my condition. Today, after 8 years following the program, my life is so much better. My ability to do daily activities continues to improve and I am still able to do my job as a news anchor. I believe that no matter how hard our life is sometimes, God always works in a mysterious ways. Everything works itself out in its time, especially with faith in our chosen path of healing and recovery.

<u>Testimonial</u>
You've probably heard the song, "I've Been Everywhere Man"; well I changed the words to, "I've <u>Tried</u> Everything Man", and I feel like I have. Twenty five years ago, after being super stressed while my mum was in hospital, my ST/CD slowly started. When I would ask family/friends if my head was shaking/turning they would say, "No", because they didn't want to worry me more. Consequently, I thought I must be going nuts which was even worse!

I have tried many things - homeopathy, acupuncture, gluten-free diet, physiotherapy, nutritional supplements, meditation, Botox, EFT, yoga, Alexander Technique, craniosacral massage, Feldenkrais, biofeedback - and on the list goes. About 7 years ago, I started the ST Recovery Clinic program and felt an improvement, but still far from where I wanted to be. Then there was a lot of family stress so things went by the wayside.

I'm not as self-conscious as I used to be, but go in spurts of wearing a soft cervical collar. It gives my neck a rest when I'm at ukulele class or out doing Nordic pole walking, which incidentally, I think might aggravate my neck but helps my bones; caught between a rock and a hard place. Sometimes I get very frustrated with this disorder and get extremely tired, but I am thankful that I can at least sleep well.

As of May 2013, I have re-committed to the ST Clinic program. Every time I watch their DVD I am inspired and enthused. Despite my lack of energy, dystonia does not stop me from doing things. I just try and remember to pace myself and that makes things easier.

Acupuncture
Acupuncture is a treatment based on Chinese medicine and is among the oldest healing practices in the world. It is based on the concept that the body is made up of energy (Qi) which flows through the body to keep it balanced, healthy, and whole. When this energy is blocked, it creates imbalances within the body which manifest as dysfunction or disease.

During a treatment, the practitioner inserts tiny sterile needles in the skin into specific points along the body to stimulate the flow of energy through channels known as meridians. Each meridian corresponds to one organ, or group of organs, that governs particular bodily functions. Achieving the proper flow of energy is thought to increase the body's ability to heal itself. Once the needles are in place, you rest for approximately 15-60 minutes. You'll probably feel relaxed and sleepy, and may even doze off.

You may also receive additional modalities such as Moxa, an herb that is burned; "cupping", where a vacuum is created inside a glass cup and then placed on different parts of the body; Guasha, a form of bodywork where a Chinese porcelain spoon is massaged over specific body areas; and Chinese herbal formulations for consumption. Other modalities may be used, but these are among the most common.

Acupuncture has numerous general health benefits and is also used to treat a host of specific health conditions. It is beneficial for ailments including, but not limited to, acute and chronic pain conditions, addictions, asthma, constipation, headaches, irregular menstrual cycles, menopausal symptoms, irritable bowel syndrome, stroke rehabilitation, sports injuries, sciatica, allergies, tinnitus, high blood pressure, insomnia, sensory disturbances, drug detoxification, depression, anxiety, and other psychological disorders. Acupuncture is also used to help the body better handle damage from other treatments, such as powerful medications, chemotherapy, and radiation.

In a 2010 acupuncture journal, authors discuss a patient who was diagnosed with idiopathic cervical dystonia and had been treated with regular Botox injections for a year and half. She was then referred for a course of acupuncture. Her treatments resulted in reduced pain and muscle spasm relief. She continued to get treatments every 8-10 weeks and requirements for Botox injections had decreased.[29]

I began seeing my acupuncturist in 2010 for chronic pain in my right rhomboid muscle. I had been to all kinds of doctors and she was the only person who was able to significantly reduce the pain. To my surprise, I began to notice other benefits as well. I had less muscle spasms and contractions, increased mobility, better sleep, less anxiety, a clearer mind, I felt more grounded, I was more comfortably active, and I had more energy. Not only did my rhomboid pain practically disappear, the rest of my body and mind was in less distress. Less tension in my muscles accompanied with less anxiety resulted in a reduction in dystonia symptoms. I was so happy with the results that I now get treatments twice a month.

It is unknown whether acupuncture can help with your dystonia, as is the case with all forms of treatment. Some benefit, some get worse, and some see no change. It depends on the individual and the practitioner. To me it was worth trying to see if I could get relief.

You can search for an acupuncturist in your area or consult the National Certification Commission of Acupuncture and Oriental Medicine at www.nccaom.org. You can also consult the American Academy of Medical Acupuncture (AAMA) at www.medicalacupuncture.org.

Chiropractic
Chiropractic is the manual treatment of restricted joint movement within the vertebral spinal column. The purpose is to improve biomechanical and neurological function to restore normal motion to the spine, relax tight muscles, improve coordination, and inhibit pain. There are numerous techniques being used by chiropractors today, too long to list here.

When it comes to chiropractic and dystonia, there is significant debate about its safety and efficacy, particularly when it comes to cervical dystonia. Neck adjustments where the head and neck are rotated, accompanied by a short quick thrust, are typically ill-advised because it tends to further aggravate dystonic muscles. If you read my story in chapter 2, the chiropractic techniques used on me made my symptoms exponentially worse. I was none the wiser since at the time I had yet to be diagnosed and was under the impression that I had a musculoskeletal problem. I strongly believe that had I not gone to those two chiropractors, I would have never had such a severe case of dystonia. I also believe that I went to the wrong kind of chiropractor for my condition. There are some chiropractic techniques that can be helpful.

The two doctors I saw did neck adjustments and different forms of traction where my head was put into extreme extension (head pulled back so I was looking at the ceiling). They also put weights on my head to engage the muscles on the opposite side of my neck that were pulling. Weights were also draped over my shoulder to try and straighten me out. These therapies may be fine for someone with acute torticollis (and other conditions), but for spasmodic torticollis/cervical dystonia, it could be very dangerous.

I saw my first chiropractor a few days a week for four months. He did a technique called Chiropractic Biophysics, a technique I was familiar with and found benefit for other conditions in years past. Unfortunately, it made me worse so he referred me to another chiropractor who practiced a technique called the Pettibon System, which I was unfamiliar with but heard good things. Within two weeks of seeing him, I was nearly crippled. My symptoms went through the roof to where the pain and spasms were so bad I could barely stand up. I attribute this to the head harness with weights, over the door traction (see chapter 2), and volatile neck adjustments. In fact, I have never had my neck adjusted in such a violent manner.

Even though my neck was stuck in a locked, turned position, the doctor still tried to adjust it. It was so hard for him to do that he had to put me in a headlock with his forearms to adjust my neck. All of this was done without a diagnosis or the doctor's recognition that I was getting worse after each visit. He still felt very strongly that I would get better if I stuck with it. As embarrassing as it is to say, I did too. I also heard glowing testimonies from other patients who told me they looked just like I did and were fixed up in a matter of a few visits. What was I to think other than, "this makes sense and I should be fine based on everything I am being told." Within about two weeks, I went from functional with a little pain, to disabled on my floor in so much pain I could barely move.

To this day, it is sometimes difficult for me to talk about. My life might have been very different had I never been to these chiropractors, the second one in particular. I kick myself for allowing this to go on, but I was desperate and vulnerable. I was also given constant reassurance that this technique would help me get better. I was in so much pain that I was grasping so hard to any shred of hope that I didn't see what it was really doing to me.

Despite this horrible experience, I think chiropractors do amazing things. I just don't think too many techniques are helpful for people with dystonia, especially cervical dystonia. The only technique I am familiar with that has received positive feedback from the dystonia community is Upper Cervical Chiropractic. According to the National Upper Cervical Chiropractic Association (NUCCA), their focus is on the relationship between the upper cervical spine and its influence on the central nervous system and brain stem function. This technique may or may not involve adjustments, depending on the doctor and your particular condition. Upper cervical treatment is more passive than what you might get from another type of chiropractor. The goal is to resolve postural imbalance to return the head to a more balanced position on top of the neck. To locate a NUCCA doctor, visit www.nucca.org.

I do not promote or discourage chiropractic care for dystonia. For me it was not helpful, while others find it to be a useful treatment. I still go to a chiropractor from time to time for back and hip adjustments, but I will not let him adjust my neck. This is a different chiropractor than the previous two. He is someone I know and trust who is very familiar with my medical history. He won't do anything that either of us even remotely feels might aggravate my symptoms.

As with any treatment, be very diligent about who you see and what they know about dystonia. If you ever feel uncomfortable with anything that a chiropractor (or any doctor) does or proposes doing, even if they say they have helped many other people with the same problem, ask to speak with those people before you have them treat you. Keep in mind that torticollis and spasmodic torticollis/cervical dystonia are very different, and your chiropractor may not know the difference. This is where your homework comes in handy. Be diligent when it comes to your personal health care.

While I only discuss upper cervical chiropractic, there are certainly other chiropractic techniques that can and do help with dystonia and related problems. Treatment efficacy varies depending on who you are.

Inversion Therapy/Gravity Table
One of many tools that might be helpful for dystonia and dystonia related conditions is an inversion/gravity table. The theory behind using this table is that by inverting your body, you are able to unload the bones, joints, and discs in the back and neck. This is thought to create a traction force through the spine. It has been theorized that this form of traction can decrease back, neck and shoulder pain, among other things. Another name for inversion therapy is gravitational traction.

Gravity is a compression force which is constantly affecting our upright frame. Over the course of the day, gravity compresses the spine and weight-bearing joints, which can cause pain, poor posture, and a host of other problems. While inverted, progressive decompression allows each joint to be decompressed by the same weight that compresses it while upright. Inversion allows your joints and spine to elongate, creating space between your ligaments and discs. This helps relieve some of the pressure accrued over the course of your daily activity (or inactivity). The image below illustrates compressive forces on the body in different positions.

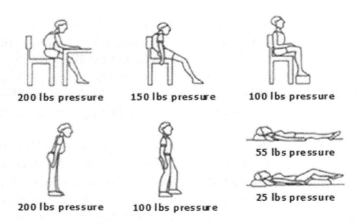

200 lbs pressure   150 lbs pressure   100 lbs pressure

200 lbs pressure   100 lbs pressure

55 lbs pressure

25 lbs pressure

Reprinted from: www.careclinic.info, Retrieved September 2, 2013 from:
http://careclinic.info/Rehabilitation.php

Daily sessions of inversion therapy for just a few minutes might make a big difference in how you feel. Proponents of inversion therapy claim that it helps relieve back, shoulder, neck, and joint pain caused by the compressive force of gravity, improves circulation, promotes lymphatic drainage, relieves the discomfort of varicose veins, eases stress on the heart, improves posture by counteracting the downward pull of gravity, revitalizes and tones facial tissue, and enriches the brain and eyes with oxygen rich blood.[30, 31]

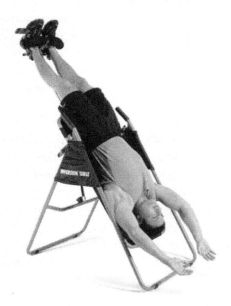

Retrieved on September 26, 2014 from: http://aprilpedia.com/stamina-gravity-inversion-table-vs-lumbar-extender-back-stretcher/

Risks using inversion/gravity table

If you are pregnant, have heart disease, acid reflux, glaucoma, high blood pressure, or cardiovascular disease, check with your doctor before attempting inversion therapy. This is recommended regardless of your health condition. In addition, the first time anyone tries inversion therapy, they should have someone standing by in case assistance is required to get out of the apparatus, or if health problems are experienced.[32]

When I first began using my inversion table, I was very uncomfortable just lying flat on the table. It took me some time to get used to the unstable "flip-flop" motion of the table. When I was lying flat, it felt like I was already inverted. In the beginning I had to have someone hold the table so I could get used to the sensation. I then had to have someone lower me back until I was comfortable doing it on my own.

The reason I began doing inversion therapy was because I had severe neck spasms in 2008 whenever I would lie down (see images below). The first image is similar to how I used to look years ago when I was sitting or standing up; actually, this is how it looked no matter what I was doing. My neck was never straight. A few years later it only twisted like this when lying on my back. Not only was I twisted, but I also had severe pulling and spasms that never stopped unless I rolled onto my side. Strangely, once I stood up the pulling ceased and my neck was straight again, as you can see in the second picture. None of my doctors or therapists had any idea why this phenomenon occurred.

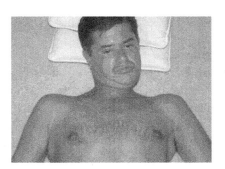 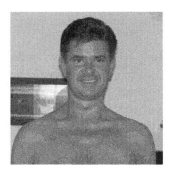

After about 3 weeks of using the inversion table roughly 3-5 minutes twice a day, I was able to lie down on my back without any twisting, pulling, or spasms. I was amazed at how little it took to relieve this problem. While some people invert a full 90 degrees, I never go beyond a maximum of 60 degrees. Usually no more than around 45 degrees is sufficient for me.

As with any treatment, inversion therapy is not for everyone. For those who it is good for, it can be dangerous if you do too much; too much meaning going back too far and/or hanging for too long. I once made the mistake of doing too much too soon and developed severe pain in my neck and upper back. It was restricted to the point where I was unable to turn my head in either direction for about a week. I think it is a great device for a variety of reasons, but please slowly build up how often and for how long you use it. Also check with your doctor to determine if it is right for you.

Oral orthotic
There are a handful of specialized dentists around the country who are using an oral orthotic as a treatment for dystonia and other movement disorders. I know several people who had an oral orthotic fit for them by specialists, some with great results and some not as much, no different than every other treatment and how we all respond differently.

There are a few doctors in the US who specialize in this orthotic for movement disorders, chronic pain, Tourette syndrome, etc. There are also a lot of doctors who try it without the background and experience and hurt people, so if you venture down this path, be sure to find a doctor who does this extensively.

The device is uniquely designed for each patient and then adjusted over a period of months until the desired results are achieved. How much it helps depends on the person and the doctor treating them. I find it to be very intriguing. As doctors continue with their research and practice, it might have a promising future as a treatment for many of us.

According to the doctors who are using this procedure, there are a great number of pain patients who have an underlying TMJ condition that has never been explored. By using an oral orthotic, it increases the vertical dimension and decreases the neuropathy within the temporomandibular joint (TMJ). It is believed that TMJ disorders can cause a variety of conditions including, but not limited to, movement disorders, muscle spasms, clicking, popping, grating, difficulty opening and closing the mouth, chewing, and speaking difficulties.

The doctors who do this work do not simply insert an orthotic as some other doctors might, and the orthotic itself is not the only factor providing relief. It is the combination of the orthotic and a very skilled doctor making fine adjustments to the orthotic, both when the device is first made for the patient and as the patient continues to progress through the treatment.

According to Dr. Gary Demerjian in Los Angeles, CA, research studies show that motor activity in specific muscles of the neck is present when the TMJ is stimulated. This stimulus causes the head and neck muscles to turn toward the same side as the stimulation. It may be the case that cervical dystonia in some people is a result of chronic activation of the reticular formation due to overstimulation of the nerves within the TMJ. When the stimulus is relieved in the TMJ, the stimulus in the reticular formation is also relieved, which then relieves the turning of the head to that side. With the compression relieved, there is a gradual reduction of CD in some patients, and the muscles of the head and neck begin to return to normal with a decrease in pain.[33]

By using this specially fit orthotic to balance the jaw, some patients are experiencing a reduction to complete elimination of symptoms. When the jaw is placed into a better anatomical position, painful TMJ symptoms are alleviated. Upon examination of the jaw joint under x-ray, doctors are finding an irritation or compression of the trigeminal nerve, which plays a crucial role in the nervous system. Its path goes all over the head area; the face, the eyes, the cheek, the lower jaw, and one of the branches goes inside the jaw joint. A painful condition that stems from irritation of this nerve is trigeminal neuralgia (tic douloureux) which causes sharp, shooting pain in the face.

An important feature to better understand the inner workings of the temporomandibular joint and this revolution in medicine is a large nerve bundle called the trigeminal nucleus. The trigeminal nucleus acts as a chief network or relay system in the brain stem. This is significant because cranial nerves run so closely together that they may be accessed at this large bundle or relay point. There are several specific nerves passing very close to this area. The main one is the vagus nerve which plays many roles in the body such as breathing regulation, control of muscle movement, regulation of the digestive system, and many other key functions.

The proximity to which these important nerves run in the cranial space allows them to be positively impacted by proper alignment of the TMJ. According to Dr. Demerjian, due to the fact that the trigeminal nucleus extends down to the C-3 level of the cervical spine, use of an oral orthotic to align the TMJ can have a significant impact in relieving symptoms for dystonia patients.

As this has become a more popular treatment over the past few years, more and more dentists have attempted it without adequate experience. In many cases, orthotics are made for patients and then not properly adjusted. There are some patients who make the mistake of going to a specialist for the orthotic and then a different doctor for a minor adjustment because it is close to their home. Unfortunately, these doctors are often unable to make the adjustments successfully. This is why it is so important to have a very skilled doctor working with you throughout the entire oral orthotic treatment process.[34]

I have never been diagnosed with a TMJ disorder or been fitted for an oral orthotic, but I've done something for years that has a similar effect. I noticed long ago that if I have something in my mouth, such as the earpiece to my sunglasses, a straw, or a toothpick, my symptoms decrease. It not only helps my dystonia, it also reduces anxiety. I don't go anywhere now without a toothpick. If it's not in my mouth, it's in my pocket or behind my ear for easy access when I need it. I would rather not walk around with a toothpick in my mouth, but if it helps reduce my symptoms I don't mind. Sometimes just chewing gum helps. I am amazed how doing these small things can make such a big difference, keeping me optimistic about the future of this treatment.

Below are the three most prominent doctors in the US using an oral orthotic:
- Dr. Gary Demerjian (Glendora, CA) www.tmjconnection.com; 626-852-1865
- Dr. Anthony Sims (Columbia, MD) www.absimsdds.com; 410-872-0872
- Dr. Brendan Stack (Vienna, VA) www.tmjstack.com; 703-821-1103

Testimonial

I developed dystonia, secondary to Reflex Sympathetic Dystrophy (RSD), just before my 29th birthday. I am now 40. I also have hypothyroidism, thoracic outlet syndrome (TOS), TMJ, cardiac ischemia, and intestinal ischemia. I had endometriosis also, but had a full hysterectomy so that is no longer an issue for me. My hand and foot were curled up, and my foot turned in to the point of being in a wheelchair to get around and not being able to wear a shoe. I also couldn't type so I used speak to text software. It has been a tough 11 years, but I fight to make my daily living better. I use whatever tools I can find to accomplish what I can, including the oral orthotic Dr. Demerjian fit for me.

I got some improvement from infusion therapy in December 2009. Follow up boosters do help some of my symptoms, but not all. I was able to begin walking with a more normal gait for more than a few steps at a time and get out of my wheelchair almost full time, but was still not able to tolerate constricting shoes on my feet. Nor did I have the balance to wear anything but a flat flip-flop shoe.

Once I got the oral orthotic, I went from doing okay physically to doing great. My life got a whole lot better with the challenges I was facing being reversed. For example, before the infusions, my hand grip strength was 0 on the right and 8 on the left. After IV therapy it improved to 17 on the right and 24 on the left. After I got the oral orthotic, it improved to 36 on the right and 37 on the left. Now I can even wear heels and tennis shoes again!

My quality of life was okay before the oral orthotic, mainly because I am a very positive person and try to face challenges as life moments. I was settling for the improvement I was getting, not knowing that there could be more to getting better. I had been undergoing IV-Infusion therapy for just over 3 years. Little did I know how much the oral orthotic was going to benefit me. Symptoms that the infusions didn't help with were greatly reduced or totally eliminated by using the oral orthotic.

I chose to get the oral orthotic after meeting a dentist who specializes in it and watching how he helped other dystonia patients. Although I didn't realize that I had TMJ at the time, the benefits I got from doing the "stick test" let me know that I was a perfect candidate for the oral orthotic. Those benefits included help with my dystonia, migraines, full body pain, increased strength, and improved coordination.

I have to remember that I still need to take life moment by moment, but now I am able to do more activities and my daily living is much more enjoyable. Not only did the oral orthotic help with my dystonia, it also helped with my concentration, strength, and coordination. I can even wear shoes again! It has been life changing. - Barby Ingle

About Barby
Barby Ingle is chairman of the Power of Pain Foundation. She is also a motivational speaker, pain patient advocate, and best selling author of two books: RSD In Me!: A Patient and Caretaker Guide to Reflex Sympathetic Dystrophy and Other Chronic Pain Conditions (2009) and ReMission Possible: Yours, If You Choose To Accept It (2011). To learn more about Barby and all the work she is doing, please visit www.barbyingle.com.

The mission of the Power of Pain Foundation is to educate and support chronic pain patients by promoting public and professional awareness of chronic pain conditions; educating those afflicted, as well as their families, friends, and healthcare providers; and provide action-oriented public education and pain policy improvement to eliminate the under treatment of chronic pain and increase proper access to care.

The foundation demonstrates its commitment to the chronic pain community by promoting new knowledge in the cause and treatment of chronic pain conditions. Its ultimate goal is to help chronic pain patients perform their regular activities in the community and to bolster society's ability to provide full opportunities and appropriate supports for its pain citizens. To learn more about the Power of Pain Foundation, please visit www.powerofpain.org.

Yoga

Yoga is considered a type of complementary and alternative medicine practice by joining the body, mind, and spirit. It originates from ancient Indian philosophy and brings together physical and mental disciplines to achieve peacefulness of body and mind, helping you relax and manage stress. In the classic written discourse on yoga philosophy, "The Yoga Sutras", the Indian sage Patanjali defined yoga as, "that which restrains the thought process and makes the mind serene." He emphasized that yoga provides a psychological approach to healing the body and achieving self-realization.

By performing physical postures, known as asanas, and by practicing breathing exercises, known as pranayama, it is believed that individuals are able to cleanse their bodies' organs and systems, and achieve a higher state of consciousness. As a therapy, the asanas are believed to affect every gland and organ in the body.

Yoga has many styles, forms, and intensities. People can benefit from any style of yoga so it is all about your personal preference. The potential health benefits of yoga include stress reduction, improved fitness, balance, and flexibility, and management of chronic conditions. Yoga's focus on strength, balance, and flexibility can be applied to dystonia since these are areas where most of us tend to have trouble.

Regardless of which type of yoga you practice, you do not have to follow it to the letter and do every posture/pose/meditation. Everyone's body is different so if any aspect of yoga is uncomfortable for any reason, do not do it or modify it to suit your needs. Find your personal limits. Good instructors will understand and encourage you along the way. Be sure to speak with your instructors about dystonia, as well as the particular style of yoga they teach to see if it is the right fit for you. Selecting an instructor who is experienced and attentive to your needs is important for safe and effective yoga practice.

For some guidance, there is a book on yoga and movement disorders that has received rave reviews called, <u>Yoga for Movement Disorders: Rebuilding</u>

Strength, Balance, and Flexibility for Parkinson's Disease and Dystonia, by Renee Le Verrier and Dr. Lewis Sudarsky.

Tai Chi

Originally developed for self-defense, tai chi has evolved into a graceful form of exercise that is now used for stress reduction and a variety of other health conditions. Often described as meditation in motion, tai chi promotes serenity through gentle, flowing movements.

Tai chi is a self paced system of gentle physical exercise and stretching. Each posture flows into the next without pause, ensuring that your body is in constant motion. There are many different styles of tai chi. Each style may have its own subtle emphasis on various tai chi principles and methods. There are also variations within each style. Some may focus on health maintenance, while others focus on the martial arts aspect.

Tai chi is low impact and puts minimal stress on muscles and joints, making it generally safe for all ages and fitness levels. In fact, because tai chi is low impact, it may be especially suitable if you are an older adult or have movement limitations due to conditions such a dystonia. You may also find tai chi appealing because it is inexpensive, requires no special equipment, and can be done indoors or out, either alone or in a group.

Tai chi may help decrease stress and anxiety, increase aerobic capacity, energy, and stamina, increase flexibility, balance, agility, and muscle strength, improve quality of sleep, enhance the immune system, lower blood pressure, and improve joint pain.

You can find tai chi videos all over the internet and classes are available in many communities. To find a class near you, contact local fitness centers, health clubs, and senior centers. Tai chi instructors do not have to be licensed or attend a standard training program so be sure to ask about an instructor's experience, and get recommendations if possible.

A tai chi instructor can teach you specific positions and how to regulate your breathing. They can also teach you how to practice tai chi safely, especially if you have injuries, chronic conditions, or balance and coordination problems. Although tai chi is slow and gentle, like anything else, it is possible to get injured if you do not do it properly.[35]

Several years prior to the onset of dystonia, I studied karate and achieved the level of brown belt. I was unable to continue taking classes because other responsibilities came about that didn't provide enough time. However, in recent years I have adapted some of my karate forms/movements into my own style of tai chi. Instead of doing movements in a forceful way, as most karate moves are done, I adapted them into slow, rhythmic motions similar to the speed at which tai chi is practiced. Not only does it revive my love for martial arts, it also provides me with greater muscle relaxation and mental peace.

Music Therapy[36-39]

If you enjoy listening to music, you already know that turning on the tunes can help calm your nerves, reduce stress, pump you up during a workout, bring back fond memories, as well as prompt countless other emotions. Listening and singing to music provokes responses due to the familiarity, predictability, and feelings of security associated with it. Our favorite songs are like best friends. When I go on YouTube, turn on the radio, or use my iPod to listen to music, I often find myself singing out loud as if I am at a concert. I have a big smile on my face and feel a sense of calm come over me.

According to Oliver Sacks, author of <u>Musicophilia: Tales of Music and the Brain</u> (2007), "Music occupies more areas of our brain than language...humans are a musical species." When we listen to music, much more is happening in our body than simple auditory processing. Music triggers activity in parts of the brain that release the feel-good chemical dopamine. At the same time, the amygdala, which is involved in processing emotion, and the prefrontal cortex, which makes abstract decision-making possible, are activated. Listening to music may also lower cortisol levels (stress hormones).

Psychologist Dr. Victoria Williamson states, "There's a very wide range of reactions in the body and mind to music, and brain imaging studies have shown that various parts of the brain may be activated by music. There is a real causal relationship between music and the reward system, a core part of the brain that reacts to stimuli which are good for us (e.g. food, light, sex) and reinforces these behaviors, meaning that we do them more."

Research has found that music can be so physically and mentally beneficial that there is now an established health profession called Music Therapy. Music therapy is used to address physical, emotional, cognitive, and social needs of individuals. Qualified music therapists provide treatments including creating, singing, moving to, and/or listening to music. Through musical involvement in the therapeutic context, clients' abilities are strengthened and transferred to other areas of their lives. Music therapy also provides avenues for communication that can be helpful to those who find it difficult to express themselves in words.

Research in music therapy supports its effectiveness in many areas such as facilitating movement and overall physical rehabilitation, increasing people's motivation to become engaged in their treatment, providing emotional support for clients and their families, and providing an outlet for the expression of feelings. Research results and clinical experiences attest to the viability of music therapy even in those patients resistant to other treatment approaches.

Music therapy programs are based on individual assessment, treatment planning, and ongoing program evaluation. Frequently functioning as members of an interdisciplinary team, music therapists implement programs with groups or individuals to address a vast number of issues including anxiety, stress management, respiration, chronic pain, physical rehabilitation, oncology treatment, diabetes, headaches, cardiac conditions, medical and surgical procedures, as well as communication and emotional expression.

Musical preference varies widely between individuals, so only you can decide what will effectively put you in a particular mood. With all the electronic devices we have available to us today, we can take music with us anywhere. Turn on the tunes. It does the body good!

Our muscles respond to music even when the brain is in neutral.
Anger, loneliness, longing, sorrow, frustration, and even confusion
respond positively to music and action. Music is your best ally.
- Bonnie Prudden -

Emotional Freedom Technique (EFT)
Emotional Freedom Technique (EFT), founded by Gary Craig, is a form of acupressure based on the same energy meridians used in traditional acupuncture to treat physical and emotional ailments, but without the use of needles. Instead, simple tapping with the fingertips is used to input energy onto specific meridians on the body while you think about a specific problem (a traumatic event, an addiction, chronic or acute pain, an illness) and say positive affirmations. This is thought by practitioners to treat a wide variety of physical and psychological disorders, and has the advantage of being a simple, self-administered form of therapy.

As described by doctors, this combination of tapping the energy meridians and voicing positive affirmations works to clear the emotional blocks from your body's bio-energy system, thus restoring your mind and body's balance, which is essential for optimal health and healing physical disease.[40]

All of our thoughts have an effect on our autonomic nervous system which creates a feeling within us (happiness, joy, fear, shame, anger, frustration, etc). Tapping certain points in the body can reduce negative nervous system reactions. For example, if we think about how our dystonia keeps us from going out with friends for dinner on a particular day, it can bring up any number of emotions, most of which are unpleasant because we want to be able to go out with our friends. If we tap in this moment, it is believed that it can decrease the emotional pain we are experiencing, as well as the physical pain that may have been the reason for us not going out in the first place. In other words, it is possible to shift the energy in our body that can affect physical and emotional trauma and pain.

Whether EFT will help with your dystonia or associated symptoms, such as anxiety and difficulty sleeping, is unknown. There have been times I have done it with success and other times where it bothered me. The tapping is very gentle, but sometimes it would irritate my muscles if I was having a bad day. For me it is most effective when I do it consistently and when my muscles are calm. Everyone is different so do what works best for you.

The Alexander Technique

Named for its founder, Frederick Matthias Alexander (1869-1955), the Alexander Technique is an educational method for becoming more aware of how we move and how we think about how we move. It also helps us become more aware of how we stay still, breathe, and learn, and how we choose our reactions in demanding situations.

Offered in wellness centers and health education programs worldwide, the Alexander Technique works to re-establish the natural relationship between the head, neck, and back, considered the "core" of the body. It is appropriate for people with chronic back pain, neck pain, migraines, repetitive stress injuries, balance and coordination problems, and for depression and anxiety that often accompanies chronic pain and stress. It is also used for skill enhancement in athletes, actors, singers, dancers, and musicians.

A leading factor in musculoskeletal pain is unrecognized patterns of excess tension. People tend to respond to pain by tensing further, which usually exacerbates discomfort. This is very common with dystonia, but can occur in anyone. In the case of dystonia, while the problems we have are felt in our muscles, it is really a problem with malfunctioning parts of the brain. For whatever reason, the brain wants parts of the body to contract, turn, twist, spasm, tremor, etc. Over time, if we do not break this pattern the brain thinks these movements are normal and then takes on these abnormal movements and postures.

By using the Alexander Technique, and similar techniques, it is possible to train the brain to change motor (movement) programming that may help relieve physical symptoms. In other words, we can re-program the brain to think that having a straight neck (in the case of cervical dystonia), no tremors, no twisting or turning, and no muscle spasms is normal. We have the ability to send messages through the nervous system from the brain to our muscles which enables us to improve mobility and posture, and relieve chronic stiffness, tension, and stress.

The characteristics of dystonia (sustained and/or involuntary muscle contractions and spasms which result in abnormal postures and movements) describe the field with which the Alexander Technique is concerned. Learning how to consciously inhibit unwanted actions is central to the Alexander Technique. It is not a series of postures or exercises; nor does it set out to cure any specific defect. It is an education of the mind-body relationship which can help release tension, prevent injury, and allow the body to move freely, poised, and balanced.

With a teacher's guidance, as you learn to refrain from or inhibit habitual patterns which are not useful, you will become more aware of tendencies towards unnecessary muscular patterns of tension. Undoing these habitual patterns provides the opportunity for natural movement and fluidity to occur. It also involves changing habits and a big part of this is habits of thinking. Many of our assumptions about how we move and act in the world are re-examined during lessons. The potential for health and improvement in learning to gain conscious control over the way we do things is highly probable. The only prerequisite to learning is an open mind and a willingness to change.[41-44]

The Feldenkrais Method
The Feldenkrais method is based on the principles of physics, biomechanics, physiology, and the connection between mind and body. Frequently used to

help ease stress and tension, the Feldenkrais method has demonstrated success in the rehabilitation of stroke victims and others living with neurological injuries (brain tumors, head trauma, multiple sclerosis, and ataxia) that cause disordered movement or a lack of coordination. Feldenkrais is gentle, non-invasive, and teaches how to improve our capabilities to function better in our daily lives.

The Feldenkrais method is named after Dr. Moshe Feldenkrais (1904-1984), a Russian-born physicist, judo expert, mechanical engineer, and educator. After a major knee injury, Feldenkrais was given a 50 percent chance of recovery and possible long-term confinement to a wheelchair. Unsatisfied with the prognosis and conventional treatments available, he developed a program of therapeutic movement.

Improving posture due to problems in bones and joints, and changing poor movement habits that may cause pain, are a large part of the Feldenkrais method. Movement therapies like Feldenkrais can also benefit people who live with distorted body images that contribute to eating disorders and other conditions, such as depression and anxiety. The exercises can re-educate the brain and nervous system to develop new ways of moving and perceiving the body, as well as elevating mood and increasing overall feelings of well being.

Practitioners use gentle movement and directed attention with the aim of increasing ease in range of motion, improving flexibility and coordination, and ultimately rediscovering an innate capacity for graceful, efficient movement. Therapies such as massage, manual manipulation, and acupuncture can often be used in conjunction with the Feldenkrais method, especially when chronic pain is involved. Movement therapies that improve balance and help prevent falls such as yoga, tai chi, and qigong, can also be used with Feldenkrais to help regulate and coordinate movement within the nervous system. Physical and occupational therapy can be used to strengthen and stretch muscles, and increase stamina.

Feldenkrais practitioners work with both individuals and groups. Group sessions, called Awareness Through Movement (ATM), involve verbal instruction by a Feldenkrais teacher who leads a series of movements with clients sitting, lying on the floor, or standing. A lesson generally lasts from 30 to 60 minutes and consists of comfortable, easy movements that gradually become more complex when the client is ready. The emphasis is on learning which movements work better and noticing the quality of positive changes in the body. Many of these movements are based on ordinary functional activities that occur during a regular day (reaching, standing, lying down, sitting, looking left and right, etc.), whereas some are based on joint, muscle, and postural dynamics. There are hundreds of ATM lessons varying in difficulty and complexity for all levels of ability.

Individualized sessions known as Functional Integration (FI) are performed with the patient usually lying on a table or in a seated or standing position. At times, various props (pillows, rollers, blankets) may be used to support posture or facilitate movements in patients who have limitations. Through gentle touch and a series of guided movements, a practitioner will develop lessons that are tailored to a patient's unique structural needs with the goal of expanding flexibility and coordination.

Dr. Andrew Weil, a world renowned integrative medical doctor, often recommends trying the Feldenkrais method for the treatment of neurological issues, especially since it claims success in training the nervous system to develop and utilize new pathways around areas of damage. Feldenkrais has demonstrated success in helping to rehabilitate stroke victims and is also effective with head injuries and other neurological conditions such as cerebral palsy and multiple sclerosis. Feldenkrais can be an effective part of an integrative medicine approach for any painful condition from degenerative arthritis to fibromyalgia.

The International Feldenkrais Federation (IFF) is the coordinating organization encompassing most of the Feldenkrais Guilds and Associations and other key Feldenkrais professional organizations worldwide. To find a qualified Feldenkrais practitioner, contact the Feldenkrais Guild of North America at 800-775-2118 or www.feldenkrais.com.[45, 46]

The Trager Approach[47, 48]

The Trager Approach, also known as Trager Work and psychophysical integration therapy, was developed by Milton Trager, M.D. Dr. Trager developed the system as a way to treat his own chronic back pain, which was the result of a congenital spinal deformity. He was fascinated by how the body coordinated its patterns of movement in response to chronic pain and injury.

The Trager Approach is a form of movement education and mind-body integration. It is based on the premise that discomfort, pain, and reduced function are physical symptoms of accumulated tension that result from accidents, poor posture, fear, emotional blockages, and daily stress. It focuses on reducing these unnatural patterns of movement and eliminating neuromuscular tension.

The Trager Approach is effective for back and neck pain, as well as other joint irritation and soft tissue discomfort. It has also been successfully used to facilitate rehabilitation from physical injuries and neurological events like a stroke. Tension headaches, stress-related disorders, and other emotional imbalances may also be relieved by the Trager Approach. Overall it is best used for postural problems, mobility issues, pain relief, and mental clarity.

There are two phases in the Trager Approach. The first is known as table work. During a table work session, a client is passive and lying on a comfortably padded table. The practitioner moves the client in ways they naturally move, and with a quality of touch and movement such that the recipient experiences the feeling of moving effortlessly and freely on his/her own. The movements are never forced so that there is no induced pain or discomfort to the client.

The practitioner will work to achieve a state known as "hook-up" - a deep state of relaxation and connection between practitioner and client. As the client reaches these deeper states of relaxation, it is thought to help facilitate the release of unhealthy patterns of tension between mind and body at an unconscious level. By teaching the mind to unlearn these patterns of "blockage", the body can also release chronic states of tension and become more flexible with less pain. A typical session lasts from 60 to 90 minutes.

The second phase is a self-care set of exercises called "Mentastics" (mental gymnastics). The client is taught certain movements to perform at home to prolong the positive effects of the table work session. These simple, active, self-induced movements can be done on your own during your daily activities. They have the same intent as the table work in terms of releasing deep-seated patterns. For many people, Mentastics become a part of their daily living to relieve themselves of stress and tension. One of the most potent aspects of the Trager Approach is the ability to recall the feeling of deep relaxation, and how it feels to move freely and easily.

Counseling/Therapy
Millions of people worldwide live with chronic conditions that interfere with their daily lives. As these conditions persist and become prolonged, the ability to cope begins to deteriorate, causing a variety of distressing and often harmful

emotional responses. With appropriate comprehensive medical care that addresses physical needs and a solid support system that addresses emotional/psychological needs, chronic conditions can be successfully managed so people can live healthy, vibrant lives.

Chronic conditions are multi-layered and the most successful treatment for coping and healthy living involve both physical and emotional support. Since our physical symptoms are often most prominent, it can be easy to ignore the emotional components.

Some of us have unfortunately been told that dystonia is "all in our head." To be fair, this does hold some truth considering that the source of our dystonia is due to a malfunction of neurotransmitters in the brain, but this is not what doctors and other people mean when they say, "It's all in your head." They are usually saying, "You are making it up for attention" or "You are a hypochondriac" or "You have anxiety or some mental disturbance that manifests into physical symptoms." If it were all in our head, wouldn't we slip up sometimes and forget the symptoms were there? Perhaps people say "It's all in your head" because they do not understand it or what to do to help us. It could simply be denial on their part.

While dystonia is not "in our head", sometimes we need to address our head. More specifically, we might need seek out a counselor or psychologist to help us better deal with the thoughts, feelings, and emotions that accompany a chronic condition. Dystonia can dramatically change our lives, making it difficult to cope with the mental and emotional pain. Many of us need and deserve help. Living with dystonia can be a mental nightmare.

Dystonia is so traumatic for some people that it can cause a major change in their work life, relationships with friends and family, and social life, all of which can lead to mood swings, isolation, depression, and suicidal thoughts. The limitations resulting from changes in our physical ability challenge how we see ourselves. This can cause an identity crisis, as what we previously knew ourselves as being disappears, such as a valued worker, an avid outdoors person, or someone others could depend on for anything. These changes can be extremely hard to deal with.

For years I always believed that with dystonia, and probably other chronic health conditions, there is a disease within the disease. What I mean is that along with physical symptoms, there is a mental component that accompanies the condition which can alter our personality, affecting our inner and outer dialogue, and how we relate to the world. This can change who we are or who we want to be. It is easy to lose our way when dealing with pain and other chronic, disruptive physical symptoms.

Since adjusting to a new life can be challenging, getting help from a counselor could be an excellent decision. Patients and doctors talk so much about physical treatments, which are of course important, but it is just as important to address the non-physical symptoms. They can often be more painful and difficult to deal with than the physical symptoms.

I have always felt that it is in our best interest to speak to other people about the things that are bothering us (as well as the things that bring us happiness and joy) whether it is with a professional therapist or trusted friend or family member. I went to school for a masters degree in counseling and also became certified as a life coach, so I clearly feel very strongly about the benefit of talk therapy.

People too often view asking for help or going to a therapist as a weakness. This couldn't be further from the truth. It takes courage to ask others for help. There is absolutely no shame at all in speaking with a therapist. We owe it to ourselves to seek out help when needed to clear out emotional baggage so we can be more mentally healthy. Holding in our feelings can be detrimental to our overall well being, particularly when we have physical health issues.

Consider the symptoms of dystonia, the main one being tight muscles. Think about some of the things that cause muscles to tighten; mental and physical pain, anger, frustration, resentment, bitterness, depression, etc. The longer we allow things to fester inside, the more it can affect our muscles.

Benefits of counseling
Meeting with a counselor gives you a place to talk freely about your feelings. There are countless online forums and support groups where people can go to talk with others, all of which can be very helpful. However, often times being with another human being having a face to face conversation is more effective and therapeutic than using a computer or other communication device. For one, it gets you out of the house and two, it gets you in front of another person where you can see and feel things that are not possible to see and feel when you are looking at words on a screen.

Addressing the implications of a chronic condition with a counselor begins with an understanding of both the physical and emotional consequences and limitations of the pain or illness. It is important for the therapist to understand that we are often unable to continue with recreational, vocational, and social activities that were once a regular part of our daily lives that brought us joy and a feeling of self worth. If counselors can identify with the profound impact these losses have on us and other challenges we face every day, they can help us work through our emotions and assist us in creating a new version of ourselves we can be proud of.

Counselors look at how psychosocial variables interact to affect our quality of life or mood states. They take many things into consideration, such as the role of stress, depression, anxiety, attitudes towards illness, factors influencing quality of life, the ways in which the illness intrudes on our lives, and the ways in which the illness affects cognition. Although dystonia does not impair cognition, when someone is in chronic pain and/or has other chronic symptoms, cognition can become altered. Dystonia can become such a major distraction that it can reduce our ability to focus and concentrate, causing mental lethargy and forgetfulness. Many of us also take medications which may alter cognition.

Counseling helps us redefine ourselves and develop a new sense of self worth and identity. Part of the counseling process involves going through the grieving process for the parts of life that have been lost as a result of the chronic condition. While there is always hope that our physical symptoms will improve, counselors help us work towards a realistic expectation and acceptance of our ability to resolve the conflict between what we want to do and what our body is able to do. This mind-body connection helps us get a better understanding of self and how we identify with our unique pain or illness.[49]

Testimonial

The visible symptoms of my ST/CD (continually twisting to the left) came on so suddenly that it turned my world upside down. My social life took a nose dive and work became extremely difficult. There was a lot of upheaval in my life and mentally I suffered. I was very lucky to have an extensive and supportive family, but I've always been the kind of person that doesn't like to burden others so I took on most of the responsibility for my condition myself. I struggled for nearly 2 years and my quality of life wasn't getting much better. I had some physical improvement, but I was emotionally distraught. I decided I would probably benefit from therapy.

I tried hypnotherapy in the early stages of my condition, but it didn't have much effect so I opted for counseling. I sampled a couple of counselors until I found someone I could talk to that put me at ease. She was near retirement age, inexpensive, and in no rush to get me out the door. She had all the time in the world to listen and help me work through the problems that I built up after developing dystonia.

I went to see her every week for about 3 months until we both thought that I'd reached the stage that I probably wouldn't benefit much from more sessions. My life had improved so much, mainly because I was cutting myself a bit of slack, accepting my condition, and relaxing more. The main thing she taught me was to accept myself as I was and to start loving myself again.

In autumn 2012, I went to see an osteopath for pain in my lower back. After the first session my back was doing better. I then mentioned I had dystonia so he asked if I wanted to try acupuncture. I decided to give it a go but it didn't help. He also did hypnotherapy so I thought I'd have a go at that again.

I don't think I'm one of the more suggestible people in the world and I was aware and conscious of most things he said, but I really benefitted from the sessions. He didn't talk about my condition much; mainly about my confidence in general and stuff about relaxation. When the money for the sessions with him ran out, I downloaded a few hypnotherapy programs and I fall asleep listening to them at night.

As a result of everything I've done, I'm probably more confident now than at any time in my life, despite feeling the effects of dystonia daily. Therapy was very instrumental in helping me make massive improvements in my life.

Vision Therapy

Vision is an amazing sense that is so important because it completes the other senses. It gives information to the body about everything in daily life and plays a major role in how our mind and body perceive the world, including the position of our head and neck.

To feel how much our eyes and neck are connected, do the following: lightly place your fingers along the back of your neck, just below your hairline. Imagine a fly buzzing around in front of your face. Without moving your head, follow the imaginary fly with just your eyes. What you should feel under your fingers is a subtle twitching as your neck muscles adjust to the movements of your eyes. Also take notice of any other muscles in your body moving or tightening. You may find that you want to move your shoulders or other parts of your upper torso. Ideally, you should only move your eyes while all the other muscles remain still. You should also be able to do this without getting dizzy. Dizziness may be a sign of weak eye muscles or a vestibular (balance) disorder.

The muscles you feel in the back of your neck when you move your eyes connect at the base of your skull with your upper cervical vertebrae. They are responsible for the orientation of the sensory organs that tell you where you are in space and what is going on around you. Considering how little it took for you to activate these muscles, imagine how much the neck is involved with much more significant eye movements and conversely, how much the eyes are involved with head and neck movement.

The receptors in the cervical spine have important connections to our vestibular (balance) system and visual apparatus, as well as several areas of the central nervous system. Dysfunction of the cervical receptors in neck disorders (e.g. dystonia) can alter sensorimotor control. Sensorimotor refers to the integration of our senses and motor (body) movements. In other words, our senses play an integral role in our movements. Changes in head position, as in the case of dystonia, may affect eye movement control and postural stability, resulting in dizziness and disorientation. It can also take place in reverse, meaning that weak eyes or one eye being more dominant than the other may affect head and neck position, as well as balance and stability.

To experience a more obvious connection between our sense of sight and body position, stand on one leg with your eyes open. Stand on two legs if you can't balance on one leg. Close your eyes and notice how unstable your body becomes after only a few seconds. When we lose visual perception of the world around us it affects our spatial orientation and balance. On a positive note, if you did this exercise everyday, over a period of time your brain would better acclimate to having your eyes closed and your balance should improve (there are many other similar exercises that improve balance). This can improve spatial orientation when you have your eyes open and may positively affect your dystonia and accompanying symptoms, such as stability and coordination.

When the head and neck muscles are tight and/or forcing the head and neck to move away from a straight position, the rest of the body has to compensate, including the eyes to a significant degree. This can alter visual balance leading to an increase in physical imbalances; all the more reason to do balance therapy. Vestibular therapists can be very helpful in this regard.[50-52]

When I consciously use my eyes when I want to turn my head, I have much better head and neck control. In other words, if I look with only my eyes in the direction I want to turn my head before turning (which is maybe a second or two before), I am able to turn my head more fluidly. My head and neck usually follow in line with my eyes.

Something that fascinates me is what happens when I eat. When I open my mouth to put food in, my head tilts/pulls to the right. If I look to my left with only my eyes as I am doing this motion, the tilt/pull is either reduced or eliminated. Also, if I quickly move my eyes to the left and right just before I take a bite, the tilt/pull decreases.

Another phenomenon I find interesting is that my dystonia symptoms decrease when I am not wearing my glasses or contact lenses. It seems that the less stimuli my eyes have to process, the more calm my neck muscles.

If you do the exercises and tips mentioned above, along with the ones described in the testimonial below, with enough practice you may be able to calm down dystonic and compensatory muscles. You may also reduce dizziness and balance problems, as well as improve head and neck stability.

Testimonial

When I was diagnosed with Spasmodic Torticollis/Cervical Dystonia, my neck significantly turned to the left and slightly tilted towards my right shoulder. I was in a great deal of pain, but what was even more distressing was the overwhelming sensation of feeling disorientated and off balance.

A few weeks before my first Botox injections, I saw a neurological physiotherapist. Understanding how vision and the vestibular (balance) system are closely linked, lying on her couch she held her finger a short way from my face and told me to follow the line of her finger while she moved it. I was absolutely taken aback that I could not do this simple exercise. I could make no connection at all with my eye muscles to track her finger. I was in a state of constant disorientation because of eye muscle imbalance.

Since this was so difficult for me to do and because my neck was so contracted to the left, she suggested I do some eye exercises at home. The eye tracking exercises I was told to do were to tone up my eye muscles so my eye movements would become normal again. Here is what to do:

Sit in a high back chair so the head is well supported and you can look straight ahead. The chair needs to be in a position so you are looking at a straight horizontal line. The line can be a window sill, a mantle piece, or similar. Without turning your head, slowly move just your eyes to follow the straight line to the right. It doesn't have to be a long line. Doing just part of a line can be hard in the beginning. Then track the eyes back to the middle and then along to the left and back again to the middle.

If this is difficult, limit how many eye tracks you do at this early stage, but try to do it a few times each day. If sitting in a chair is too difficult to look straight ahead, try lying on the floor instead and use the ceiling to track along.

When tracking becomes easier, build up to longer horizontal lengths, as well as looking up, down, and diagonally, and a doing quick tracks from one direction to another. When you are outside you can use the horizon for really long movements. In the bath or shower, tile lines are great for doing a long maze; but don't slip, be safe!

I find that when I walk, my head wants to turn. With concentration, I can help counteract this turn by looking in the opposite direction using my very strong eye muscles. Thinking back, I realized that my neck turning was not new. An activity I enjoyed with my husband was sea kayaking along beautiful coastlines. I had been aware that when I kayaked with the coast on my left, I always looked at the cliffs and beaches. But on the return journey, it was easier to look out to sea! It was not just my neck pointing one way; my eyes were naturally looking that way too.

When we look forward, the eye muscles are equally balanced. When the head is constantly looking sideways, the eyeballs are turned in their sockets. The muscles on one side of the eye become dominant. My eye muscles on one side had become so dominant that the opposing side had little to no power at all.

We move our eyes to see, which is obvious, but we can also use our eyes to turn our head. We can turn our head to "turn our head", but by using our eyes, we use a different brain pathway to turn our head; the head follows the eye in the direction it wants to look.

My dystonia is a combination of parts that are not working properly. Each separate part has its own problems. Any one of these parts might be interacting with another part, either being caused by it, or making each other worse. As each part becomes even worse, other bits deteriorate further.

Just improving one bit may make little difference to the overall dystonia because it is part of a bigger failing neurological system. Because everything is interconnected in one way or more, the fixed bit may begin to fail again if other issues are not addressed. My eye tracking exercises are hugely beneficial, but it is done in concert with managing other failing parts at the same time. It took me a few weeks before my eyes were back to normal. And once so, I made sure I continued with the exercises. A comprehensive approach to managing my dystonia is most effective for me and eye tracking has been a critical puzzle piece.

Relaxation breathing exercises
Breathing is obviously necessary for our survival. Without oxygen, our bodies would die. Along with keeping us alive, breathing has many health benefits such as detoxification, it releases tension, relieves emotional problems, relaxes the body and mind, massages organs, strengthens the immune system, improves posture, improves digestion, balances the nervous system, boosts energy, improves cellular regeneration, and elevates moods, to name a few. In this section we will focus on breathing exercises for relaxation, all of which benefit the other things listed. Before practicing any type of breathing exercise, consult your doctor to see if it is safe for you to do.

There are countless ways to work on breathing for relaxation. I am going to touch on a few exercises that I find helpful. The first thing to do is to determine if you are breathing correctly (i.e. breathing through your stomach and not your chest).

1. Stand, sit or lie down with your back straight. Do not cross your legs or arms. Put one hand on your chest and the other on your stomach.
2. Breathe in through your nose. The hand on your stomach should rise. This is your diaphragm pushing into your belly. The hand on your chest should move very little or not at all.
3. Exhale through your nose and mouth. The hand on your stomach should move in as you exhale and the hand on your chest should move very little.
4. Continue to breathe normally in through your nose and out through your mouth, only being mindful of which hand rises and falls.

In stomach breathing, also called belly, abdominal, or diaphragmatic breathing, you use your entire lung capacity. The diaphragm and abdominal muscles pull down on the abdominal cavity to fully inflate the lungs. Breaths are slow and deep, taking longer to inhale and exhale, which delivers a larger amount of oxygen to the bloodstream. This larger amount of air intake also allows you to exhale a larger amount of carbon dioxide, eliminating it from your body at a faster rate.[53]

Chest breathing tends to be short and quick, using only a small portion of the lungs and delivering a relatively minimal amount of oxygen to the bloodstream. Chest breathing is often associated with hyperventilation and a sensation of feeling out of breath, as you attempt to take in oxygen quickly despite the low air volume from each breath.

Progressive muscle relaxation
- Get in a comfortable position sitting in a chair or lying down. You may want to loosen your clothing and take off your shoes.
- Close your eyes.
- Take a few minutes to get comfortable and practice abdominal breathing as described above.
- When you are relaxed and ready to begin, shift your attention to your right foot. Observe any tension that may be present.
- Breathe in and tense the muscles in your right foot. Hold for a count of 3-5 seconds. As you exhale, relax your right foot and visualize your breath pushing the tension away, making it feel limp and loose. Try to not tense muscles other than the one you are focused on at the moment.
- Stay in this relaxed state for a moment, breathing normally.
- Shift your attention to your left foot. Follow the same sequence of muscle tension and release.

Move slowly up through your body, contracting and relaxing the muscle groups as you go. You can start anywhere you would like. I like to follow this progression: right foot, left foot, right calf, left calf, right thigh, left thigh, hips and buttocks, stomach, chest, back, right hand and arm, left hand and arm, shoulders and neck, face, eyes, and head. There are times when I will only focus on one or two areas where I feel tension or have spasms. It is not uncommon with dystonia to hold extra tension in certain areas. Be mindful of these areas so you can give them extra attention.

You can also focus on even more specific body parts, such as your fingers, wrist, forearm, elbow, upper arm, shoulder, neck, throat, jaw, chin, lips, tongue, nose, cheeks, eyes, forehead, temples, scalp, back of the head, top of the head, etc. When you reach the very top of your head, imagine yourself hovering above yourself in total and complete relaxation.

A variation of this breathing exercise is to do it without tensing your muscles. For some people with dystonia, tensing can sometimes exacerbate symptoms. Practice and see what works best for you. Instead of tensing, simply breathe in and out while focusing on a single body part. On your out breath, visualize tension flowing away from that area.

I can't stress enough the importance of breathing and breathing properly. Practicing just a few minutes a day can really make a big difference in how we feel, mentally and physically. Be good to yourself and take those few minutes. You'll be glad you did.

Neuroplasticity (Farias Technique)
Neuroplasticity, also known as brain plasticity, refers to the brain's ability to change throughout its lifetime. Scientists once thought that the brain stopped developing somewhere between 20 to 40 years of age. They thought that connections formed between the brain's nerve cells early on and were then fixed in place as we aged. If connections between neurons developed only during the early years of life, then only young brains would be "plastic" and thus able to form new connections and learn new tasks. This has proven to be untrue (think of the saying, "you can't teach an old dog new tricks", which is erroneous).

Throughout its entire lifetime, the brain has the ability to reorganize itself by forming new connections between brain cells. The term neuroplasticity is derived from the words neuron and plastic (neuro = neuron; plastic = moldable). A neuron refers to the nerve cells in our brain. The word plastic means to mold, sculpt, or modify. Neuroplasticity refers to the potential the brain has to reorganize by creating new neural pathways to adapt as it needs. In other words, the brain is an organ that is capable of changing/learning as long as it is alive. In fact, neuronal change is the basis for memory and behavioral change resulting from experience. Plasticity takes place constantly, whether we are undergoing intense training or doing absolutely nothing.

What does this mean for dystonia and other movement disorders? In simplest terms, it means that the malfunctioning circuits in the brain that cause unwanted, involuntary movements may be reprogrammed/rewired to restore normal movement, done through a variety of means, often unique to the individual depending on their physical and behavioral patterns. The most well-known practitioner to date utilizing this information with dystonia patients is Dr. Joaquin Farias.

Dr. Farias is the director of the Neuroplastic Training Institute Toronto and researcher at the University of Toronto. He utilizes neuroplasticity to treat individuals with focal dystonia. According to his website (www.fariastechnique.com) he discovered that most people affected by dystonia experience some unexpected moments of freedom of movement due to unknown reasons. He realized that both proper coordination and dysfunctional coordination coexist simultaneously. This made him hypothesize that the body is naturally able to restore proper coordination by itself. As a result, the goal of his training is to facilitate this process of reorganization (neuroplasticity). Dr. Farias considers dystonia to be a temporary lack or loss of accuracy and precision in brain activity. For this reason, his neuroplastic training aims to retune the brain and restore proper function of cognitive processes, perception, and motor functions.

References
1) www.drugs.com, Retrieved May 12, 2014 from: http://www.drugs.com/sfx/botox-side-effects.html
2) www.xeomin.com, Retrieved May 12, 2014 from: http://www.xeomin.com/
3) www.rxlist.com, Retrieved May 12, 2014 from: http://www.rxlist.com/botox-side-effects-drug-center.htm
4) www.webmd.com, Retrieved May 31, 2013 from: http://www.webmd.com/digestive-disorders/tc/difficulty-swallowing-dysphagia-overview
5) www.upmc.com, Retrieved December 2, 2013 from: http://www.upmc.com/patients-visitors/education/neurology/pages/phenol-benzyl-alcohol.aspx
6) Truong, D., Pathak, M., Frei, K. (2010) Living well with Dystonia. New York: Demos Medical Publishing, p. 57-59.
7) NIH – National Institute of Neurological Disorders and Stroke. Retrieved April 28, 2013 from: http://www.ninds.nih.gov/disorders/dystonias/detail_dystonias.htm
8) Dystonia Medical Research Foundation (DMRF), Retrieved on February 15, 2014 from: http://www.dystonia-foundation.org/pages/more_info___dopa_responsive_dystonia/64.php
9) Ashton, H. Benzodiazepines: How They Work & How to Withdraw. www.benzo.org.uk/manual/
10) Net Doctor, www.netdoctor.co.uk, Retrieved May 2, 2013 from: http://www.netdoctor.co.uk/diseases/facts/dystonia.htm
11) ST/Dystonia, Inc. http://www.spasmodictorticollis.org, Retrieved May 2, 2013 from: http://www.spasmodictorticollis.org/index.cfm?pid=60 and http://www.spasmodictorticollis.org/media/pdf/Broch-Meds.pdf

276

12) www.lifeinpain.org. Retrieved May 2, 2013 from: http://lifeinpain.org/node/3
13) Chou, K., Grube, S., Patil, P. Deep Brain Stimulation: A New Life for People with Parkinson's, Dystonia, and Essential Tremor. Demos Medical Publishing, 2011.
14) UCSF, Retrieved April 23, 2013 from: http://neurosurgery.ucsf.edu/index.php/movement_disorders_dystonia.html
15) Dystonia Medical Research Foundation (DMRF), Retrieved April 23, 2013 from: http://www.dystonia-foundation.org/pages/deep_brain_stimulation/151.php
16) www.aetna.com, Retrieved on May 3, 2013 from: http://www.aetna.com/cpb/medical/data/400_499/0401.html
17) www.wemove.org, Retrieved on May 3, 2013 from: http://www.wemove.org/dys/dys_sur.html
18) Retrieved December 5, 2013 from: http://www.healthcommunities.com/dystonia/treatment.shtml
19) www.wemove.org, Retrieved on May 3, 2013 from: http://www.wemove.org/dys/dys_sur.html
20) www.healthcommunities.com, Retrieved December 5, 2013 from: http://www.healthcommunities.com/brain-surgery/parkinsons-disease-surgery.shtml
21) Dystonia Medical Research Foundation (DMRF) http://www.dystonia-foundation.org/pages/generalized_dystonia___intrathecal_Baclofen/145.php. Retrieved April 22, 2013
22) www.michiganmedicalmarijuana.org, Retrieved on March 30, 2014 from: http://michiganmedicalmarijuana.org/page/articles/caregivers/what-cg-do
23) Franson KL, Nussbaum AM, Wang GS (February 2013). "The pharmacologic and clinical effects of medical cannabis". Pharmacotherapy (Review) 33 (2): 195–209.
24) www.medicalmarijuana.procon.org, Retrieved on March 30, 2014 from: http://medicalmarijuana.procon.org/
25) www.wikihow.com, Retrieved on March 30, 2014 from: http://www.wikihow.com/Get-a-Medical-Marijuana-ID-Card
26) Silverman, Jacob. "How Medical Marijuana Works", 11 August 2008. HowStuffWorks.com, http://science.howstuffworks.com/medical-marijuana.htm, 30 March 2014. Retrieved March 30, 2014
27) www.drugabuse.gov, Retrieved March 30, 2014 from: http://www.drugabuse.gov/publications/drugfacts/marijuana-medicine
28) www.mayo.edu. Retrieved on August 19, 2013 from: http://www.mayo.edu/mshs/careers/physical-therapy
29) Deepak R, Mathew H, Koshy M. Effectiveness of acupuncture in cervical dystonia. Acupunct Med. 2010 Jun;28(2):94-6
30) www.relaxtheback.com, Retrieved August 21, 2013 from: http://www.relaxtheback.com/fitness-therapy/inversion-tables.html
31) www.naturalhealthway.com, Retrieved August 21, 2013 from: http://www.naturalhealthway.com/articles/inversiontherapy.html
32) www.physicaltherapy.about.com, Retrieved August 21, 2013 from: http://physicaltherapy.about.com/od/devicesandorthotics/f/Inversion-tables.htm
33) Demerjian, G. Retrieved May 6, 2013 from: http://www.tmjconnection.com/dystonia.html
34) Power of Pain Foundation (POPF), Retrieved May 6, 2013 from: http://patientawareness.org/2012/12/09/dr-gary-demerjian-on-tmj-and-oral-orthotics/
35) www.mayoclinic.com, Retrieved May 10. 2013 from: http://www.mayoclinic.com/health/tai-chi/SA00087.
36) www.musictherapy.org, Retrieved September 17, 2013 from: http://www.musictherapy.org/assets/1/7/MT_Medicine_2006.pdf and http://www.musictherapy.org/about/musictherapy/

37) Mercola, J. www.mercola.com, Retrieved September 17, 2013 from: http://articles.mercola.com/sites/articles/archive/2013/07/04/13-mind-body-techniques.aspx

38) Ramsey, A. www.netdoctor.co.uk, Retrieved September 17, 2013 from: http://www.netdoctor.co.uk/healthy-living/wellbeing/health-benefits-of-music.htm

39) www.musictherapy.org, Retrieved September 17, 2013 from: http://www.musictherapy.org/assets/1/7/MT_Pain_2010.pdf

40) Mercola, J. Retrieved May 5, 2013 from: http://eft.mercola.com/

41) www.amsatonline.org, Retrieved October 22, 2013 from: http://www.amsatonline.org/faq

42) www.abigailalbaugh.com, Retrieved October 22, 2013 from: http://www.abigailalbaugh.com/The_Alexander_Technique.html

43) www.stat.org.uk, Retrieved October 22, 2013 from: http://www.stat.org.uk/pages/general.htm

44) www.alexandertechniqueatlantic.ca, Retrieved October 22, 2013 from: http://www.alexandertechniqueatlantic.ca/resources/articles/Dystonia.pdf

45) www.feldenkrais.com, Retrieved October 23, 2013 from: http://www.feldenkrais.com/method/the_feldenkrais_method_of_somatic_education/

46) www.drweil.com, Retrieved October 23, 2013 from: http://www.drweil.com/drw/u/ART00467/Feldenkrais-Method.html

47) www.drweil.com, Retrieved on November 22, 2014 from: http://www.drweil.com/drw/u/ART00473/Trager-Approach-Dr-Weils-Wellness-Therapies.html

48) www.trager.com, Retrieved on November 22, 2014 from: http://www.trager.com/approach.html

49) www.theravive.com, Retrieved on July 15, 2013 from: http://www.theravive.com/services/chronic-pain.htm

50) Bond, M. *Building good posture for healthy living*. www.healhyourposture.com, Retrieved September 13, 2013 from: http://healyourposture.com/2011/11/stiff-eyes-and-neck-pain/

51) www.vestibular.org, Retrieved September 13, 2013 from: http://vestibular.org/understanding-vestibular-disorder/human-balance-system

52) Treleaven J. *Sensorimotor disturbances in neck disorders affecting postural stability, head and eye movement control*. Man Ther. 2008 Feb;13(1):2-11. Epub 2007 Aug 16. Retrieved September 12, 2013 from: http://www.ncbi.nlm.nih.gov/pubmed/17702636

53) www.healthyliving.azcentral.com, Retrieved on February 17, 2014 from: http://healthyliving.azcentral.com/chest-vs-stomach-breathing-5640.html

Chapter 16
Working and Dystonia

There is great pride in having a job. It gives us confidence and makes us feel worthy. Getting paid for an honest day's work is a rewarding experience, not to mention the decreased stress of having money to pay bills and the financial freedom to do the things we enjoy. Many jobs in and of themselves are also very rewarding, which is why not having one or having to leave one can be so distressing.

We are conditioned to complain about work (TGIF is a popular saying for a reason), but when our body, the source of our pain and struggle, is letting us down, work can be a place where we can continue to feel good about ourselves because we have something to offer the world. However, we have to keep good balance. Our body doesn't just request our time and attention. It demands it. Phone calls, appointments, procedures, and self care are time consuming and draining. Work can soon become very challenging.

It has been over 12 years that I have been out of work. It is actually quite shocking and a little embarrassing that I have been out of work for so long. Even though I have good reason, I still carry around some guilt. When I am having a good day, I think to myself, "I could be working, even if only for a few hours," and then I might get hit with symptoms that knock me on my tail and I only feel well enough to get up from lying down to get something to eat. The day to day uncertainty is very unsettling.

I have always been a go getter and give my all to everything I do. When I had to stop working, I gave my all to learning how to survive the unbearable pain and neck contractions/spasms/twisting, as well as the anger, frustration, and depression that came with it. Hands down, the toughest job I ever had has been living day to day with dystonia. It's also the longest "job" I ever had and it doesn't include days off or vacations.

My last job was working as an intern at the Career Development Center at the university where I was studying for my master's degree. That was when my symptoms began and progressively worsened over the next several months. About two weeks into my second semester, I had to quit school and my job because my dystonia became so severe that I couldn't handle the workload. I could barely get out of bed in the morning to make breakfast, let alone shower, shave, and drive a mere mile to school for class and work. It was devastating.

For the prior six years I was in private business as a partner in several health related companies where I pretty much worked every day of the week and did a good amount of travelling around the country. I never thought twice about how much I was doing. My health was intact and I was having fun. The last job I had before beginning school was managing a water park on a beach on a lake in the mountains. I was also one of the project managers for the construction of the new park and family fun center. I worked my tail off seven days a week in a demanding job that required a lot of responsibility. Little did I know that within 6 months of working full time that I would be disabled to the point that I could barely get out of bed. It's amazing how life can turn on a dime.

Since 2002, when I dropped out of the work force, I still made efforts to make money. I was not well enough to go and work for someone; nor would I put an employer in a position where they didn't know if they could count on me from hour to hour, day to day. As you all know, we can't predict our symptoms. One day we may be well enough to do our job as well as anyone else, while other days half as much and some days barely at all. Because of the severity of my symptoms early on and even what they are now which is much improved, the unpredictability of my symptoms makes it uncomfortable for me to put an employer at risk for a potentially lame duck worker. I can do most jobs, but I don't know how much I can work from one day to the next, if at all.

Instead of getting a job, I opted to start an at home business using my computer skills to do customized printing. I then did some work setting up a website business. I also sold things on eBay and Amazon. I even sold Avon. Unfortunately, I didn't make enough money with any of those businesses that made up for the physical toll they took on my body.

I then decided to get certified as a life coach in the area of health and wellness so I could build a business around my communication and helping skills. It also allows me to work around my dystonia by being able to set my own hours. Having flexible hours allows me to schedule clients when I feel well enough to give my all. It also provides me the opportunity to work with dystonia clients.

Since everyone doesn't have the opportunity to work from home and set their own hours, there are challenges that come with getting a job and sustaining a job while managing a chronic health condition. Do we tell our employer or potential employer about our condition? How do we explain our limitations? How do we hide our dystonia if that is required in order to get or keep a job? What and how much do we tell our co-workers? The questions are endless.

Unfortunately, I don't have the answers. I have ideas and opinion as it relates to my life, but each of us is different so there really are no clear answers.

There are many ways that disabilities can affect the ability to perform effectively on the job, all of which are unique to the individual. It is also increasingly difficult these days when jobs are at a minimum for everyone. We not only have to navigate a competitive job market, but also compete with able bodied people.

Some concerns about working include: will I be well enough to do the job; will my dystonia get worse; how can I work when I am in so much pain; will I get fired because I won't be able to keep up with the demands; do I tell people I work with what is wrong with me; will my co-workers think less of me because of my dystonia (when we have something "wrong" with us, sometimes we are not viewed as a valuable worker because people may not believe that a person with a condition like dystonia is capable); how do I keep working but at a slower pace or less hours per week; will I get special treatment and if so, will that impact my working relationship with others; how can I work when I don't know if I will be functional one day to the next; can I ask for certain compensations to help me do my job better; who do I talk to about my concerns; should I not say anything at all and just do my job. This is a lot to think about and still just a partial list of concerns.

Applying for a job[1,2]

When applying for a job, be confident about your abilities and be clear about your objectives working with the company. If the topic of dystonia comes up and you are asked if you can handle the responsibilities, one of the best answers I have seen is, "Of course no one can guarantee what their health will be like in the future and I am no different. However, I understand your expectations and am confident I can do the job." This answer is concise, positive, and unambiguous. It shows you are confident in your work abilities and health management, while at the same time reminding the employer that no single person can make guarantees about the future. If our symptoms are effectively managed then we should approach our job search with confidence, knowing that any prediction beyond any time frame is actually unrealistic for anyone to make.

No one ever really knows the best thing to say in an interview because each job is different and each interviewer/employer is different. Honesty is the best policy, unless your symptoms are mild enough to where they can't be seen and/or do not impair your ability to work. If they don't, then say nothing about your dystonia unless you feel you should. If visible, then it is only fair be honest with your employer if they ask why your body is doing something that seems out of the ordinary. Be confident and frame what you say in a way that shows you are already finding ways around obstacles in order to achieve excellence.

Just because we have dystonia does not mean we are unable to work. Not only are we as good as others, in many cases we may be better. Thanks to the health challenges we face each day, we place great value on our work because we know the price it takes to sustain a job even in the best of circumstances. After what we have been through, our passion and desire to work trumps that of a lot of people. Use all you have learned from dystonia as a source of motivation for making the job world take notice of your drive and determination, as well as the value you bring to the table.

The U.S. Equal Employment Opportunity Commission (EEOC) is responsible for enforcing federal laws that make it illegal to discriminate against a job applicant or an employee because of the person's race, color, religion, sex (including pregnancy), national origin, age (40 or older), disability, or genetic information. It is also illegal to discriminate against a person because the person complained about discrimination, filed a charge of discrimination, or participated in an employment discrimination investigation or lawsuit.

Most employers with at least 15 employees are covered by EEOC laws (20 employees in age discrimination cases). Most labor unions and employment agencies are also covered. The laws apply to all types of work situations, including hiring, firing, promotions, harassment, training, wages, and benefits. The EEOC has the authority to investigate charges of discrimination against employers who are covered by the law.

Maintaining your job
If you already have a job and feel as though you are unable to fully withstand the demands, there are options. For example, you can speak with your employer about taking more breaks during the day to sit or lie down, you can cut your hours back, or you can swap hours with another employee. Ask your employer what ideas they have and what your options are.

Just because you are having difficulty does not mean that you and your employer can't make adjustments to make your job more tolerable. You also need not be afraid to let people you work with know that you are having difficulty. People will probably find out anyway. It is better to be honest than ignore the obvious. Most people are understanding and want to help. We just need to give them a chance. Strong co-workers will back you up when your body lets you down.

I understand how embarrassing it can be to look different and require special accommodations. I know how disappointing it is to have to cut back hours and also leave a job for health reasons. I've been there. I remember clear as day all of the conversations I had with my co-workers over 12 years when I had to resign. I was met with compassion, which was surprising to me because I felt like a failure even though I had done nothing wrong. I felt I was letting them and myself down, but mainly it was because I was so scared about what was to come next. Everything I had worked so hard for was slipping through my fingers and I had no idea what to do about it.

Coming to the decision to leave work can be a humbling experience, but we need to be smart about how we balance our work, family, and health, and do the very best we can with no regrets. We have to do what is best for us and our family.

If you are unable to work but still have some good hours during the day, volunteering is a great option. Also, if you are not confident at this point to make the transition back to work, volunteering may be a great start to get your feet wet. You are not only helping others, you are preparing yourself for the next step into paid employment. There is also the option of going on disability. Please see the information on Social Security Disability Insurance (SSDI) and Supplemental Security Income (SSI) in Chapter 17 to learn more.

Job protection[3, 4]
To protect your health and job, carefully navigate an employer's policies. There are two laws that offer some relief. The Family and Medical Leave Act allows employees to take up to 12 weeks off each year for medical or family emergencies, but without pay. The Americans with Disabilities Act requires that employers make reasonable accommodations and adjustments for disabled workers, often in the form of additional time off. Ask for adjustments if your condition meets the definition of a disability. If you are a valued employee, your employer will hopefully work with you. If you feel you are being unfairly treated, speak with your supervisor. If that doesn't work, go to the human resources department.

Your employer does not have to provide an accommodation if it would impose significant difficulty or expense. According to the Society for Human Resource Managers, the top five accommodations under the disability act provided by employers are parking or transportation modifications, making existing facilities accessible, offering new equipment to workers, restructuring jobs, and modifying the work environment.

If you are not sure what type of accommodations you are entitled to or how to ask for them, contact the Job Accommodation Network (800-526-7234), a service provided by the federal Department of Labor.

Also speak with the human resources department about the company's time off policies. Some companies have short and long-term disability plans. Disability policies typically allow you to take a specific time off at reduced or no pay.

Find out if the company has a corporate or employee health department. It can help to speak with an occupational health representative who can provide guidance for handling your job and health condition. It is also important to speak to the people with whom you work to help them better understand how they can help with your condition. Share with them only what they need to know. It is important to make them aware without creating excessive concern.

If the hours are too long or the work is too taxing, find out if you can work part time or take a different job in the company. If neither is feasible, you may need to explore other career options.

Testimonial

Twenty years ago, at age 42 and after 22 years of continuous employment, I exited the workforce. I had been living with a diagnosed illness and then a second one for 13 years, but I never made any conscious choices regarding my career plan based on my increasingly limited health. Within a matter of weeks, I left a job that I loved because I was too sick to even get myself to work.

When I made that decision, and for a short time after, all I felt was tremendous relief that I had at least eliminated one source of stress in my fragile world. But 'retirement' didn't produce the desired results. Although I had a full and satisfying life with two young children, a husband, friends, and extended family, I sorely missed what I no longer had; my life as a 'worker'. That person had a predictable schedule, daily socialization with colleagues, and was valued and compensated for her ideas and performance.

No longer employed, I volunteered in ways I hoped would be rewarding and give me the flexibility I needed. I found the former but not the latter. I still had to show up when I made a commitment and volunteer work felt like a 'job' rather than the career to which I had always aspired.

I became desperate to return to the workforce in whatever way I could. It seemed like my lifeline to improving my overall well being. This time I approached my career with care and thought, thinking strategically about my limits and my options, and setting clear intentions around my purpose.

Over the following years, I developed a business coaching people with chronic illness around career challenges. My clients' stories reinforced my own experience regarding the value of working, particularly when you live with chronic health challenges. That notion propelled me to write my book, <u>Women, Work and Autoimmune Disease: Keep Working, Girlfriend!</u> (2008).

While doing research for the book, I found several studies to support my experience that working promotes better psycho/social health outcomes in those living with chronic illness. Recently I found a study that says, "Retirement results in the drastic decline in health in the short and long term."

Specifically, the study found that retiring may "increase one's risk of developing clinical depression by 40% and the risk of suffering from a physical ailment by 60%." These risks increase with each year of retirement. Researchers recommend that people consider staying in the workforce beyond the average retirement age for health and economic reasons.

Most people who are not at "retirement age" think of retirement as a choice. Unfortunately, too often that is not the case. Many organizations have mandatory retirement ages and others have expected (not required but it is obvious) retirement ages. If you keep working when you are an older worker and have difficulties doing a job the way you once did, you can easily feel like you are being forced out. There are striking similarities among the healthy, but aging population, to those who leave the workforce due to debilitating health problems.

Clearly, it is a different story if the work you do or the place that you work is toxic - a highly pressured or extremely negative environment; the tasks are deadly boring or too difficult. If that's the case, then leaving, even if you don't have another employment opportunity, may be the best way to promote your well being.

If you live with a chronic condition, it is typically a gradual increase in symptoms and debilitation. Actual aging is more predictable. Thus, it is in anyone's best interest, healthy or not, to look at your future and prepare. Consider all of your options, create plans that offer you flexibility and maximize your sense of resilience, before you reach a dead end. - Rosalind Joffe

About Rosalind Joffe

Rosalind holds a Master's Degree in Education, is an International Coaching Federation accredited coach, a certified mediator, and has completed training in Focusing Practice. Rosalind has proven successes in coaching nearly 1,000 people for 15 years. Co-author of <u>Women, Work and Autoimmune Disease: Keep Working, Girlfriend!</u> (2008), Rosalind is recognized as a national expert on chronic illness and work. She has been quoted in The Wall Street Journal, The New York Times, The Washington Post, The Boston Globe, msnbc.com, WebMD, and ABC Radio, to name a few. As a leading career coach who focuses on chronic illness, she is a sought after speaker and workshop leader, and is published in dozens of disease organizations and health journals. She also writes a widely acclaimed blog, www.WorkingWithChronicIllness.com.

Contact Information:
Email: RosalindciCoach@gmail.com
Website: www.cicoach.com
Blog: www.WorkingWithChronicIllness.com

References
1) www.eeoc.gov, Retrieved September 8, 2013 from: http://www.eeoc.gov/eeoc/
2) www.sickwithsuccess.com, Retrieved September 7, 2013 from: http://sickwithsuccess.com/do-job/
3) www.nytimes.com, Retrieved September 8, 2013 from: http://www.nytimes.com/2009/06/20/health/20patient.html?ref=health
4) www.webmd.com, Retrieved on September 8, 2013 from: http://www.webmd.com/epilepsy/features/how-to-handle-chronic-illness-at-work

Chapter 17
Disability (SSDI and SSI)

The transition from a work environment to an extended period of disability or unplanned retirement can be challenging. To go from being physically able to work and financially provide for yourself and your family, to receiving a check each month from the government can be demoralizing and rob us of our dignity and independence. Most of us with dystonia are go getters. We are active, hard working people, and even with our limitations, we still do as much as we can each day to live as normal a life as possible. We are persistent, independent people. It is not easy for us to be physically limited to such a degree where we become financially dependent on others. It can alter our identity and make us question our self worth when we are unable to make a living.

Without the knowledge of what resources are available, the thought of the road ahead without work can often be frightening. Applying for disability can also be a confusing and humbling experience. Just like learning to live with a chronic health condition is difficult, going on disability, and perhaps receiving food stamps and other government support, is a big adjustment for many people. On top of that, the application process itself can often be very grueling.

However, despite problems with the system and the challenges navigating the application to approval process, the system is in place to help those in need. If you are someone who truly needs assistance, please accept and understand that you deserve the help and there is no shame in receiving it. It can be a life saver. Keep in mind that disability benefits need not be permanent. If your health improves to where you can work again, you do not need to stay on disability.

When it was proposed to me in the very beginning when my dystonia set in, I refused to go on disability. At the time, to me it was saying that I had a condition that I would never recover from and my getting disability was akin to giving up. Even at my worst I did not want to even consider disability as an option. I did not want to set the intention in my mind that I was sick, even though I had never been sicker in my life. I also didn't want to be a burden to an already burdened welfare system. Looking back, I realize how much easier things would have been financially had I not been so stubborn.

Disability defined

"Disability" under Social Security is based on your inability to work. The Social Security Administration (SSA) considers you disabled if you cannot do work that you did before, you cannot adjust to other work because of your medical condition(s), and your disability has lasted or is expected to last for at least one year or result in death. If you cannot adjust to other work, your claim will be approved. If you can adjust to other work, your claim will be denied. Along with your medical condition, SSA also considers your age, education, past work experience, and any transferable skills you may have.[1]

What this all means is that your condition must interfere with basic work-related activities for your claim to be considered. If it does not, SSA will find that you are not disabled. You must not be able to engage in what SSA calls "Substantial Gainful Activity" (SGA) because of your medically-determinable physical or mental impairment(s). SSA uses the term SGA to describe a level of work activity and earnings. Work is "substantial" if it involves doing significant physical or mental activities, or a combination of both. For work activity to be substantial, it does not need to be performed on a full-time basis. Work activity performed on a part-time basis may also be substantial gainful activity. "Gainful" work activity is work performed for pay or profit, work of a nature generally performed for pay or profit, or work intended for profit, whether or not a profit is realized.[2]

For each of the major body systems, SSA maintains a list of medical conditions so severe that automatically qualify you for disability. If your condition is not on the list, they have to decide if it is of equal severity to a medical condition that is on the list. If it is, they will find that you are disabled. Dystonia is not on this list, so it is imperative that you use words to describe your condition that Social Security understands or get a disability attorney/representative who can do this for you.

Applying for disability benefits

To begin the application process, you can go to your local SSA office or their website to complete the necessary forms. You can also contact a disability attorney/representative for instructions on how to begin the process. I suggest the latter, as it can be somewhat difficult to traverse the application process without help, as well as any appeals or hearings that may be forthcoming.

Upon receipt, the SSA will review your application to make sure you meet some basic requirements. "Basic requirements" include a medical condition that meets Social Security's definition of disability and if you worked long enough to earn "work credits" in jobs covered by Social Security (where you paid FICA taxes - Federal Insurance Contribution Act tax).

Work credits are based on your total yearly wages or self-employment income. You can earn a maximum of 4 credits each year. The amount needed for a credit changes from year to year. In 2020, you earn one credit for each $1,410 of wages or self-employment income. In 2019, a person received a quarter of coverage (work credit) for every $1,360 earned.

The number of work credits you need to qualify for disability benefits depends on your age when you become disabled. Generally, an individual must have at least 20 quarters of earnings (20 credits) within the 10 year period prior to becoming disabled. Younger workers may qualify with fewer credits. Whatever your age, you must have earned the required number of work credits within a certain period ending with the time you become disabled. If you do not meet the required number of work credits you are not eligible for SSDI, but you may be eligible for Supplemental Security Income (SSI).[3]

If you meet the basic requirements, your application will be sent to the Disability Determination Services office in your state. Doctors and disability specialists in the state agency will ask your doctors for information about your condition, when it began, how your medical condition limits your activities, what medical tests have shown, and what treatments you have received. All medical evidence from doctors, hospitals, clinics or institutions where you have been treated, as well as all other applicable information, will be used in determining your disability.

Social Security will also ask doctors for information about your ability to do work-related activities such as walking, sitting, lifting and carrying things, and remembering instructions. However, your doctors are not asked to decide if you are disabled. The state agency staff makes the determination. Sometimes they may need more medical information before they can decide if you are disabled. If more information is not available from your current medical sources, the state agency may ask you to go for a special examination. The SSA prefers you ask your own doctor, but sometimes the exam may have to be done by someone else, usually of their choosing. Social Security will pay for the exam and for some of the related travel costs.[4]

Social Security Disability Insurance (SSDI/SSD)

Social Security Disability Insurance is a program that pays monthly benefits if you become disabled before you reach retirement age and are not able to work. It is designed to provide income supplements to people who are physically restricted in their ability to be employed because of a disability. SSDI can be supplied on either a temporary or permanent basis, usually directly correlated to whether the person's disability is temporary or permanent.

According to the Americans with Disabilities Act, a disabled person of any income level can theoretically receive SSDI. Most Supplemental Security Insurance (SSI) recipients are below an administratively-mandated income threshold, and these individuals must stay below that threshold to continue receiving SSI. This is not the case with SSDI.[5]

If you are eligible for SSDI, the amount you receive each month will be based on your average lifetime earnings before your disability began. It is not based on how severe your disability is or how much income you have. The amount received on a monthly basis is unique for every individual. The Social Security Administration uses a complex weighted formula in order to calculate benefits for each person.

Most SSDI recipients receive between $800 and $1,800. The average monthly SSDI benefit in 2020 is $1,258, while the maximum SSDI monthly payment is $2,788. Your SSDI benefit may also be supplemented by a benefit from the Supplemental Security Income program. The SSI benefit is based on financial need and not your past earnings.[6]

To continue receiving benefits, you must remain medically disabled and unable to work at the Substantial Gainful Activity (SGA) level. However, SSDI rules allow you to work and receive earnings above SGA along with your SSDI benefit during specified periods, such as Trial Work Period and Extended Period of Eligibility, incentive programs to help you re-enter the work force.

Supplemental Security Income (SSI)

Supplemental Security Income (SSI) is a federal income supplement program designed to help aged, blind, and disabled people who have little or no income and do not meet the requirements for Social Security Disability Insurance (SSDI). Unlike SSDI, benefits for Supplemental Security Income (SSI) depend on the current income of the disabled individual.

In most states, as soon as you are approved for SSI you will automatically receive Medicaid. Medicaid is a needs based program that provides for a certain number of doctor visits and prescriptions each month/year, as well as nursing home care under certain conditions. Check with your local Medicaid office to find out about eligibility. You may also be eligible for food stamps (SNAP – Supplemental Nutrition Assistance Program) and Section 8 housing. This also applies to people receiving SSDI, as long as they meet income requirements.

The monthly payment amount for the SSI program is based on the Federal Benefit Rate (FBR). The FBR increases annually if there is a cost-of-living adjustment. For example, in 2019, the maximum FBR was $771 per month for individuals and $1,157 for married couples that were both receiving SSI. In 2020, the maximum FBR is $783 per month for individuals and $1,175 for couples. Income you receive during the month, minus certain exclusions, may be subtracted from your monthly SSI payment. However, you are allowed to deduct a portion of that income before it is subtracted from your SSI payment.

If you receive SSI benefits and someone provides you with shelter and/or food that you do not pay for, the Social Security Administration will count this as income and subtract it from your SSI payment. It is called "In-Kind Support and Maintenance." It reduces your monthly SSI payment because the SSA decides that you do not need the full SSI payment since you are receiving some food and/or shelter for free.[7]

Back Pay
In almost every case where you are awarded SSI or SSDI benefits, you will receive "back pay" in addition to your monthly payment. Back pay is for past due disability benefits from when the disability application was filed, or sometimes earlier. Since most claims are denied one or more times before you are approved for benefits, the disability application process is usually lengthy; months or years can go by waiting for approval. Back pay is just another term for past due benefits that have accrued during the approval process.

One of the factors that will determine when your disability starts is your application date. For SSDI benefits, you can receive benefits back to your date of application and also potentially receive retroactive benefits during the year prior to your application date (this does not apply to SSI). For SSI, you may potentially receive benefits back to the first month after you filed the disability application. This is known as the "alleged onset date" (AOD).

When you have been approved for benefits, you will be given an "established onset date" (EOD). The EOD will be based entirely on your medical records and work history. In other words, how far back your disability is determined to have begun will be decided according to the evidence available from doctor reports, lab results, and other information you provide on the disability application.

All SSDI retroactive payments and back pay are paid as one lump sum. For SSI, small amounts of back pay (under a couple of thousand dollars) are paid in a lump sum, but larger amounts of back pay are split into three payments, six months apart.[8]

Medicare and SSDI

Medicare is a health insurance program for people 65 years of age and older, disabled people under 65 years of age, and people with End-Stage Renal Disease (ESRD). Everyone eligible for SSDI is also eligible for Medicare. When you become eligible for disability benefits, The Social Security Administration (SSA) will automatically enroll you in Medicare.

You will receive Medicare benefits two years after the time you are deemed eligible for SSDI. This does not mean that Medicare benefits become available two years after you are approved for SSDI or two years after your monthly payments have started. Instead, you will receive Medicare benefits two years after your eligibility for benefits has been established. In other words, two years after your date of entitlement. In many cases, since the SSA takes so long to decide cases, you'll be approved for Medicare at the same time you are approved for SSDI benefits.[9]

Medicare has four parts:

1) Hospital insurance (Part A) helps pay hospital bills and some follow-up care. The taxes you paid while you were working financed this coverage so it is premium free.

2) Medical insurance (Part B) helps pay doctor bills and other services. There is a monthly premium you must pay for Medicare Part B. You have the option to refuse this coverage.

3) Medicare Advantage (Part C) plans generally cover many of the same benefits a Medigap policy would cover, such as extra days in the hospital after you have used the number of days Medicare covers. People with Medicare

Parts A and B can choose to receive all of their health care services through one of the provider organizations under Part C. There might be additional premiums required for some plans.

4) Prescription drug coverage (Part D) helps pay for medications doctors prescribe for treatment. Anyone who has Medicare hospital insurance (Part A), medical insurance (Part B) or a Medicare Advantage plan (Part C) is eligible for prescription drug coverage (Part D). Joining a Medicare prescription drug plan is voluntary and you pay an additional monthly premium for the coverage.

If you have questions about this coverage, you can contact Medicare toll-free at 1-800-MEDICARE (1-800-633-4227).[10]

Benefits outside the United States
Countries other than the United States have similar benefit programs. For example, Canada has a program called Employment Insurance (EI) and the UK has a program called Employment and Support Allowance (ESA). Employment Insurance (EI) provides temporary financial assistance to unemployed Canadians who have lost their job through no fault of their own, while they look for work or upgrade their skills. Canadians who are sick, pregnant, or caring for a newborn or adopted child, as well as those who must care for a family member who is seriously ill with a significant risk of death or who must provide care or support to their critically ill or injured child, may also be assisted by Employment Insurance. There are several types of benefits available to Canadians depending on their situation.[11]

In the UK, if you are ill or disabled, Employment and Support Allowance (ESA) offers you financial support if you are unable to work and personalized help so that you can work if you are able. You can apply for ESA if you are employed, self-employed, or unemployed. You might be transferred to ESA if you have been claiming other benefits like Income Support or Incapacity Benefit. In 2008, ESA replaced Income Support and Incapacity Benefit programs for new claims.

Another benefit is called Disability Living Allowance (DLA), which was replaced by Personal Independence Payment (PIP) in April 2013. PIP helps towards some of the extra costs arising from a long term ill-health condition or disability, and is based on how a person's condition affects them; not the condition they have. It is not means tested or subject to tax, and it is payable to people who are both in and out of work. How much money you receive is not based on your condition, but how your condition affects you.

Other benefits in the UK for which you may be eligible include: Carer's Allowance, Carer's Credit, Access to Work, Attendance Allowance, Blind Person's Allowance, Disability Premiums (Income Support), Disabled Facilities Grants, Disabled Students' Allowances (DSAs), Incapacity Benefit, Independent Living Fund, Reduced Earnings Allowance, Severe Disablement Allowance, and Work Choice.[12]

In the United States, depending on the state in which you live as well as other factors that vary according to your condition, prior work experience, and who is handling your application, the disability process can be grueling. It is almost as if the system is designed to make us sicker than we already are. The stress can have harmful affects on our body as we wait for the process to unfold. Very few people I know are approved the first time. It often takes one or more appeals and perhaps a hearing in front of a judge before you are approved.

Be prepared at the outset that it may take a great deal of patience on your part. You may get denied a couple of times and may also need to go to doctors for various assessments as deemed necessary by the government. Do your best to go with the flow. Getting frustrated will not make the process move any faster, but it will make your stress levels go up which will probably exacerbate your dystonia. There are many people who can help you with your disability case. Please find a reliable person, preferably one who understands dystonia, to represent your case and take some of that stress and workload from you.

References
1) www.ssa.gov, Retrieved on August 3, 2013 from: http://www.ssa.gov/dibplan/dqualify5.htm#a0=4
2) www.ssa.gov, Retrieved July 22. 2013 from: http://www.ssa.gov/redbook/eng/definedisability.htm#a0=0
3) www.ssa.gov, Retrieved August 3, 2013 from http://www.ssa.gov/dibplan/dqualify2.htm
4) www.socialsecurity.gov, Retrieved July 30, 2013 from http://www.socialsecurity.gov/hlp/radr/10/ent001-app-process.htm
5) www.ssa.gov, Retrieved July 22. 2013 from: http://www.ssa.gov/redbook/eng/definedisability.htm#a0=0
6) www.disabilitysecrets.com, Retrieved on July 24, 2013 from: http://www.disabilitysecrets.com/how-much-in-ssd.html
7) www.disabilitysecrets.com, Retrieved on July 24, 2013 from: http://www.disabilitysecrets.com/question18.html
8) www.disabilitysecrets.com, Retrieved on July 25, 2013 from: http://www.disabilitysecrets.com/back-pay.html
9) www.disabilitysecrets.com, Retrieved on July 30, 2013 from http://www.disabilitysecrets.com/question19.html
10) www.ssa-custhelp.ssa.gov, Retrieved August 3, 2013 from: http://ssa-custhelp.ssa.gov/app/answers/detail/a_id/155/~/receiving-medicare-and-disability-benefits

294

11) www.servicecanada.gc.ca, Retrieved on July 27, 2013 from:
http://www.servicecanada.gc.ca/eng/sc/ei/index.shtml

12) www.gov.uk, Retrieved on July 27, 2013 from: https://www.gov.uk/employment-support-allowance/overview, https://www.gov.uk/browse/benefits/disability, https://www.gov.uk/pip, http://www.disabilityrightsuk.org/personal-independence-payment-pip

Chapter 18
Tips, Tricks, and Tools for Daily Living

Some of these tips and tricks for daily living with dystonia apply to all people, but they are mainly for those with cervical dystonia.

Finding ways to go about our daily activities with as little pain, muscle spasms, pulling, twisting, tremors, etc., is a great challenge. For a lot of us, many common, everyday activities we never gave a second thought to before dystonia have become very difficult.

While we all pretty much have a baseline of relatively consistent daily symptoms, some activities exacerbate our symptoms because of how our body reacts when we engage or disengage certain muscles. Some people are so severe that they spend much of their day in bed or in a wheelchair. Then there are those with mild symptoms who are living their lives as they once did prior to developing dystonia. Most people fall somewhere between these extremes.

Some common questions you might find yourself asking are, "How can I do this or that particular activity more easily?" or "Why does my neck (and other body parts) spasm, jerk, and pull when I do this activity and not when I do that activity?", or "How can I do things differently so my overall symptoms do not get worse?" This section will give you answers to these questions by providing a variety of tips and tricks for common daily activities.

I learned most of these things through trial and error since my symptoms first appeared in 2001, as well as information I gathered from friends. Some suggestions might seem silly and trivial, but sometimes the smallest changes to the way we do things can make a significant difference in how we feel.

While it is not possible to cover every activity and all the various tips and tricks that can help everyone, I have identified the things I believe are most relevant to a good majority of us. If you are unable to find specific tips that are of benefit, at the very least, I hope they give you ideas for other things to try that will help you with daily activities. There is no one size fits all, so experiment to see what helps you. You may already be doing these things and possibly more. It is also possible that some or all of these are of no help, while for some, they will be of significant help.

Antagonistic gesture - "geste antagoniste" - sensory trick
It is common for people with cervical dystonia to hold their neck, head, or face with their hand to reduce spasms and keep it from pulling, turning, and twisting. It also helps with pain. When my symptoms started, I cupped my chin in my hand. As I got worse, I held my hand against the side of my face in the opposite direction my head turned. This progressed to pushing the side of my chin with my fingers as hard as I could. I pushed so hard that I developed a red welt on my face. There had to be a better way!

I then learned about a sensory trick called an antaganostic gesture or "geste antagoniste." By lightly placing your hand or finger on your cheek, chin, nose, forehead, or other part of the face/head, it may help reduce neck muscle spasms. Others find that touching their eyebrows helps alleviate contractions in the eyelids, especially for those with blepharospasm. These are just a few of many sensory tricks. In all cases, the brain is somehow tricked or distracted, causing the muscles to relax.

Researchers from a Dystonia Coalition research project found that there is a physiological basis for sensory tricks involving motor cortex excitability; in particular, the sensory trick "produces its effect by inhibiting the over activity of the motor cortex." That such tricks work suggests that dystonia is not just a motor-function disorder, but involves other neuronal processes, researchers suggest.[1] "Neuronal" meaning any of the impulse-conducting cells that constitute the brain, spinal column, and nerves.

When I had bad symptoms, I used an antagonistic gesture when I was sitting at the computer, watching TV, eating, reading, driving, and talking on the phone. Pretty much all the time. I remember the very first time I was able to take my finger off my face and have my head stay in place. I was playing solitaire on the computer and listening to relaxing music before bed. I felt very at ease so I decided to take my finger away to see what would happen. Usually my head would pull hard to the right. This time it stayed in place! The excitement I felt is indescribable. This was the biggest breakthrough I had up to that point.

I did the same thing the next several nights and it still worked. I would start by lightly touching my cheek with a finger for a few minutes and then take it away. I would keep my finger close to my face in case of a spasm, but without touching it. Within a couple weeks, I was able to take my finger away and rest my arm to the side with my neck staying in place. As strange as it may sound, this was one of the most joyous moments of my life.

This sensory trick has a different level of affect for everyone who tries it. The exact location where to touch is different as well. Try a few spots and see if it helps. It worked best for me when I was in a very relaxed environment. Once I began to trust that it worked, I was able to get the same effect in other environments. As my symptoms changed over the years, I found different sensory tricks that help. I don't use them much anymore, but it's nice to have them in my bag of tricks when needed.

Walking

A big challenge for many people is walking without their neck muscles pulling, turning, shaking, etc. When I was in rough shape (with my neck stuck to the right and pulling with the slightest breath or movement), the mere thought of walking was almost as painful as walking itself. I was basically bedridden so my walking consisted of going from the bed or the floor to the bathroom or kitchen. I avoided walking as much as possible.

When I had to sit, stand, or walk, I would push my face with my hand to hold my head straight. If I had to use both hands for something, like preparing food, I rested my head against the cabinets or a wall to reduce the pain and neck twisting. I made food as fast as I could and then ate it lying down on my side, sliding the food from my plate into my mouth. I will discuss tips for eating (at a table) later.

As my symptoms improved, walking became easier, but it came with practice. I had to relearn how to walk so my neck wouldn't turn so violently. Walking eventually became easier, but my neck still pulls off center a little if I walk too much, so I have to temper this activity.

Practice walking can be a helpful exercise to retrain your brain. Set up an area in your house, driveway, or garage about 10-20 feet. You can put tape on the ground or just measure out a comfortable distance using objects on each end. Stand in as upright posture as possible and practice walking the designated distance until you can do it with less involuntary movements. When your brain gets used to comfortably walking this distance, increase it another 10-20 feet. Slowly progress to where you can walk further with more comfort. The moment you feel an uncomfortable symptom, stop in your tracks, breathe, visualize normal walking movements (whatever that means to you), and then begin again. If this is too much, stand in place and practice walking with your arms and legs as if you were moving forward.

In 2007, because of significant weight gain from being sedentary for several years, I began to walk for exercise. I started by walking to the end of my driveway once a day for about a week. I then walked to the end of my street (about 100 yards) once a day for a couple of weeks. I then increased this distance as long as my neck did not turn, pull off center, or spasm. With practice, I gradually got up to 2-3 miles twice a day. However, my excitement about losing weight and being active again caused me to overdo it, which increased my dystonia again. My neck began pulling uncontrollably with more frequency and severity. My head would turn and pull way off to the side which caused intense upper back pain. The pain got to the point where I had to stop walking entirely.

After a few months of getting my symptoms under better control, I had to relearn to walk without my neck pulling. I started in my garage walking 10-20 feet as described above. I then went to the end of my driveway (about 50 feet); then to the end of my street and so on. Now I can walk further distances with less discomfort, but I only do so until I feel my back and neck start to contract. Then there are days when my neck pulls when I only walk a few feet. On those days, I rest my body. I then continue the next day making modifications if necessary. Listen to the signs your body gives you and do not push your limits.

One of the things I learned with many activities that helps reduce symptoms is to "trick" the muscles by doing some other activity, similar to an antagonistic gesture as described above. For example, when I walk and simultaneously toss a tennis ball back and forth from one hand to the other or bounce it in front of me, it prevents my neck from pulling as much. The act of tossing/bouncing the ball seems to disengage some dystonic muscles. As soon as I stop tossing or bouncing the ball, my neck contracts and pulls off center. If I don't have a ball, I will pretend I do and "throw" it back and forth as I walk. This also helps.

I also use something called a "shepherd's crook." It is a long, curved, metal hook with rubber on both ends designed for working on hard to reach trigger points. When I put pressure on certain spots on my back, or sometimes just hang the crook over my left shoulder, the muscle pulling decreases. When I walk, I will often put one end on a spot on my back and then pull forward to put pressure on that spot. This reduces the tension in the muscle allowing me to walk more upright with less pain and spasms.

Tips to help you walk with more ease:

- Do shoulder shrugs as you walk. If I shrug one of my shoulders every few feet, it prevents my neck from pulling to the right. Shrugging either shoulder helps; sometimes I need to shrug both.
- Keep your eyes focused on one spot in front of you.
- Move your eyes left and right and/or up and down.
- Lightly shake or sway your head as you walk. In other words, instead of letting your neck move on its own involuntarily, voluntarily move it slowly on your own. This will sometimes shut off the muscles that make your neck contract.
- Slightly tuck in your chin and lightly pull your neck back so it is flat. This is called a cervical brace (or military brace) position, without the use of an actual cervical brace or neck collar.
- Swing your arms a little more quickly or slowly than you would with your normal gait (walking motion).
- Swing one arm more than the other.
- Put one hand in your pocket or hold it to your side while the other one swings.
- Breathe through your stomach (abdominals) and not your chest. Chest breathing will cause your body to tense up more than it already is. To make sure you are breathing properly, place one hand on your chest and one on your stomach. Now breathe normally. The goal is to have your stomach expand and not your chest. If your chest expands rather than your stomach, then you need to practice your breathing. Proper breathing will decrease stress, improve blood circulation, and relax tight muscles, so it is a good idea to do anyway.
- Distract yourself by listening to music, reciting a favorite quote, mantra, affirmation, or prayer to keep your attention off walking.
- Put something in your mouth like a toothpick, a straw, the earpiece to your sunglasses, or a piece of gum. For some people, having something in their mouth will reduce their symptoms. It is believed by some that cervical dystonia is partly due to a problem with the temporomandibular joint (TMJ) and having something in our mouth apparently relaxes the jaw which relaxes the neck muscles.
- Use a cane or walker.
- Stop walking as soon as you feel any contraction or spasm beyond what is normal. Once you are comfortable, begin walking again.

Miscellaneous activities

For so many activities, it is a strain to hold our neck in a position that is comfortable. When we cook, clean, look/reach into the refrigerator, cabinet, and oven, do laundry, and vacuum, we often have to put our neck into positions that cause pain and exacerbate symptoms.

Vacuuming

Instead of pushing the vacuum back and forth and side to side, stand as upright as possible in good posture and walk around with the vacuum as if you were cutting the lawn. Move in as linear a pattern as possible. Keep the vacuum close to your body so you do not have to extend your arms. Anytime we extend our arms we put strain on our neck. While this may not be the most efficient way to vacuum, it is more back and neck friendly. Doing things in a hurry can often make symptoms worse, so it is sometimes better to take extra time to do things that are dystonia friendly.

Picking up objects below us

- Keeping your back and neck in as straight a posture as possible, put one leg in front of the other and crouch down to one knee. Keep your head from jutting forward. Pick up the object and stand up while maintaining this posture.
- Get into a crouch position like a baseball catcher (keep neck neutral as possible).
- Spread your legs wide and squat down (keep neck neutral as possible).

Reaching for objects above our head

One of the positions most of us should avoid is extending our neck (looking upwards) because it puts too much pressure on the external occipital protuberance (EOP). This is the bony ridge at the base of the skull where the muscles of the head and neck attach to hold the weight of the head upright. Many neck muscles meet here so it can get "congested", causing a lot of us to experience tightness, spasms, and pain. Putting pressure on this area by looking upwards will more than likely exacerbate these symptoms.

If you need to reach for an object above your head, find the object with your eyes; then reach up to the object while you let your head rest neutral or down towards your chest the best you can. This alleviates stress on the EOP. You can also use a chair or ladder so you can stand with good posture and not extend your neck, and/or use a grabbing tool that has an extended arm.

Carrying bags/objects

It is best to avoid carrying heavy objects whenever possible. However, this is sometimes unavoidable. Even carrying light objects can put strain on our necks. The best way I found to carry any object is to hold it close to my body. When carrying more than one thing, like grocery bags or luggage, for example, balance your body out using both arms to carry the load.

For women, carrying a purse/pocketbook over your shoulder can often cause a problem because it unbalances the body, pulling it to one side. This being the case, it would be best to carry a small bag that you can keep in your hands rather than draped over your shoulder. Bring only the essentials so you don't have a heavy bag. There are also pocketbooks that have straps like a back pack. This allows you to carry more and have the weight evenly distributed. It's good for every day use and for travelling. It's probably a better option than carrying your luggage or dragging it behind you.

In the grocery store, always use a cart no matter how many items you have to buy. The cart takes away the burden of carrying anything. Also, if you hold your neck, head, or face with your hand, you have the cart to put your other hand. It also helps to have a cart to hold onto if you have balance problems. If you need to use a motorized cart, please don't be ashamed to do so.

Tying your shoes

All of the ideas for picking up an object can be used for tying your shoes. I try to wear shoes that don't have laces so I can just slide them on and off without bending over. With my sneakers, I put the laces in the shoe itself and they turn into loafers with laces. If you want to try this, in the top eye hole, put the laces in facing towards the shoe so it will be easier to put them in your shoe.

Brushing your teeth

Use an electric or battery operated toothbrush. Rather than using your arm to do the brushing, which will often make your neck pull more, let the brush do the work for you. This reduces stress on your shoulders and neck. You can also try brushing while lying down in bed on your back with your head propped up on a pillow. When I rinse my mouth out, I use a cup with a straw. I never fill my cupped hands with water to rinse because leaning my head down into the sink makes my neck spasm and twist, as does drinking from a cup. Instead, using a cup with a straw allows me to stand in good posture so I have better control of my neck.

Flossing

Flossing is more difficult for me than brushing. Instead of using dental floss, I use a combination toothpick and floss tool. The brand I use is called Plackers. One end has about a half inch piece of floss and the other end is a tooth pick. This tool puts far less stress on my neck than dental floss. You can purchase them from any grocery store or pharmacy.

Washing your hair

Showering in general wears my body out. For some reason, standing and moving around to wash ignites all the muscles in my body. It takes almost an hour before they calm down. Washing my hair is the worst part. It makes my neck pull more and I get so dizzy that I feel like I am going to fall. This being the case, I much prefer to shower before bed than in the morning because I can lie down afterwards. In the morning I can just get up, wash my face, brush my teeth, get dressed, fix my hair, eat, and get on with my day. When I was at my worst, I washed my hair using one hand while I held my face/neck with my other hand. I would also sometimes lean my head against the wall as I washed it. Both are fine if you can't handle the pain and pulling when using two hands.

Hair washing tips:
- If you are able to tolerate using two hands, rest your head down towards your chest as you wash and rinse. This will take pressure off the top of the neck in back (where the neck muscles meet the head).
- Stand in as good a posture as possible. Slightly tuck your chin down and pull your head flat back a little so you are standing straight as you can. Then proceed to wash and rinse.
- Sit on a shower seat to wash your hair using one of the ideas above. You can also sit in a chair to wash the rest of your body if standing is too uncomfortable.
- Use a hand held extension shower device. This allows you to wash and rinse your hair with one hand if you need to hold your head with the other hand. This is also a great device for washing/rinsing your body.
- Wash it in the sink. While standing, lean over and have someone wash it for you. You can also do it on your own this way if you are able. I prefer this over the other options, unless I have a very tall shower head where I can stand upright and rest my back against the wall.
- When you go for a haircut, never have them wash your hair using their salon sink. This is one the worst positions for your neck. This is something that people without ST/CD should never even do. Instead, stand over the sink and let your head hang down to have it washed.

Shaving

I can really only speak for men on this one, but I can offer some advice for woman that might help. For men, try shaving your face with an electric razor instead of a blade razor. It may reduce cuts if you have spasms. I went from a blade razor to an electric razor which helped a lot. However, I started to develop a painful rash so I went back to a blade razor. I would lather and shave one side at a time while holding the dry side of my face. This helped reduced spasms so I wouldn't cut myself. When I gained better control over my neck, I was able to lather and shave my entire face without having to hold it.

It also helps to find a good time of the day to shave. Since shaving can sometimes take a lot out of me, I prefer to do it in the evening. This way I can deal with any increased symptoms when I have nothing else I need to do except go to bed. If I shave in the morning and it exacerbates my symptoms, it makes getting on with the day much more difficult. You may be the opposite so find the time when you are most comfortable.

For women, I imagine shaving your legs is no fun even without dystonia. The only tip I can offer is based on how the neck muscles work in cervical dystonia. One of the best ways to stretch the neck and get relief is to let it hang straight down. If you do this while shaving your legs, it might make it easier. To be more specific, bend at your waist (either sitting or standing) as if touching your toes. With your head hanging down, shave your legs. You not only get a nice stretch in your neck and back, it may also be a comfortable position to shave your legs more easily. You can also shave while sitting in a bath tub if getting in and out of the tub is something you are able to do. How you shave other parts of your body are up to you as to the best way to do it without exacerbating your symptoms.

Cooking

For some, cooking is a relaxing activity. For others, it can be a major undertaking; in fact, one that is dreaded. There was a time when I didn't make anything that I couldn't quickly put in the microwave and then take to the floor or bed with me to eat. It was too painful to stand and use my hands to prepare food. I needed my hands to hold my head to reduce spasms and pain. I didn't care how unhealthy the food may have been. My only concern was how to get through a meal with as little pain as possible. Thankfully, this is no longer the case. For the most part, I enjoy cooking now. I don't make anything extravagant, but I can stand and prepare meals unlike I used to.

One of the things that helped me when it was difficult was to rest my head against the wall or cabinet when I was cleaning (both food and dishes), cutting, and cooking. Something else I found helpful, and still do, is making several meals at once. Instead of making food for one day, I make enough to last me a few days. For example, when I make chicken breast I bake three breasts at a time. This way I have one for dinner and then two more I can take from the refrigerator for lunch or dinner the next couple of days. I pretty much do this with anything I make. It is much easier for me to cook a lot one day so I have little to nothing to do on other days. When I feel up to it, I also make my lunch for the next day (or several days depending on what I make) so I don't have to worry about that either. Leftovers are my key to stress free cooking and eating.

It really helps to take the time to plan and prepare your meals for a few days or the week if you are able. Having something ready that you can take from the refrigerator or freezer will make it easier on you when you are having a particularly tough day and cooking is too challenging. Ordering take-out is also a great option, but it can get pricey if you are not careful.

Eating
When my ST/CD was at its worst, I had to push my head in order to open my mouth to put food in. When I was ready to swallow, I pushed even harder so my throat would open wide enough to swallow. There were times when I choked merely trying to drink water, so the only way for me to swallow safely was to push my head as straight as I could. I then added the tips below to make eating a little easier.

- Eat from a bowl or a plate with high sides. I almost always put what I eat into a bowl so it is easier to scoop out the food using the side of the bowl as an aid for getting food on my fork or spoon.
- Cut everything up beforehand so you have less work to do when eating.
- Use a spoon. It depends on what you are eating of course, but I find it easier to eat most food with a spoon. Less food spills with a spoon than it does with a fork.
- Use your non-dominant arm. For me that would be my left arm because I am right handed and my neck pulls to the right. Often, lifting the arm opposite to the side my neck pulls will balance out the other side so I don't pull as much. The muscles on the right side from my mid back up to my skull feel "over weighted", so when I use my right arm for things, it feels like I add more weight to that side, causing my neck to pull. Using my opposite arm helps offset the pulling.

- Use your eyes. Look in a certain direction as you bring food to your mouth. If I look down, my neck pulls. If I look straight ahead and slightly up (with just my eyes, not my head) my neck does not pull as much, regardless of which arm I use. It also doesn't pull as much if I look to the opposite side to which my neck wants to pull, which for me would be to the left since I pull to the right. This is all with just my eyes. Not my head. I prefer to look straight ahead with my eyes (rather than to the left) because I always try to reinforce "straight and centered" in my brain. You can also try closing your eyes just before putting food in your mouth.
- Sit in an erect posture with your chin down and head slightly pulled back. Good posture in all things we do promotes a reduction in overall symptoms.
- Sit close to the table so you don't have to jut your head forward.
- Put something under your plate to raise it closer to your mouth so you don't have to lift your arms too far.
- Slightly shake your head left and right as if saying "no" right before you put the utensil in your mouth. For some reason, just as I am lifting my arm and opening my mouth, a very slight shake of my head seems to deactivate the muscles that contract. Also try nodding up and down.
- Practice eating. When you are sitting at your desk, at a stoplight in the car, watching TV, etc., practice as if you are actually eating. This might help program your brain to move your arm so that your neck no longer pulls, or pulls as much. Our brains learn through repetition, so we can either train it to repeat an activity that yields a desired result or an undesired result.
- Eat standing up. When I used to sit and eat, my neck pulled more, so unless I was at a restaurant or other place where I had to sit, I would stand. I stood at the kitchen counter and moved around a little in between bites. This helped keep me loose and less symptomatic.

Drinking

If your neck is twisted, turned, pulling, in spasm, or shaking, drinking from a regular glass can be difficult. I have spilled on myself more times than I like to admit. If you have a similar problem drinking from a glass, use a straw whenever possible. It reduces how much you have to move your neck and ensures that the fluid gets into your mouth rather than on your face and clothing. It also prevents you from putting your neck into extension (looking up) which places pressure on the top of the neck at the base of your skull.

306

Another option is to use a bottle. With a bottle, you don't have to put your neck into extension. You only need to use your wrist to manipulate the bottle to drink. The small opening prevents spilling, which can occur when we drink from a glass or cup with a wide opening. Using cups that have a top with a small opening are also a good choice, similar to the lids that are put on coffee cups. It looks like a child's "sippy cup." There are also specially designed water bottles that have a nipple top that only release liquid when you suck on it.

Sitting
Good posture in all activities is critical for people with dystonia because our body positions can either exacerbate or relax our symptoms. Sitting is especially important to pay close attention to since a lot of us spend a great deal of time in a chair. Sitting is also when many of us tend to get lazy. A chair itself is a good visual for how we should sit. If you look at the way a chair is shaped, this is how our bodies should be shaped when sitting. Below is an example of how to sit in good posture.

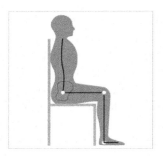

The knee and hip joints should both make a 90 degree angle. Feet should be flat on the floor. Do not cross your legs. If your feet don't reach the floor, use a foot stool. Your shoulders should be relaxed and resting under your ears, and your hips should be lined up under your shoulders. Depending on your condition, this may not be possible so do the best you can within your ability.

When we sit, body weight is transferred from the pelvis onto the chair. On the bottom of the pelvis there are two bones called "sitting bones", technically called the ischial tuberosity. To get on top of your sitting bones, rock back and forth on them and stop in the center. If your chair is cushioned you may not be able to feel your sitting bones as well as if you sit on something hard. Notice if your weight is in front, back, or on top of your sitting bones. If your weight is forward, your low back may be arched. If your weight is back, you are probably slouching. If you over arch, let the pelvis drop into a neutral position so that you are on top of the sitting bones. If you slouch, you may benefit from a lumbar cushion. The diaphragm plays a role in upright posture so take some deep breaths through your stomach to help you get into a good position. Avoid chest breathing. It can make your muscles tighter.

Sit on a chair that does not have a dip or slant in the seat. A dip will encourage you to slump your low back and a slant creates an unhealthy angle. If your seat is not level then sit close to the edge. Sitting close to the edge provides you with a balanced, stable platform on which to find your sitting bones and practice good posture.[2] If you would like, use a pillow or other back support. I use an Obsuforme which helps support my back and neck, and promote good posture.

Desk/Office set up
When my symptoms were severe, I had to push my head straight to see the computer screen and was only able to type with one hand. Suffice to say, I did not spend much time at the computer. The pain and muscle pulling was too much to handle. As my symptoms improved, my time at the computer increased. My desk setup also changed to meet my needs. For those of you that need to hold your head for support, by all means do so. Putting a pillow or a book under the arm you use to hold your head might make it easier so you don't slouch or lean to one side. This is how I started. I then got to a point where I could lightly touch my chin using an antagonistic gesture to keep my neck from pulling. I then got to where I didn't need to hold my head or rest it in my hand. I have full use of both hands now which is such a treat compared to how things were.

People complain a lot about increased pain and fatigue when working at the computer. One of the reasons of course is that dystonia causes pain and fatigue. The other reason is poor posture and using desk setups that promote pain and fatigue. One of the main culprits is improper use of arm rests or not using them at all. Resting our arms at certain angles or holding them up to type puts stress on the neck, shoulders, and back. Even people without dystonia develop problems in these areas when they don't use arm rests or when they use them improperly (too high or too low), so it especially important for us.

Many of us have laptops, smart phones, tablets, iPads, etc., making it so we can sit, stand, or lay down wherever we want to do our work. However, we tend to get lazy and find the most comfortable position, which is usually one that promotes poor posture. Some people will put their gadget on a desk or table where they have to lift their arms up and/or out to reach the keys to type. Some put them on a coffee table or bed and then lean forward to type. All of this puts too much strain on the body since the arms, shoulders, and neck are not supported. Even sitting with computers on our laps can promote poor posture, typically one that is slumped or rounded. This shortens/tightens our muscles, potentially increasing symptoms.

Below is an image showing one of the ways to not sit at the computer. At first glance it looks like he is in a good position, but notice the amount of space (in white) between his elbow/arm and arm rest, keeping him in a chronic shrug position. Although he is sitting in good posture and not reaching for the keyboard, holding his arms in the air to type strains his neck, shoulders, and back. Also notice the upward angle of his arms to the keyboard, the opposite they should be for a relaxed working position.

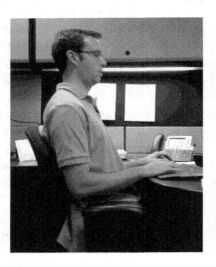 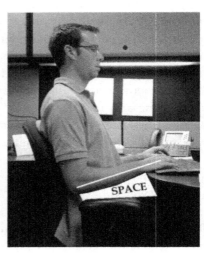

This gentleman lives with dystonia. His primary area of pain and tightness is his neck, shoulders, and base of the skull. When he modified his work station that allowed him to rest his arms, it reduced his pain and tightness. Compare this to your work station and you might find that adjustments need to be made. Remember that even though he is sitting in good posture, it still caused him great discomfort because of his arm angle and not using the arm rests.

I have experimented with many different desk setups over the years and finally found one that works great for me. It is comfortable and safe for my dystonia, causing little to no symptom flare ups. I still have to get up and move around because sitting for too long bothers me, but I can endure far more hours than I used to.

I have a laptop. Since I don't like to type on a laptop keyboard and can't find a comfortable position to sit and work without reaching for the keys and straining my neck and shoulders, I bought a wireless keyboard and mouse. I also bought a desk that has a slide out keyboard tray. I put the wireless keyboard and mouse on the slide out tray and the laptop on the desk. I have a desk chair where the arm rests slide right up to the keyboard tray. My arms are at a level that when I am typing my hands sit comfortably on the keys. There is a slight downward angle from my elbows to my hands to the keyboard, which keeps my shoulders relaxed. My screen is a little below eye level so I don't have to strain to hold up my head or lean it forward or back. I raised the screen about four inches so my head is more upright and my eyes are not looking in a steep, downward angle. My chin is slightly pulled back and tucked, keeping my head and neck in a neutral position. I also use an obusforme back rest to help with posture.

Below is an image of my work station. I don't have the best posture in the world and my core is not as engaged as well as it should be, but notice how my elbows sit comfortably on the arm rests and my arms angle downward toward the keyboard, taking stress off my neck and shoulders. A line is drawn to illustrate my relaxed arm position.

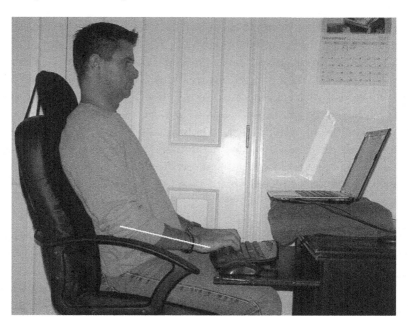

Talking on the phone

I used to talk exclusively on a phone that I held to my ear. This increased my existing neck spasms, causing my chin to hit the numbers while I was talking as if I were dialing the phone. I also had intense pain from lifting my arm and holding the phone to my ear. I then began to use a headset which helped tremendously. I bought a hands-free headset phone for the house and use a headset or Bluetooth when I talk on my cell phone. This has been a lifesaver. It allows me to spend more time on the phone with far less pain.

If I don't have a headset, I put the person on speaker phone. If I am around other people where speaker phone is inappropriate, I will talk for a few minutes with the phone to my ear and then tell the person that I have to call them back some other time. I will of course take emergency calls, but those that can wait until I have my headset are going to wait. It might seem like a trivial thing to use a headset or speaker phone all the time, but whenever I hold the phone to my ear, it causes more problems than it's worth. I really try to do my best to avoid anything that might exacerbate my symptoms.

Sleeping

Sleep is so important to our overall well being and it also gives our dystonic muscles a chance to rest. While it may not be the most comfortable way to sleep, I believe the best position is on our back. If we sleep on the same side that our neck is tight or the direction it turns (short side), we create an isometric position which will more than likely aggravate the muscles. If we sleep on the opposite side that our neck is tight or turns, this is a bit safer but it might cause spasms where you feel your neck jumping off the pillow. When we sleep on our stomach we have to turn our head one way or the other, forcing us to either favor our dystonia or fight against it, both of which can be problematic. It is also bad for posture. The only time I recommend sleeping on your stomach is if you are on a massage table with a head cradle where you can rest your neck. There were nights when the only place I could get comfortable enough to sleep was in my massage chair.

When we are sleeping, we don't want to be in any position that makes our muscles work. Thus, sleeping on our back with our chins slightly tucked down is probably the safest way to sleep. It is also the best position for good posture and it lightly stretches the muscles in the neck that attach at the base of the skull. Side and stomach sleeping tend to tighten this area of the head/neck in an unbalanced way which will more than likely cause interrupted sleep and more pain upon waking. It may take time to become a "back sleeper", but it is worth the practice because it offers the least chance of aggravating your muscles. It took me many months to learn how to sleep on my back and it has paid dividends.

Driving
Driving is a dangerous activity if you are unable to keep your neck straight, have difficulty turning your head, and/or have tremors. This being the case, please drive only when you have to and opt to have someone else drive you whenever possible. I know this reduces our independence, but consider the consequences of an accident where you put yourself and others on the road in danger. If you must drive, find a comfortable way to position your seat that controls your symptoms as much as possible. Wear a neck brace if need be, use a back support to promote good posture, and get attachments for your mirrors that expand your vision so you don't have to turn your head too much.

When I was in really bad shape, I bit down on the seatbelt shoulder harness to keep my head straight. I learned this from a friend who did it when she was having trouble. I also reversed my head rest. It was angled too far forward, pushing into my head, which caused more spasms. With it reversed, my head is free to move and I can also comfortably rest my head on it if need be. Make any necessary adjustments to your vehicle that suits your needs.

Drive only short distances. Plan your trip ahead of time. Do not take unnecessary risks. Stay in your lane and always have a place in mind to turn off the road if your symptoms get bad. Think about what you are doing. Minimize as many lane changes and windy roads as possible, even if that means changing your route. Prior to each car ride, no matter the distance, map it out in your head beforehand so you are better prepared. Put your defensive driving skills to work.

Clothing/Dressing
Unless you have reason to wear certain clothing for work or an event, dress as comfortably as possible. It matters not what others think. Your comfort is priority number one. For me, loose clothing is most comfortable. I do not like anything that is too tight or touches my neck. It is very sensitive to fabric so certain shirts will make it spasm. Whenever possible, I avoid high collared shirts, turtlenecks, a shirt and tie, and scarves. They all cause more neck tightness and muscle contractions. Other people find the opposite to be the case so they wear turtlenecks, collared shirts, and scarves; to hide their symptoms or because it is simply more comfortable. Wear whatever makes you feel best.

Tools for pain and other symptoms

TENS Unit (Transcutaneous Electrical Nerve Stimulation): Pocket sized, portable, battery-operated device that sends electrical impulses to certain parts of the body to block pain signals. The electrical currents produced are mild, but they can prevent pain messages from being transmitted to the brain and may raise the level of endorphins (natural pain killers produced by the brain).

Electrodes are attached to the surface of the skin over or near the area where you are experiencing pain. Before using your personal TENS unit, it is important that you learn how to properly place the electrodes, adjust the controls and settings (frequency and voltage), and set the proper duration and intensity of the stimulation (depending on the location and type of pain).

Bodo: Handheld device for trigger points that you can reach by hand. There are many handheld trigger point tools you can use. Find what best suits you.

Shepherds crook: The shepherd's crook is a long, curved, metal hook with rubber on both ends designed for working on hard to reach trigger points. The bodo and shepherd's crook can be purchased from Bonnie Prudden Myotherapy at www.bonnieprudden.com. A similar product is called the *Back Buddy*, which can be purchased at a variety of online stores.

Another way to work on trigger points in your back that you can't reach by hand is to put a tennis ball (or ball of your choice) into a long sock or stocking. Throw it over your shoulder and lean against the wall putting pressure on the area(s) that bother you. You can also lay on a bed or floor with golf balls or marbles under your back to access trigger points.

Obusforme: Backrest support that transforms ordinary chairs into ergonomically correct seating. It puts your spine into a more anatomically correct position to enhance overall posture by supporting proper spinal alignment.

Kneading Fingers: Massage machine made by Clark Wellness that has two rotating balls that work on the neck and back. It is designed to duplicate the firm kneading action of a massage therapist (www.clarkenterprises2000.com).

Cervical collar: When I had a "floppy" neck early on with my dystonia and for about a month after it became severe, I wore a cervical collar. One was a soft collar and the other was a hard plastic collar that is similar to what is used to immobilize someone who is in an accident. Both gave me some relief, but my symptoms got worse when I took them off. My neck would involuntarily turn and spasm more. I soon found out from some other people with cervical dystonia that they had a similar experience.

A cervical collar can certainly help relieve symptoms for a short period of time and I think a wise thing to wear when doing activities where you need extra neck support, but I do not believe it to be helpful to wear on a regular basis. It weakens neck muscles. Weakening muscles may seem like a good idea since we have strong, overactive muscles in cervical dystonia, but the collar will weaken the non-dystonic muscles that are working hard to support the neck. This will more than likely make symptoms worse. Thus, it is probably best to only wear for short periods of time when absolutely necessary.

Epsom salt: Epsom salt pulls harmful toxins out of the body and allows magnesium and sulfates enter into the body. Magnesium plays a critical role in over 325 enzymes, helps improve muscle and nerve function, reduces inflammation, and improves blood flow and oxygenation throughout the body. Sulfates are necessary building blocks for healthy joints, skin, and nervous tissue. Regular baths with Epsom salt replenishes the body with magnesium and sulfates, helps flush toxins from the body, reduces inflammation, and builds key protein molecules in the brain tissue and joints.[3]

Ice: For pain, inflammation, spasms, and swelling. It may also relax tremors.

Heat: For many of the same uses as ice. I find heat to be most beneficial before I do my stretching, get a massage, when I am extra tight and/or sore, and when I have spasms due to cold weather. Hot baths and whirlpools also relax tight muscles. I like the ice products from Core Products (www.coreproducts.com) and heat/aromatherapy packs made by BodySense (www.ebodewell.com).

There are so many things we can do to make our daily lives a little more tolerable. It may take trial and error, but never give up looking for safer and more comfortable ways to do things.

References
1) www.medpagetoday.com, *Sensory Tricks' in Dystonia Examined*, May, 1, 2014. Retrieved on May 12, 2014 from: http://www.medpagetoday.com/MeetingCoverage/AAN/45548
2) www.backandneck.about.com, Retrieved on April 26, 2014 from: http://backandneck.about.com/od/ergonomics/ht/goodsittingposture.htm
3) www.healthy-holistic-living.com, Retrieved on January 26, 2015 from: http://www.healthy-holistic-living.com/benefits-of-epsom-salt-baths.html

Afterword

Dystonia is a challenge unlike anything many of us have ever faced. While it may seem like we are victims of a cruel disorder, I believe there is a power greater than us that is a source of infinite love. Anything that comes from a place of love such as this is not intended to hurt us or make us suffer. Everything happens for us so we can learn and grow. There is no way I could ever survive dystonia if I didn't believe that there is an important reason it is part of my life, or anything else in my life, no matter how challenging.

Our response to what happens in life determines our mindset. We can choose to live a suffering life or we can choose to live one with passion and joy, regardless of our circumstances. If you want to be happy, work on living with the mindset that life is happening for you and not to you. Living in gratitude for all that is happening for you will open doors that will make your life more joyful, more meaningful, and more peaceful.

Find the courage to live your life the way you want to the very best of your ability. It can get messy at times, but nothing in life defines us and how we live unless we let it. Choose to live your life the way you want regardless of any obstacle that comes your way.

Remember that with every obstacle comes opportunity. Look for the many opportunities in your life. They are all around you waiting for you to take advantage. Dystonia is not the story of your life. It is just one of many chapters.

As Ralph Waldo Emerson said, "When you were born you were crying and everyone else was smiling. Live your life so at the end, you're the one who is smiling and everyone else is crying."

Thank you for taking this journey with me. Peace and happiness to you all.

The True Meaning of Life
We are visitors on this planet.
We are here for ninety or one hundred years at the very most.
During that period, we must try to do something good,
something useful with our lives.
If you contribute to other people's happiness,
you will find the true goal, the true meaning of life.
- Tenzin Gyatso, 14th Dalai Lama of Tibet -

Appendix
Dystonia Organizations and Support Groups

Bachmann-Strauss Dystonia & Parkinson Foundation
Fred French Building
551 Fifth Avenue at 45th Street, Suite 520
New York, NY 10176
Phone: 212-682-9900
Email: info@bsdpf.org
Website: www.dystonia-parkinsons.org
The Bachmann-Strauss Dystonia and Parkinson Foundation was established in 1995 to find better treatments and cures for dystonia and Parkinson's disease, and to provide medical and patient information.

Benign Essential Blepharospasm Research Foundation (BEBRF)
637 North 7th Street, Suite 102
PO Box 12468
Beaumont, TX 77726-2468
Phone: 409-832-0788
Email: bebrf@blepharospasm.org
Website: www.blepharospasm.org
The mission of the Benign Essential Blepharospasm Research Foundation (BEBRF) is to fund and promote medical research in the search for the cause and cure of blepharospasm, Meige's Syndrome, and other related disorders of the facial musculature; to provide support, education and referrals to persons with these disorders, and to disseminate information and serve as an authoritative resource to the medical community and the general public.

Canadian Movement Disorder Group
Website: www.cmdg.org
To support a network of movement disorder clinics across Canada to provide the appropriate facilities to treat patients with movement disorders, and to conduct clinical research trials in movement disorder patients.

Dystonia Advocacy Network (DAN)
1 East Wacker Drive, Suite 2810
Chicago, IL 60601
Website: www.dystonia-advocacy.org

DAN is a grassroots organization that brings dystonia-affected individuals together to speak out with a single, powerful voice on legislative and public policy issues which impact the dystonia community.

Dystonia Coalition
Website: www.rarediseasesnetwork.org/Dystonia
The Dystonia Coalition is a collaboration of medical researchers and patient advocacy groups that is working to advance the pace of clinical and translational research in the dystonias to find better treatments and a cure. Emory University in Atlanta, GA (Druid Hills, GA) serves as the Central Coordinating Center for the Dystonia Coalition's activities.

Dystonia Europe
Square de Meeus 37 - 4th Floor
Brussels, 1000 Belgium
Phone: 447-736-625450
Email: sec@dystonia-europe.org
Website: www.dystonia-europe.org
Dystonia Europe was formed in 1993 as European Dystonia Federation, the European umbrella organization for national dystonia groups. The aims of Dystonia Europe are to provide an international platform at the European level to improve the lives of people with dystonia, stimulate research for more effective treatments, and to ultimately find a cure.

Dystonia Ireland
33 Larkfield Grove
Harold's Cross, Dublin 6W Ireland
Phone: 00 353 (01) 4922514
Email: info@dystonia.ie
Website: www.dystonia.ie
The mission of Dystonia Ireland is to promote and encourage scientific research into the causes and treatments of dystonia, raise the level of awareness amongst the general public and the medical profession, and offer support and information to all people with dystonia and their families nationwide.

Dystonia Medical Research Foundation (DMRF)
1 East Wacker Drive, Suite 2810
Chicago, IL   60601-1905
Phone: 312-755-0198
Email: dystonia@dystonia-foundation.org

Website: www.dystonia-foundation.org
The mission of the DMRF is to advance research for more treatments and ultimately a cure, to promote awareness and education, and to support the needs and well being of affected individuals and families.

Dystonia Medical Research Foundation Canada (DMRFC)
121 Richmond Street West, Suite 305
Toronto, Ontario M5H 2K1 Canada
Phone: 800-361-8061
Website: www.dystoniacanada.org
The mission of the Dystonia Medical Research Foundation Canada (DMRFC) is to advance research for more treatments and ultimately a cure; to promote awareness and education; and to support the needs and well being of affected individuals and families. DMRFC is a registered non-profit Canadian charity governed by a volunteer Board of Directors.

Dystonia Network of Australia
Email: info@dystonia.org.au
Website: www.dystonia.org.au
Providing a pathway to support, information, literature and community awareness for adults and children living with dystonia and their carers and health providers.

National Organization for Rare Diseases (NORD) - Connecticut Office
55 Kenosia Avenue
Danbury, CT 06810
Phone: 744-0100; 800-999-6673
Website: www.rarediseases.org
The National Organization for Rare Disorders (NORD), is a federation of voluntary health organizations dedicated to helping people with rare "orphan" diseases and assisting the organizations that serve them. NORD is committed to the identification, treatment, and cure of rare disorders through programs of education, advocacy, research, and service.

National Organization for Rare Diseases (NORD) - Washington Office
1779 Massachusetts Avenue, Suite 500
Washington, DC 20036
Phone: 202-588-5700
Website: www.rarediseases.org

National Spasmodic Dysphonia Association (NSDA)
300 Park Boulevard, Suite 415
Itasca, IL 60143
Phone: 800-795-6732
Email: NSDA@dysphonia.org
Website: www.dysphonia.org
The mission of the NSDA is to advance medical research into the causes of and treatments for spasmodic dysphonia, promote physician and public awareness of the disorder, and provide support to those affected. The NSDA is the only organization dedicated solely to the spasmodic dysphonia community.

National Spasmodic Torticollis Association (NSTA)
9920 Talbert Avenue
Fountain Valley, CA 92708
Phone: 714-378-9837; 800-487-8385
Email: NSTAmail@aol.com
Website: www.torticollis.org
The mission of the NSTA is to support the needs and well being of affected individuals and families, to promote awareness and education, and to advance research for more treatments and ultimately a cure.

New Zealand Dystonia Patient Network
Website: www.dystonia.org.nz
To support dystonia patients with information, advice about living with dystonia and networking opportunities. To increase awareness about dystonia, both among the medical community and the general public. To encourage and facilitate research, with the aim of seeking better treatments, prevention, a cure.

NIH/National Institute of Neurological Disorders and Stroke
P.O. Box 5801
Bethesda, MD 20824
Phone: 301-496-5751; 800-352-9424
Website: www.ninds.nih.gov
The NINDS conducts, fosters, coordinates, and guides research on the causes, prevention, diagnosis, and treatment of neurological disorders and stroke, and supports basic research in related scientific areas. It provides grants-in-aid to public and private institutions, and individuals in fields related to its areas of interest, including research projects, program projects, and research center grants. It operates a program of contracts for the funding of research and research support efforts, provides individual and institutional fellowships,

conducts a diversified program of intramural and collaborative research in its own laboratories, branches, and clinics, and collects and disseminates research information related to neurological disorders.

The Dystonia Society UK
89 Albert Embankment, 2nd Floor
Vauxhall London, SE1 7TP United Kingdom
Phone: 084-545-86211; 800-084-545-86322
Email: angie@dystonia.org.uk
Website: www.dystonia.org.uk
The Dystonia Society is a charity in the United Kingdom providing support, advice and information for anyone affected by dystonia. Its aim is to ensure that everyone affected has access to the most appropriate treatments and support to achieve the best possible quality of life.

Tyler's Hope for a Dystonia Cure
13351 Progress Blvd
Alachua, FL 32615
Phone: 386-462-5220
Email: tylershope@intermed1.com
Website: www.tylershope.org
Tyler's Hope for a dystonia cure was created to passionately pursue solutions and a cure to the pain and limitations caused by DYT1 dystonia (early-onset primary dystonia). While raising global awareness of this disease, it is committed to funding the research required to find a cure for dystonia and develop treatments while on this task.

Made in the USA
Coppell, TX
04 February 2020